Principles and Practice of
High Dependency Nursing

For Elsevier:

Senior Commissioning Editor: Ninette Premdas
Project Development Manager: Mairi McCubbin
Project Manager: Andrew Palfreyman
Design Direction: George Ajayi
Illustrations Manager: Bruce Hogarth

Principles and Practice of High Dependency Nursing

SECOND EDITION

Edited by

Mandy Sheppard

Training and Development Consultant, Kent, UK

Mike Wright MBA RN DMS CHSM ENB100

Executive Nurse Director, Bromley Hospitals NHS Trust, London, UK

Foreword by

Sheila Adam

Nurse Consultant, Middlesex Hospital, London, UK

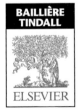

BAILLIÈRE TINDALL

ELSEVIER

EDINBURGH LONDON NEW YORK OXFORD PHILADELPHIA ST LOUIS SYDNEY TORONTO 2006

BAILLIÈRE
TINDALL
ELSEVIER

© Harcourt Publishers Limited 2001
© 2005, Elsevier Limited. All rights reserved.

The right of Mandy Sheppard and Mike Wright to be identified as editors of this work has been asserted by them in accordance with the Copyright, Designs and Patents Act 1988.

First edition 2000
Second edition 2006

A060076
WB 300.1

ISBN 070202712X

British Library Cataloguing in Publication Data
A catalogue record for this book is available from the British Library

Library of Congress Cataloging in Publication Data
A catalog record for this book is available from the Library of Congress

Notice
Knowledge and best practice in this field are constantly changing. As new research and experience broaden our knowledge, changes in practice, treatment and drug therapy may become necessary or appropriate. Readers are advised to check the most current information provided (i) on procedures featured or (ii) by the manufacturer of each product to be administered, to verify the recommended dose or formula, the method and duration of administration, and contraindications. It is the responsibility of the practitioner, relying on their own experience and knowledge of the patient, to make diagnoses, to determine dosages and the best treatment for each individual patient, and to take all appropriate safety precautions. To the fullest extent of the law, neither the publisher nor the editors assumes any liability for any injury and/or damage.

The Publisher

Printed in China

Contents

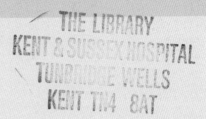

Contributors

Helena Baxter MSc BSc(Hons) RGN
Service Improvement Manager, Hinchingbrooke Healthcare NHS Trust, Huntingdon, UK
11 Pain management

Pauline Chinn RGN PGDip ENB100 N53
Acute Pain Nurse Specialist, Peterborough Hospital NHS Trust, Peterborough, UK
11 Pain management

Mary Currie BSc(Hons) DipMgnt RGN ENB124
Nurse Consultant, Department of Cardiolgy, Bromley Hospitals NHS Trust, Princess Royal University Hospital, Kent, UK
6 Cardiac care

Nigel Davies BSc MSc Certed RGN ENB254
Chief Nurse/Director of Patient Services, Papworth Hospital NHS Trust, Cambridge, UK
6 Cardiac care

Deborah Dawson BSc(Hons) RGN ENB100
Head of Nursing, Critical Care, Royal Sussex County Hospital, Brighton, UK
7 Neurological care

Debbie Field BSc(Hons) MSc DipNurs ENB249 RGN
Debbie Field, Network Respiratory Weaning Coordinator, Surrey Wide Critical Care Network, UK
5 Respiratory care

Susan Laight BSc(Hons) MSc RGN ENB100
Nursing Practice Facilitator (Critical Care), Buckinghamshire Hospitals NHS Trust, High Wycombe, UK
6 Cardiac care

Wayne Large RGN BA(Hons) MA
Nurse Consultant Critical Care, BUPA Hospitals, London, UK
10 Fluid and electrolytes

Paul Mulligan BSc RN DipNurs(Lond) PG Dip HE MA
Risk Manager, Guy's and St Thomas' Foundation Trust, London, UK
4 Social issues in high dependency care

Helen O'Keefe BSc(Hons) RGN, ENB100
Assistant Director of Nursing, East Kent Hospitals NHS Trust, William Harvey Hospital, Kent, UK
9 Clinical emergencies

Rebecca Purdy MSc BSc(Hons) DipN, RGN, ODP
Deputy Theatre Manager, Surrey & Sussex NHS Trust, UK
8 Post-anaesthetic and post-operative care

Sarah Shah BSc DipMgt ENB100, 148, 998
Practice Educator Neurocritical Care Unit, St George's Hospital, London, UK
7 Neurological care

Mandy Sheppard
Training and Development Consultant, Kent, UK
2 The fundamental principles of high dependency care

Chris Wilkinson BSc(Hons) MSc RGN DipNEd ENB100
Director of Nursing, Peterborough and Stamford Hospitals NHS Foundation Trust, Cambridgeshire, UK
3 Interpersonal issues in high dependency care

John Allen Wilkinson BSc(Hons) MSc RGN RMN DipNEd ENB100
Regional Officer, Royal College of Nursing Eastern Region, UK
3 Interpersonal issues in high dependency care

Mike Wright MBA RN DMS CHSM ENB100
Executive Nurse Director, Bromley Hospitals NHS Trust, London, UK
1 The development, growth and context of high dependency care

Guy Young MSc RN ENB100
Director of Nursing, Homerton University Hospital NHS Foundation Trust, London, UK
8 Post-anaesthetic and post-operative care

Foreword

One of the most profound changes in approach to critically ill patients in hospital has occurred in the last 5 yrs. The publication of Comprehensive Critical Care (DH 2000) ensured that the provision of critical care skills and the access of patients to critical care staff knowledge and expertise would no longer be confined by geographical location. Instead, staff working in acute hospital wards would be educated to recognise and respond to the acutely unwell patient and be empowered to call directly for assistance from critical care outreach services. Development of this approach has been led in many cases by Nurse Consultants, which has further empowered nurses. The change has enabled many patients to receive more appropriate and timely care in emergencies as well as facilitated transfer to higher levels of care. Early studies have shown this to be associated with decreased readmission to intensive and high dependency care (Ball and Kirby, 2003), decreased length of stay (Priestley et al 2004) and improved mortality (Priestley et al 2004).

One of the major impacts of this change on nurses working in acute areas has been the increased contact with and knowledge about caring for patients with increased levels of critical care need. In addition, nurses in many clinical areas face an increased requirement to become familiar with the skills, knowledge and competencies necessary to nurse these patients. This book provides the underlying physiological, social and technical knowledge to allow nurses in many areas to develop the confidence and skills they need. If used in conjunction with clinical exposure to high dependency patients, it will be invaluable in developing expertise. While many nurses may only consider using such a book when working in a designated high dependency (level 2 critical care) area, it is likely that most trained nurses and student nurses working with the acute hospital in-patient will find relevant information and useful clinical advice from this book. In particular, the respiratory and fluid status chapters are applicable to many general hospital patients.

As the level of acuity in ward patients increases due to the increasing age of patients, frequent co-morbidity, more use of day surgery for uncomplicated procedures and faster discharge, it is likely that most nurses will require an understanding of the needs of high dependency patients.

This book benefits from a holistic approach to the high dependency patient including psychological and social issues allowing the reader to develop an understanding of context. The combination of recognised clinical experts and more senior nurses with a broad healthcare view allows the text to cover both the micro and macro spectrum.

Sheila Adam, London

References

Ball C, Kirkby M, Williams S. Effect of the critical care outreach team on patient survival to discharge from hospital and readmission to critical care: non-randomised population based study. British medical journal 2003; 327:1014-1017

Priestley G, Watson W, Rashidian, A. et al Introducing Critical Care Outreach: a ward-randomised trial of phased introduction in a general hospital. Intensive Care Medicine,

Story D.A, Shelton A.C, Poustie, S.J. et al The effect of critical care outreach on postoperative serious adverse events. Anaesthesia, 2004; 59: 762-766

Preface

We are delighted to welcome you the second edition of this book. It is relevant to nurses at all levels, whether as a student nurse or later in your career as a qualified nurse working in any general or specialist area, where you may be required to care for patients requiring level 1 and/or level 2 critical care.

The old adage states that the only constant in life is change. What is certain is that acute hospital environments are changing constantly; the introduction of minimally invasive technologies, much more emphasis on treating patients on a day case basis, advances in chronic disease management and reductions in hospital length of stay being prime examples. As these dynamics continue to change and people continue to live longer on the whole, so the profile of the hospital inpatient population changes. By definition, this population is more likely to suffer from multiple pathologies and have more complex or multi-faceted needs. In turn, this is increasing the level of sophistication of the care that these patients need, with more of this care now taking place outside formal intensive care and high dependency units. The result is that nurses working in all areas need not only to deliver high-quality basic or fundamental care, but also to acquire the necessary expertise to achieve optimum outcomes for the sicker inpatient population.

It is essential that patients who require high dependency care are placed in an appropriate setting, where resources, skills and expertise are available and focused. In recent years this has resulted in the growth of areas that can provide level 2 critical care. These include more formalized high dependency units – either as stand-alone units or as part of general wards, accident and emergency departments, recovery units or intensive care units. In addition, there are occasions when patients deteriorate suddenly and unexpectedly, and need rapid and skilled intervention either to resuscitate them or to prevent further deterioration, where possible. These are patients who are more likely to require level 1 critical care. This is when more competent and skilled nursing assessment, care and evaluation become essential; either to prevent deterioration to the point of emergency in the first instance, where possible, or to ensure on-going high-quality care until transfer to a more formal high dependency area takes place.

This book captures the expertise of professional leaders, academics, managers and practitioners who are both passionate about this important and growing area of patient care and have been involved in the development of the high dependency concept in the UK in recent years. The authors have been committed to:

- reflect the diversity of high dependency care and its many care settings;
- provide a foundation for clinical application of the principles and demystify some of the terminology and concepts;
- focus on high dependency care as an entity in its own right;
- support the development of sophisticated assessment, planning, implementation and evaluation of care skills in nurses to assist with the development of their confidence and competence in this subject area.

Some chapters are devoted to specific clinical systems or circumstances. Other chapters address broader issues such as the history and context of high dependency care, and the social and interpersonal issues therein.

We would like to thank the chapter authors for their hard work, commitment and attention to detail when writing this book. We hope that it will be a valuable resource for nurses working in all areas and for managers who may have to develop or manage such a facility. Whatever your area of work or professional setting, we wish you every success with whatever you do.

Mandy Sheppard
Mike Wright
Kent & London 2005

SECTION 1

General issues in high dependency care

SECTION CONTENTS

Chapter 1

The development, growth and context of high dependency care

Mike Wright

KEY LEARNING OBJECTIVES

- To appreciate how the historical development of high dependency care has led to the current status of the service in the UK
- To understand the complex and variable nature of high dependency care with specific reference to:
  - what constitutes high dependency care
  - which patients need high dependency care
  - where high dependency care is undertaken
  - its context in modern healthcare within the UK
- To utilize the background information in the ongoing development of high dependency care

INTRODUCTION

The chapter will commence with a definition of high dependency care, followed by an understanding of the types of location where high dependency-type care can be delivered. It will then consider the development, growth and context of the concept of high dependency care, from the early thoughts of Florence Nightingale to the modern day and beyond. It will also include consideration of the types of patient that may need access to high dependency care, the resources required, and the nursing and managerial considerations therein.

WHAT IS HIGH DEPENDENCY CARE?

High dependency care is not a new concept. As individuals become sicker and more dependent, a higher level of care and attention is required than can normally be provided on a general hospital ward.

Furthermore, it is often inappropriate for such patients to require the full care of an intensive care unit. It is these patients who are considered to require high dependency care.

High dependency care has been recognized, albeit informally, for many years. In more recent times, there have been attempts to clarify what high dependency care is and what constitutes a high dependency care unit (HDU) (Department of Health 1996).

The HDU is not, however, necessarily synonymous with high dependency care. Patients may require high dependency care (anticipated or otherwise) at various stages of a hospital stay. For example, after a general anaesthetic, it is expected that a patient will require close monitoring and observation, usually in a recovery ward. For this period of time, the patient is undoubtedly highly dependent, and the level of nursing resource and monitoring equipment is greater than on a general ward. Although recovery wards are not generally labelled as HDUs, the nurses are, however, routinely practising high dependency care.

> The concept of a designated high dependency unit may be new, but the quality of care implied is not. Patients have always needed varying levels of care at varying stages of their illness.

Theoretically, any patient in an acute hospital setting could unexpectedly deteriorate and become highly dependent, possibly requiring transfer to a more formal critical care environment.

WHERE SHOULD HIGH DEPENDENCY CARE BE DELIVERED?

High dependency care can occur in many different areas within the acute hospital setting, be they formally established for this purpose or otherwise.

The unpredictable nature of healthcare means that 'unlikely' venues for high dependency care may suddenly be faced with a highly dependent patient; for example, a patient who collapses while in the outpatient or X-ray department. The environment, together with the sporadic occurrence, dictates that high dependency care should not be undertaken in such areas. There is a requirement, however, for *all* patient areas to have staff, equipment and the relevant protocols to deal with such eventualities, with emergency resuscitation equipment and capability as a minimum.

There are other clinical areas where the probability of high dependency care is higher; for example, a medical admission or acute assessment/acute admissions ward. Many acute hospitals have developed such facilities to relieve the accident and emergency services, and/or to maintain a more consistent workload pattern in the general ward areas. The clinical condition of a patient may not be fully appreciated until arrival on the ward and, once admitted, that condition may change rapidly. In view of this, there is a requirement for staff working in these areas to be competent in the principles of high dependency care, either to stabilize the patient and prevent further deterioration, or to care for the patient until transfer to a more appropriate location. This should be available (along with access to suitably experienced medical staff) throughout each 24-hour period.

Accident and emergency departments and standard post-operative recovery rooms are well-known examples of areas where highly dependent patients are a more common and predictable feature of the workload pattern. This is reflected by the enhanced nurse to patient ratios, the skill mix of the nurses, access to medical staff and the utilization/availability of monitoring equipment. These areas, while regularly undertaking high dependency care, would normally only do so for short periods of time, after which, if still required, the patient would be transferred to another location.

Formally designated high dependency areas can take many different forms. Broadly, these can be described in three categories, as described below.

- Those that are attached to a general or specialized ward; either geographically within the ward, perhaps as a bay of beds, or in close proximity to the ward. This could also include renal units or coronary care units (CCUs).
- Those that are attached to the intensive care unit (ICU), either geographically within the ICU or in close proximity to it, or in another part of the hospital, but still managed by the ICU.
- Those that stand alone, but are managed by surgical or medical teams. This could also include specialized high dependency areas such as CCUs, renal units or intensive recovery units (Aps 2000, 2002, 2004).

There are advantages and disadvantages associated with all of these categories and this will vary according to the exigencies of each hospital. Thompson & Singer's (1995) survey of HDUs in UK hospitals revealed the wide range in function, size, structure, venue and services available. Regardless of the geographical venue for high dependency care, however, there are principles that can underpin the effectiveness of any high dependency area.

High dependency care is part of a continuum of care for patients within a hospital; it should not be a completely segregated or isolated facility, as Figure 1.1 illustrates. This figure also serves to illustrate an important function of high dependency care, which is to provide a 'step-up' facility (i.e. for patients who become too sick for a general ward, yet are not sick enough for intensive care) and a 'step-down' facility (i.e. for patients who progress such that intensive care is no longer required but they are still too sick for a general ward). As can also be seen from the diagram,

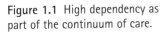

Figure 1.1 High dependency as part of the continuum of care.

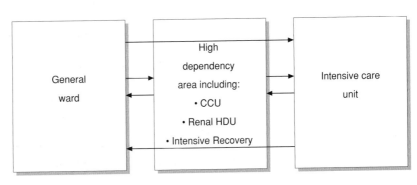

patients can also be admitted directly to and from the ICU from the ward, if it is appropriate and safe to do so. Therefore, patients do not always have to go via the HDU facility, where it is not indicated.

Patients move along the continuum according to the severity of their illness, and that movement should be as smooth and efficient as possible. Protocols that ensure effective written and verbal communication must be in place between the high dependency facility and the other clinical areas. This applies to all aspects of communication; however, of particular importance is the clear handover of information that directly relates to patient care and management. Also, it is extremely unlikely that all of the clinical areas involved in the continuum of care will be managed by the same directorate or department. Therefore, the need for effective communication is heightened, and clinical professionals should always be mindful of their professional obligations and accountability to ensure that patient care is not compromised as a result of a transfer over to another care team.

Another important factor in the successful movement of patients between levels of care, and to ensure the appropriate use of facilities, is the presence of documented and agreed admission and discharge guidelines. These should be compiled by a team that comprises membership of all relevant stakeholders, examples for which are shown below.

- Nurses responsible for the day-to-day operational management of the area (to include):
  — nurse manager(s) (including ward sisters and charge nurses)
  — nurse educators.
- Medical staff (to include):
  — those responsible for consultant cover for the area;
  — representation from 'user directorates' (e.g. surgeon, cardiologist, physician).
- Directorate/business/operations manager.
- Physiotherapists.
- Radiographers.
- Pathology/laboratory staff.
- Primary Care/Strategic Health Authority (as appropriate).
- Accident and emergency representative.
- Intensive care representative (if separate team).
- User ward/department representation.
- Clinical audit.
- Patient/relative/user groups.
- Pharmacists.
- Facilities and estates staff.

One of the key elements of high dependency care, as already discussed, is the availability of suitably skilled nursing and medical staff during the day and at night; the venue for high dependency care may have some influence upon this. Many high dependency areas have been developed as part of general or specialized wards. Under this model, nurses usually rotate from the ward area through to the high dependency area, which maintains some continuity for patients and helps to prevent the deskilling of staff. It is essential in these circumstances that staff are provided with the appropriate training and level of supervision, which will prevent any feelings of inadequacy or vulnerability within them when caring for highly dependent patients. Although part of a ward, the levels and skill mix of staff, particularly at night, should be differentiated for the high dependency area.

A potential problem that can result from the development of a number of high dependency areas within one hospital (as opposed to a single central facility) is that the caseload of highly dependent patients is diluted as the patients are spread throughout a number of areas. For staff to maintain competence, the individual high dependency areas must have a sufficient number of patients and activity patterns to enable them to retain their skills (Department of Health 1996). Although many acute hospitals utilize the directorate/divisional system of organization, a 'cross-directorate' or 'whole-hospital' approach should be taken during the planning and development of new high dependency facilities. This will help to ensure smooth inter-departmental relationships once the unit is operational.

Evidence of need will undoubtedly be required initially to set up a high dependency area and, once operational, audit processes should be in place to ensure the appropriate and effective use of the service. In addition, the future direction and shaping of the service should be based upon informed decisions and an evidence base, where this exists. For these reasons, data collection and an audit plan should be integral to the management framework of a high dependency area.

THE DEVELOPMENT AND GROWTH OF HIGH DEPENDENCY CARE

The first reference to high dependency care was probably in 1852 when Florence Nightingale wrote: 'It is valuable to have one place where post-operative and other patients requiring close attention can be watched' (Jennett 1990).

During the 1940s, post-operative recovery rooms were introduced, significantly reducing the morbidity and mortality of post-operative patients (Oh 1997). This development allowed the close observation of patients and was in fact high dependency care. The use of intermittent positive pressure ventilation (IPPV) during the poliomyelitis epidemic of the 1950s prompted the development of the concept of intensive care.

In 1967, a report from the British Medical Association asserted that the presence of an intensive care unit in a hospital would improve the care and outcome of seriously ill patients. The report also stated that, at that time, many hospitals were considering the setting up of ICUs (Hopkinson 1996). The 1960s also saw the use of continuous electrocardiogram (ECG) monitoring for patients with myocardial infarction and, subsequently, the development of specialized high dependency areas, such as coronary care units (CCUs).

In many ways, the subsequent and rapid growth of intensive care overshadowed the formal and documented development of high dependency care, which still occurred in specialized areas, such as post-operative recovery rooms and CCUs. Other specialized forms of high dependency care were also introduced, such as renal and bone marrow transplant units.

Patients in the general hospital environment requiring high dependency care were (and in some cases still are) cared for in general wards, often situated in an area of the ward that enabled close observation (i.e. at the entrance to the ward) or in close proximity to the 'nurses' station'. Sometimes these patients were 'specialled', whereby the nurse to patient ratio increased from the normal ratio for general ward patients. Although the distinction between a general ward patient and a patient of higher dependency is often blurred, there is, however, a clear recognition that certain patients require more nursing resource and closer observation – two essential elements of high dependency care. These distinctions will be considered again later in this chapter.

Some of these patients could deteriorate further and would require intensive care facilities, if available. The requirement of IPPV was a common indication for admission to intensive care but, generally, the distinction between high dependency care and intensive care was (and still is in some cases) unclear.

It was more during the 1970s and 1980s that specialized high dependency care became established and, although a few hospitals developed designated general clinical areas for highly dependent patients, the majority of such patients remained scattered throughout the hospital, being cared for in general wards. Intensive care continued its rapid development, aided by advances in technology and in response to healthcare needs.

In 1986, the government of the time proposed the Resource Management Initiative, which was introduced in six pilot hospitals, and, in 1989, the introduction of the National Health Service (NHS) internal market (Mohan 1995). This placed increasing pressure on all providers of healthcare to demonstrate cost effectiveness of healthcare services. Intensive care was no exception and the requirement to justify the high costs associated with the service increased. Cost and the rising demand for intensive care prompted closer scrutiny into the types of patient being admitted to these facilities. As part of this analysis, two categories of patients caused concern. They were those patients that could be considered to be 'too sick' and, therefore, unlikely to benefit from intensive care and, conversely, those patients that could be considered to be 'too well' to require intensive care. By virtue of occupying an intensive care bed inappropriately, both of these types of patient could possibly have prevented the timely admission of patients who genuinely required, and would likely have benefited from, intensive care. There was a growing awareness of the latter category, the high dependency patient: too sick for a general ward, yet not sick enough for intensive care. This was a predicament and still remains so today for many hospitals. Therefore, where should this category of patient be cared for?

In 1988, the report 'Intensive care services – provision for the future' (Association of Anaesthetists 1988) highlighted the need for effective use of intensive care and made recommendations about the size, location, workload and staffing of ICUs. Within this report, a definition of a high dependency care unit was given as 'an area for patients that require more intensive observation and/or nursing care than would be expected on a general ward. It would not normally include patients requiring mechanical ventilation or invasive monitoring'.

Also in 1988, an article was published showing that within 1 year of setting up an HDU, ward mortality in the hospital fell by 13.3% (Franklin et al 1988). A King's Fund Panel was then set up, which questioned, among other things, the lack of evidence that could justify which patients were most likely to benefit from intensive care (King's Fund Panel 1989). Both the Intensive Care Society in the report 'The intensive care service in the UK' (Intensive Care Society 1990) and the Association of Anaesthetists in their report 'The high dependency unit – acute care for the future' (Association of Anaesthetists 1991), highlighted the problem over this 'middle band' of patient – the highly dependent patient.

In the Association of Anaesthetists' report, a survey was published of 339 acute hospitals and a further 96 hospitals, which performed only elective surgery. Only 55 of these hospitals had a designated HDU and, of these, 48 also had an ICU. The survey also revealed that many of the patients located on the ICU in fact required high dependency care and that many of the patients on the general wards should have been cared for in an HDU.

This report went on to describe the concept of 'progressive patient care'. It noted how patients require varying levels of care during a hospital stay, and that traditional methods of providing high dependency care by 'specialling' individual patients in general wards diluted expertise and were largely inefficient and uneconomical. The report defined progressive patient care as:

a system of organizing patient care in which patients are grouped together in units depending on their need for care as determined by their degree of illness rather than by traditional factors such as medical or surgical specialty. The three usual levels of care were described as intensive, intermediate and minimal or self care.

In 1993, a study was undertaken on behalf of the Department of Health to investigate the provision of intensive care in England (Metcalfe & McPherson 1995). Although it concentrated primarily on intensive care, it also highlighted aspects of high dependency care. The report revealed a significant variation in the provision of high dependency care. Only 34 of the acute hospitals in England with an ICU also had an HDU at that time. In many hospitals, there was a complete absence of high dependency beds, while in others there would be an HDU but not an ICU. Consultants who participated in the study indicated that 65% of admissions to the ICU would have been more appropriately admitted to an HDU. The report suggested that there may well be a requirement for more high dependency beds.

In 1994, Kilpatrick and colleagues published an article that mirrored parts of the 1991 Association of Anaesthetists' report. Specifically, the article said that it made both clinical and economic sense to have ill patients confined to specialized areas and not scattered throughout the hospital. In this way, problems could be anticipated early and intervention could be timely (Kilpatrick et al 1994). Several other articles were published in relation to the demand for intensive care and how the effective use of high dependency may also enable the effective use of intensive care services (Bion 1994, Peacock & Edbrooke 1995, Ryan 1995).

In December 1995, a 10-year-old boy was transferred a total of four times in 12 hours by ambulance because of a shortage of intensive care beds. Following this, health authorities were asked to review their emergency services and to consider a national database of intensive care beds. Notably, the then Health Secretary, Stephen Dorrell MP, asked health authorities to make more use of 'intermediate, high dependency beds' (Carnall 1996). Although there had been numerous reports and medical papers, all supporting the need for high dependency care, this political statement was highly significant in the recognition of high dependency care. It prompted healthcare providers (Trusts) to examine how they proposed to care for this group of patients.

In 1995, Rennie wrote that 'at present, less than 10% of UK hospitals have HDUs' (Rennie 1995). This article also highlighted the need to make better use of intensive care facilities and argued some cost implications. 1996 was one of the early significant years in terms of high dependency care. The beginning of the year saw the publication of 'The Report of the Joint Working Party on Graduated Care' (Royal College of Anaesthetists & Royal College of Surgeons 1996). In many ways, the report reiterated but also expanded upon the Association of Anaesthetists' report, with graduated care being conceptually akin to progressive patient care. This new report had far-reaching consequences, not only for the design of modern hospitals but also the traditional method of care organization and delivery in the UK. It quoted the Report of the National Confidential Enquiry into Peri-operative Deaths (1992–1993), which had found that:

> Overall there is an inadequate provision of high dependency units across the country and this is something that should be addressed very urgently by both clinicians and managers. It is pointless to perform major surgery on patients that are physiologically compromised unless there are facilities for these patients to recover post-operatively.

By 1996, there was a significant and growing body of evidence that justified the need for formalized high dependency care. It was accepted that high dependency care was a category between the general ward and intensive care. However, whilst this category appeared to be generally recognized and accepted by some, ambiguity remained with others. In March of that year, the Department of Health published 'Guidelines on Admission to and discharge from intensive care and high dependency units' (Department of Health 1996) to help provide further clarity on this position. These guidelines were produced by a working party, which comprised clinicians (nursing and medical), health service managers and members of the NHS Executive. Their terms of reference had been:

To produce national guidelines which are evidence-based (or based on clear professional consensus) and which set out specific indications for admission to and discharge from intensive care; to produce clear and practical definitions of intensive care and high dependency units and other levels of care above that expected on a general hospital ward; and to cover in the guidelines the nature of the relationship which should exist between the different levels of such care.

The guidelines defined not only what high dependency care should provide but also for whom it was appropriate.

In March 1997, a new method of data collection was described, entitled the augmented care period (ACP) dataset (Department of Health 1997). The ACP Dataset was designed to capture information regarding the level and location of intensive and high dependency care being practised in acute hospitals, and collection of the the ACP Dataset became a mandatory requirement for all acute hospitals later that year.

The next major development within the UK was the introduction of the NHS Plan in 2000 (Department of Health 2000a). This set the strategic context for the modernization and development of the NHS over the following ten years, and the efficient and effective deployment of NHS resources. The NHS Plan confirmed that the NHS did not have the right number of beds in the right places to do its job quickly and effectively. This resulted in a pledge to increase the number of adult critical care beds by 30% over the following 3 years.

THE CONTEXT FOR MODERN HIGH DEPENDENCY CARE

The year 2000 also saw the introduction of 'Comprehensive critical care – a review of adult critical care services' (Department of Health, 2000b). This is the most significant development in relation to high dependency and general critical care in recent years. This built upon the findings and recommendations of 'Critical to success' (Audit Commission 1999), and recommended that the division into high dependency and intensive care beds be replaced by a classification that focuses on the level of care that individual patients need. This introduced the concept of 'critical care without walls'. This document also offers guidance and recommendations with regard to the resources required to care for patients in accordance with the workload generated by the condition of each specific patient, rather than by the physical environment within which each patient is being cared for. Comprehensive critical care set the blueprint for modernized critical care services into the 21st century. This set the following key challenges for acute hospital trusts:

- to adopt hospital-wide and more holistic approaches to adult critical care services that extend beyond the physical boundaries of discrete units and departments, in order to ensure the optimum use of available resources;
- to establish geographically linked critical care networks across the NHS to enable the development of common standards and protocols;

- to develop a planned approach to workforce development including the recruitment, training and retention of medical and nursing staff, and to balance the skill mix so that professional staff are able to delegate less skilled and non-clinical tasks;
- to improve data collection and audit to ensure more reliable information for analysis and to aid decision-making.

Classification of critical care patients

Comprehensive critical care also recommended that the classification of care into high dependency and intensive care categories based upon the physical location of the bed be replaced by a classification that focuses on the level of care that each individual needs, regardless of location. The new classifications are shown in Box 1.1.

High dependency as a continuing definition

In view of the developments around attempting to classify patients according to their specific critical care needs rather than by the physical location within which they are being cared for, it could be argued that the term 'high dependency' is now outmoded. This certainly looks likely in the future. However, for the purposes of this book, the term 'high dependency' will be retained as a means of describing those critical care patients who require equivalent to Level 1 or Level 2 care, particularly as many of the areas within which these types of patient are cared for are still located separately from the formal intensive care units.

Box 1.1 Classification of critical care patients

Level 0

Patients whose needs can be met through normal ward care in an acute hospital

Level 1

Patients at risk of their condition deteriorating, or those recently relocated from higher levels of care, whose needs can be met on an acute ward with additional advice and support from the critical care team

Level 2

Patients requiring more detailed observation or intervention including support for a single failing organ system or post-operative care and those 'stepping down' from higher levels of care

Level 3

Patients requiring advanced respiratory support alone or basic respiratory support together with support of at least two organ systems. This level includes all complex patients receiving support for multiorgan failure

Critical care outreach services

In order to assist with the promotion of the concept of critical care without walls, comprehensive critical care recommended the introduction of critical care outreach services (CCOs) in all acute hospitals. Critical care outreach services were charged with three essential objectives:

- *to avert admissions to HDUs and ICUs* by the early detection of patients who were either deteriorating or at risk of deteriorating, and either helping to prevent admission to a critical care bed or ensuring that admission happens in a manner that ensures the best outcome for each patient;
- *to enable discharges* through the provision of support to ensure the continuing recovery of patients discharged to wards, and the follow-up support post-discharge from hospital;
- *to share critical care skills* with staff on wards, through knowledge and information sharing, and the enhancement of training opportunities and skills acquisition.

Early warning scoring systems

Comprehensive critical care also promotes the use of early warning scoring systems (EWSs). These are tools that can be used by any member of the healthcare team to raise awareness of the early clinical deterioration of a patient. The idea behind an EWS is to capture the deterioration or potential deterioration of a patient early in order to either prevent further deterioration or, where necessary and possible, enable a more planned and structured transfer to a more formal critical care area. Other names for EWS are patient at risk scores (PAR), and physiological track and trigger warning systems (PTTWS). A variety of EWSs are in use across the UK. However, the fundamental principles are that each EWS uses either a points-based or parameter-based assessment process to trigger actions (early action, assistance, support and/or advice) based upon changes to physiological observations/dimensions.

Progress against the NHS Plan and 'Comprehensive critical care'

It is recognized that the NHS is ever changing and dynamic. Nonetheless, whilst recognizing that there is still a great deal to achieve in modernizing the nation's health services, much progress has been made since the publication of the NHS Plan and 'Comprehensive critical care' in 2000. These achievements are highlighted below, and many were mentioned in a keynote speech by Rosie Winterton MP, Minister of State for Health, at the 'Critical Care United – National Sharing Event' on 5 March 2004 (Winterton 2004):

Critical care networks

Every critical care facility in England is now part of a 'network'. The networks bring together NHS Trusts in geographical areas so that they are able to take responsibility for the planning and implementation of improvement projects, and the provision of critical care services. The sharing of critical care skills has played an important part in the 23% reduction in heart-related deaths since 1997 and the 10% reduction in the rate of premature deaths from cancer since 1997.

Critical care capacity   The NHS has exceeded the NHS Plan objective, with a 32% increase in adult critical care beds since January 2000.

Critical care transfers   The numbers of critical care transfers between hospitals is down by up to 48% (October 2003 to January 2004 compared to the same period in 2000–2001).

Critical care outreach   A total of 170 hospitals out of 220 hospitals in England with critical care services now have critical care outreach teams. Ball & Kirby (2003) highlighted that the introduction of a critical care outreach service in one hospital resulted in an improvement in survival to discharge from hospital after discharge from critical care by 6.8 % and that readmission to critical care was reduced by 6.4%.

Track and trigger warning systems   Early warning scoring systems are now in place in many hospitals. However, as yet, there is no clear evidence identifying the ideal choice of track and trigger model. Nonetheless, the NHS Modernisation Agency (2003a) recommends that post-implementation audit, evaluation and local refinement of the selected track and trigger system are essential. Further suggestions are made around the need for measuring outcomes rather than associations and for the focus to be on patient needs, and not activity. This approach is congruent with the requirements of the 'National Standards, Local Action – Health & Social Care Standards and Planning Framework 2005–2008' (Department of Health 2004), and reflects a continuing trend to measure health service performance on qualitative methods in addition to quantitative methods.

Workforce development and clinical competence issues

Whilst it would be unreasonable to expect all nurses working in general areas to be competent in all aspects of high dependency nursing, it is essential that all nurses have at least a working understanding of the fundamental principles of high dependency patient assessment and care. Following the publication of 'Comprehensive critical care', the Department of Health (2001) published 'The nursing contribution to the provision of comprehensive critical care for adults: a strategic programme of action'. This document set recommendations for all ward and departmental nurses to have access to competency-based education and training to ensure that each is able to provide Level 0–2 care with appropriate specialist support within the ward environment. The intention of this is to complement the aforementioned principles of both critical care outreach teams and early warning systems, to help to prevent further deterioration in a patient's condition, and possibly avert the need for the patient to be transferred to a more formal critical care environment. However, if such a transfer were inevitable, the nurse with the prerequisite assessment skills would be in a position to provide more appropriate and timely care until and during the transfer, thus reducing the risks to the patient.

Equally, there are many clinical areas where a significant proportion of patients require high dependency care on a regular basis, but perhaps only for short periods of time. For example, this would include the accident and emergency department, the acute admissions ward or the medical assessment ward/unit. Nurses working in these areas are not working in formal HDUs but it is nonetheless imperative that they are competent in the requisite high dependency/critical care nursing skills. A further dimension for consideration is around the rather rapid change in in-patient demographics in most acute hospitals. The continuing drive for greater efficiency in the NHS (NHS Modernisation Agency 2003b) is leading to many surgical procedures now being carried out on a day-surgery basis. This means that, by definition, the in-patient population is likely to be more highly dependent compared to 15–20 years ago, when hospital wards contained a mix of both high and lower dependency patients. This is much less likely to be the case now; hence the need for nurses to be trained not only in the fundamentals of care, but also in comprehensive patient assessment and observation skills.

Regardless of the presence of monitoring equipment, an extremely important part of nursing practice is the visual (and auditory) observation of the patient. It may often be the discrete and gradual changes in the behaviour or appearance of a patient that signal the advent of more ominous physiological changes. For example, the patient who is gradually becoming more restless and agitated may be uncomfortable in bed, or be in pain, or perhaps have a blocked urinary catheter. Of graver concern would be the possibility that the patient is becoming increasingly hypoxic or is haemorrhaging. The need for close observation dictates that high dependency care should provide a level of nursing resource (the number and the skill mix of nurses) that can provide this essential component of care.

Many hospitals are linking with their higher education providers to respond to the workforce development requirements of the modern critical care agenda. Thorne & Hackwood (2002) describe a successful approach to work-based learning, using a competency-based assessment model as the focus for critical care skills development. Other areas are employing practice development nurses to assist with the critical care skills-acquisition programme.

It is imperative, therefore, that nurse training, development and clinical supervision requirements are given due consideration in order that high-quality patient care services can be delivered in the high dependency area. The amount of time and resources required to train, develop and supervise the acquisition of advanced clinical and assessment skills in nurses should not be underestimated. For example, it is wholly unacceptable for nurses to be expected to care for patients requiring artificial ventilation if they have not had the necessary training, development and assessment to carry out this care safely and effectively. Acquiring such skills takes time, commitment from all members of the multidisciplinary team and investment, both in financial terms and with regard to access to study resources, research, etc. It is also important that any formal programme of education acquires academic accreditation that forms part of a degree programme.

It is indefensible for hospitals to expect nurses to provide high-quality care if the hospital cannot provide access to high-quality training.

Nurse and healthcare assistant staffing in critical care areas

It is clear from an understanding of the physiological, physical and emotional needs of the high dependency patient that nursing is key to effective high dependency care. In order to provide this level of observation and care, there has to be a corresponding ratio of nurses and healthcare assistants. It is a logical progression that, for any given number of patients, as the nurse to patient ratio falls, the capacity to observe/input care for each individual patient is also likely to fall.

The guidelines on admission to and discharge from intensive care and high dependency units (Department of Health, 1996) stated that:

A key distinguishing feature between intensive care, high dependency care and ward care is the nursing activity required. Nursing activity will vary with patient dependency and there is usually an association between patient dependency and nursing activity. As a result, in general, intensive care patients require the highest nursing activity. There are times, however, when a patient who has a lower dependency requires greater nursing activity, such as the spontaneously breathing, hypoxic patient who is admitted to high dependency care for close observation and may require more nursing activity than the fully ventilated and sedated patient in intensive care.

These guidelines suggested *minimum* recommended nurse–patient ratios in intensive care and high dependency as shown in Table 1.1.

Taking the example of the aforementioned hypoxic patient, it is highly possible that with the hypoxia comes confusion and probable agitation. This alone can increase the patient's nursing dependency needs greatly. In addition, it is also highly possible for this type of patient to be nursed in a general ward environment, which, in turn, can lead to significant clinical risk issues and also affect the care of other patients, particularly if the ward is not resourced adequately from a staffing perspective.

It is also important to differentiate between the patient requiring high dependency care and the patient who is only *physically* dependent. The latter may require a high input of nursing care but may not require *high dependency care* as discussed in this context. It would be an inappropriate use of acute high dependency or critical care facilities if patients were admitted as a result of their need for physical nursing care (Vandyk 1997).

Nonetheless, the concept of nurse to patient ratios of 1:1 for ICU and 1:2 for HDU no longer appear to be as robust as has previously been suggested. Endacott suggests that the 1:1 nurse-to-patient ratio required for intensive care, as stipulated by the Department of Health, is not research-based and that 'nurses need to be ready to answer the critics who suggest that such levels of staffing are not necessary' (Endacott

Table 1.1   Minimum recommended nurse–patient ratios in intensive care and high dependency areas (Department of Health 1996)

Area	Number of nurses	Number of patients	Nurse to patient ratio
Intensive care	1	1	1:1
High dependency areas	1	2	1:2

1996). 'Comprehensive critical care' (Department of Health, 2000b) suggests a move away from the use of rigid ratios to determine nursing staffing for patients requiring Level 2 or Level 3 care to the use of more flexible systems for assessing nursing workload. Such systems include the system of patient-related activity (SOPRA) and comprehensive nursing intervention score (CNIS).

However, despite these, it seems that the methodology for the calculation of ideal nursing staffing levels in critical care areas still does not exist. In the absence of anything better, it would seem that most critical care areas still use a patient category scoring system to calculate nurse–patient ratios, similar to that recommended by the Department of Health in 1996. However, Adomat & Hicks (2003) conducted an observational study that used a video recorder to document nurse activity for 48 continuous shifts in two intensive care units to determine the accuracy of the nursing workload patient category scoring system in measuring nursing workload. The results of this study demonstrated that, despite complex care needs, a high percentage of nursing activities observed in each unit consisted of low skill activity. Furthermore, it concluded that nurses spent less time with patients categorized as in need of intensive care than with those in need of those in need of high dependency care, and that existing nurse–patient ratio classifications may, therefore, be inappropriate.

Another important distinction to make is in relation to the use of acute physiology and intervention scoring systems such as:

- acute physiology and chronic health evaluation (APACHE III);
- simplified acute physiology score (SAPS II);
- sequential organ failure assessment (SOFA);
- mortality probability model (MPM II);
- therapeutic intervention scoring system (TISS).

These systems are commonly used in ICUs and some HDUs, and are useful evaluative research and audit tools for critical care environments with regard to the prediction of care and treatment outcomes (Ridley 1994, Collins 1995, Gunning & Rowan 1999). However, they are not designed to predict nurse–patient ratios or nursing workload, or to determine admission to or discharge from an intensive care or high dependency area (Department of Health 1996a,b, Endacott & Chellel 1996, Viney et al 1997).

It would seem that there is no patient dependency or nurse workload scoring system currently in existence that encompasses all aspects of nursing care and work in both high dependency and intensive care areas. With reference to Needham's work (1997), it is questionable as to whether a model will ever be developed that will become a single predictor of nursing care and work. However, it is important, in the absence of anything else, that physiological scoring systems and intervention scoring systems are not used as predictors of nurse workload and patient dependency.

So how do we get clarity on this complex subject area? In February 2003, the Royal College of Nursing produced a document entitled 'Guidance for nurse staffing in critical care'. This is probably the most useful and practical document currently available to assist nurse leaders and managers in determining the right numbers and skill mix of nurses and healthcare assistants. This document suggests that the best people to decide on nursing staffing levels are senior critical care nurses themselves, who have the requisite skills in assessing patient need. In addition, it offers very practical advice on the following topics:

- the workload and skill mix required to meet patients' needs (including patient dependency);
- the role of critical care nurses;
- staffing levels and skill mix of the multiprofessional team;
- the contribution of healthcare assistants;
- the presence of a supervisory shift leader;
- nursing work other than direct patient care;
- the critical care facilities and physical environment;
- flexible working patterns;
- professional development for nurses;
- pre-registration education for nurses;
- developing a strategic plan for the critical care workforce.

Whatever the setting for the delivery of high dependency care, the following key elements must be in place for nursing staff, if the care delivered is to be safe, of high quality and effective:

- a nurse–patient ratio that allows the close observation of patients 24 hours a day;
- a nursing establishment that is appropriately trained and competent to deliver the care required, and to the highest standards;
- a skill mix and competency base within that nursing establishment that enables all of the patients' care needs to be assessed, analysed, understood and acted upon 24 hours a day;
- ready access to suitably experienced and qualified medical staff, and other relevant members of the multidisciplinary team 24 hours a day;
- the appropriate equipment to carry out care safely and effectively.

There should be evidence of these key elements, or a plan to enable their future provision, in clinical areas that routinely undertake high dependency-type care. It is also important to realize that the success of a high dependency care area will largely be reliant upon the quality of the clinical leadership (nursing and medical) provided to that area.

CONCLUSION

The development of the concept of high dependency care, and areas where that level of care is provided, has been rapid since the 1940s. It is essential that, wherever that level of care is provided, the area is appropriately staffed and resourced in a way that ensures the delivery of safe and effective care to patients.

Such care is expensive, and it is important to monitor costs and utilization, in both human and material resource terms. However, if established and managed appropriately, with supportive nurse and medical staff development programmes, the high dependency area can be an extremely rewarding and motivating environment in which to work. In addition, such an environment can offer invaluable professional development opportunities to nurses at all levels, while providing the opportunity to deliver the ultimate objective of safe, high-quality and effective patient-care.

References

Adomat R, Hicks C 2003 Measuring nursing workload in intensive care: an observational study using closed-circuit video cameras. Journal of Advanced Nursing 42: 402–412

Aps C 2000 Operating theatres, cutting edge. Health Service Journal 110: 24–25

Aps C 2002 Critical care of the surgical patient. British Journal of Perioperative Nursing 12: 258–265

Aps C 2004 Editorial: Surgical critical care: the overnight intensive OIR concept. British Journal of Anaesthesia 92: 164–166

Association of Anaesthetists 1988 Intensive care services – provision for the future. Association of Anaesthetists of Great Britain and Ireland, London

Association of Anaesthetists 1991 The high dependency unit – acute care in the future. Association of Anaesthetists of Great Britain and Ireland, London

Audit Commission 1999 Critical to success – the place of efficient and effective care services within the acute hospital. Audit Commission, London

Ball C, Kirby M 2003 Effect of the critical care outreach team on patient survival to discharge from hospital and readmission to critical care: non-randomized population based study. British Medical Journal 327: 1014

Bion J 1994 Cost containment Europe. United Kingdom Critical Care Medicine 2: 341–344

Carnall D 1996 UK reviews intensive care and emergency services. British Medical Journal 312: 655

Collins A 1995 MPM II and SAPS II: a review of easy to use severity systems. Care of the Critically Ill 11: 73–76

Department of Health 1996a Report of the working group on guidelines on admission to and discharge from intensive care and high dependency units. NHS Executive, London

Department of Health 1996b Guidelines on admission to and discharge from intensive care and high dependency units. NHS Executive, London

Department of Health 1997 Intensive and high dependency care data collection – user's manual for the augmented care period (ACP) dataset. NHS Executive, London

Department of Health 2000a The new NHS, modern, dependable. NHS Executive, London

Department of Health 2000b Comprehensive critical care – a review of adult critical care services. NHS Executive, London.

Department of Health 2001 The nursing contribution to the provision of comprehensive critical care for adults: a strategic programme of action. NHS Executive, London

Department of Health 2004 National standards, local action – health and social care planning framework 2005–2008. NHS Executive, London

Endacott R 1996 Staffing intensive care units: a consideration of contemporary issues. Intensive and Critical Care Nursing 12: 193–199

Endacott R, Chellel A 1996 Nursing dependency scoring: measuring total care workload. Nursing Standard 10(37): 39–42

Franklin C M, Rackow E C, Mamdani B et al 1988 Decreases in mortality on a large urban service by facilitating access to critical care. Archives of Internal Medicine 148: 1403–1405

Gunning K, Rowan K 1999 Outcome data and scoring systems. British Medical Journal 319: 24

Hopkinson R 1996 General care units. In: Tinker J, Browne D, Sibbald W (eds) Critical care – standards, audit and ethics. Edward Arnold, London, ch 4

Intensive Care Society 1990 The intensive care service in the UK. Intensive Care Society, London

Jennett B 1990 Is intensive care worthwhile? Care of the Critically Ill 6(3): 85–88

Kilpatrick A, Ridley S, Plenerleith L 1994 A changing role for intensive therapy: is there a case for high dependency care? Anaesthesia 49: 666–670

King's Fund Panel 1989 Intensive care in the United Kingdom: report from the King's Fund Panel. Anaesthesia 44: 428–431

Metcalfe A, McPherson K 1995 Study of provision of intensive care in England. Revised report for the Department of Health. School of Hygiene and Tropical Medicine, London

Mohan J 1995 A national health service? The restructuring of health care in Britain since 1979. St Martins Press, London

Needham J 1997 Accuracy in workload measurement: a fact or fallacy? Journal of Nursing Management 5: 83–87

NHS Modernisation Agency 2003a Critical care outreach – progress in developing services. NHS Executive, London

NHS Modernisation Agency 2003b Annual report. NHS Executive, London

Oh T 1997 Intensive care manual. Reed Educational and Professional Publishing Ltd, London: 3–10

Peacock J, Edbrooke D 1995 Rationing intensive care. Data from one high dependency unit supports their effectiveness. British Medical Journal 310: 1413

Rennie M 1995 Strengthening the case for high dependency care. British Journal of Intensive Care January: 5

Report of the National Confidential Enquiry into Perioperative Deaths (NCEPOD) 1992–1993. NCEPOD, London (Website: www.ncepod.org)

Ridley S 1994 Scoring systems and prognosis for critical illness. Care of the Critically Ill 10(2): 666–670

Royal College of Anaesthetists & Royal College of Surgeons of England (RCA/RCSE) 1996 Report of the Joint Working Party on Graduated Patient Care. RCA/RCSE, London

Royal College of Nursing (RCN) 2003 Guidance for nurse staffing in critical care. RCN, London

Ryan D W 1995 Rationing intensive care. High dependency units may be the answer. British Medical Journal 310: 682–683

Thompson F, Singer M 1995 High dependency units in the UK: variable size, variable character, few in number. Journal of Postgraduate Medicine 71: 217–221

Thorne L, Hackwood H 2002 Developing critical care skills for nurses in the ward environment: a work-based learning approach. Nursing in Critical Care 7(3): 121–125

Vandyk R 1997 Cash and carry. Health Service Journal 1 May: 28–29

Viney C, Poxon I, Jordan C, Winter B 1997 Does the APACHE II scoring system equate with the Nottingham Patient Dependency System? – can these systems be used to determine nursing workload and skill mix? Nursing in Critical Care 2(2): 62–63

Winterton R 2004 Speech to Critical Care United – National Sharing Event

Chapter **2**

The fundamental principles of high dependency care

Mandy Sheppard

KEY LEARNING OBJECTIVES

- To understand the reasons for close observation and assessment of the highly dependent patient
- To appreciate the importance of an effective multidisciplinary team and responsive services
- To understand the factors that contribute to and influence effective patient assessment and monitoring
- To appreciate the need to detect and manage both current and potential patient problems in high dependency care

INTRODUCTION

The highly dependent patient requires an enhanced level of care and is classified as a Level 2 patient. A definition of Level 2 care is:

> *Patients requiring more detailed observation or intervention including support for a single failing organ system or post-operative care and those 'stepping down' from higher levels of care.*
>
> (Department of Health 2000)

A core feature of high dependency care is the need for more detailed observation or intervention, and a key aim of this chapter is to explore a range of factors that contribute to the rationale for this level of care.

At times, it can be difficult to distinguish between the Level 1 and the Level 2 patient. At some point, the Level 1 patient who is deteriorating will become a Level 2 patient. Equally, a Level 2 patient who is improving will become a Level 1 patient. In both cases, the point at which the patient crosses over to a different level of care is a fine line. Consequently, this chapter is applicable to both levels of patient.

THE CONTEXT OF HIGH DEPENDENCY CARE

When a patient requires high dependency care, it is not simply a matter of moving the patient into a differently named clinical area. High dependency care is a service not a location and there are certain requirements that are relevant, regardless of the location.

Close observation and assessment

As patients become sicker, it is a natural, almost automatic, response to observe them more closely and to record their observations more frequently. This takes time, hence the nurse–patient ratios are usually higher than compared to a patient at Level 0.

It is inappropriate for nurse–patient ratios to be 'set' according to the type of patient or clinical area. There are many variables that can influence the required ratio, including: the physical and psychological needs of the patient; the needs of the relatives; the presence of healthcare assistants within the nursing establishment; the presence of pre- or post-registration students, and patient safety. This dictates that staffing should be flexible to meet the individual needs of the patient (Royal College of Nursing 2003).

Close observation and assessment is required in order to detect the following.

Sudden, unexpected but noticeable changes in condition

Sudden changes can occur in a patient's condition and may also be completely unexpected (i.e. with nothing in the past medical history to alert staff to a potential problem).

Example: A 72-year-old gentleman has had a total hip replacement; he is now in his second post-operative day on the orthopaedic ward and is progressing as would be expected. When walking past his bed, one of the nurses notices that the patient appears sweaty and, on engaging him in discussion, seems disorientated. The nurse decides to perform some observations, which reveal:

- pulse is extremely rapid at 140 beats/minute (bpm), irregular and weak (normally regular between 75 and 85 bpm);
- blood pressure is 75/50 mmHg (normally 120–130/85–90 mmHg);
- respiratory rate is 26 respirations/minute (rpm; normally 12–16 rpm).

The nurse calls a doctor and, while waiting, performs a 12-lead electrocardiogram (ECG). The nurse stays with the patient allowing close observation and records the vital signs every 15 minutes. Atrial fibrillation is diagnosed, and it is decided to transfer the patient to the surgical high dependency unit for continuous ECG monitoring and treatment with amiodarone.

Discreet slower changes in condition

Sometimes the condition of a patient may change discreetly and, unlike the previous example, the change may not be sudden or overtly noticeable. There will be small changes, which, in combination, alert the nurse to observe the patient more closely and record the observations more regularly. The slight changes may not be causing current instability but will in time, if not detected and treated.

Example A 52-year-old lady has returned to the gynaecological ward following a total abdominal hysterectomy. Her vital signs on return to the ward at 2 pm are:

- pulse is 62 bpm and regular (pre-operatively 60–75 bpm);
- blood pressure is 120/75 mmHg (pre-operatively 120/80 mmHg);
- respiratory rate is 12 rpm (pre-operatively 14 rpm);
- oxygen saturation of haemoglobin in the peripheral capillaries (SpO_2) is 96% on 3 litres of oxygen;
- temperature is 35.2°C and peripherally cool to touch;
- the urinary catheter bag is emptied and 250 ml of urine is recorded on the fluid balance chart;
- there is minimal drainage from the wound drains;
- the patient is drowsy but rousable, and her pain seems well controlled with morphine patient-controlled analgesia (PCA).

At 4 pm, her vital signs are:

- pulse is 75 bpm;
- blood pressure is 110/80 mmHg;
- respiratory rate is 14 rpm;
- SpO_2 is 96% on 3 litres of oxygen;
- temperature is 36.2°C and peripherally warm to touch;
- there is an unmeasured volume of urine in the catheter bag;
- there is minimal drainage from the wound drains;
- pain remains well controlled with analgesia and she has had some sips of water.

At 6 pm, her vital signs are:

- pulse is 76 bpm;
- blood pressure is 110/85 mmHg;
- respiratory rate is 14 rpm;
- SpO_2 is 95% on 3 litres of oxygen;
- temperature 36.1°C and peripherally cool to touch;
- the urinary catheter bag is emptied and, since 2 pm, only 8 ml of urine has drained;
- there is minimal drainage from the wound drains;
- the patient seems a little restless but reports no pain; she does appear slightly paler than before.

At 6 pm, the nurse performing the observations notes that, whilst the patient's pulse, blood pressure, respiratory rate and SpO_2 are all within normal parameters, she is cooler peripherally, appears pale, slightly restless yet not in pain, and her urine output is less than 0.5 ml/kg per hour for the last 4 hours.

Although the patient is haemodynamically stable, there are some subtle changes in her condition, and the nurse decides to assess and perform observations of the vital signs every 15 minutes and calls the doctor to assess the patient. The patient's intravenous fluids are increased and her urine output measured hourly. She remains oliguric (less than 0.5 ml/kg per hour) and cool to touch. Her pulse increases slightly and her blood pressure remains at 110/85 mmHg; although her vital signs are within normal parameters, it is decided to return the patient to theatre where a bleeding point is found and a clot evacuated.

This is an example of a patient with a post-operative haemorrhage who maintains her vital signs through compensatory mechanisms. The subtle changes that alert the nurse are cool peripheries, a reduction in urine output, pallor and restlessness.

Potential problems

Well-defined potential problems   Certain clinical conditions are associated with potential problems and close observation is maintained to detect the problems.

Example: A 58-year-old gentleman is admitted to the coronary care unit with a diagnosed myocardial infarction. One potential problem post-infarction is the advent of arrhythmias and, to enable prompt detection, he is attached to a monitor that will continuously display his heart rate and rhythm.

General potential problems   For some patients, there will be a combination of events and circumstances that in combination suggest a more general, less defined potential for deterioration.

Example: A 78-year-old lady with a history of hypertension, diet-controlled diabetes and angina is admitted to the hospital for a total knee replacement. Post-operatively it is planned for her to return to the orthopaedic ward. Peri-operatively there are problems with bleeding, which require significant fluid resuscitation and the anaesthetic time is longer than had been anticipated. Now, the operative events in combination with her co-morbidities dictate that closer observation than is possible on the ward is required and it is decided to keep her in the recovery/post-operative care unit overnight.

Response to treatment

Some treatments are titrated to the patient's clinical response, and close regular (often continuous) observation and assessment is required.

Example 1 central venous pressure (CVP) measurements to assess the effect of a fluid challenge.

Example 2 ECG monitoring to assess the effect of an antiarrhythmic drug (e.g. amiodarone) in a patient with fast atrial fibrillation.

Example 3 blood pressure monitoring to assess the effect of an anti-hypertensive drug infusion (e.g. sodium nitroprusside).

The multidisciplinary team

The highly dependent patient, in addition to more detailed observation, may also require prompt intervention. This requires a well-coordinated multidisciplinary team; the nurse who is usually in more regular attendance may often be the coordinator of the team.

Examples of multidisciplinary team members could include physiotherapists, doctors, dieticians and pharmacists. The important point is that they are readily available to the highly dependent patient to provide timely intervention, which is often dictated as a result of close observation.

In addition to the availability of these staff, there are also certain services that must be available. One example is the laboratory services and the ability to provide a quick turn-around time for samples to enable prompt analysis of the results and again timely intervention, if required.

PATIENT ASSESSMENT

There are number of models for patient assessment. 'Know, see, find' (Norman & Cook 2000) and 'Airway, breathing, circulation, disability, exposure' (adapted from Smith 2000) are two models often used in combination to provide a comprehensive patient assessment (see Chapter 9). Specific assessment methods are also discussed in the relevant clinical chapters (see Chapters 5–11).

Regardless of the model, method or tool used for assessment, there are a number of underpinning principles relevant to all forms of patient assessment.

The clinical decision

One such principle is that the model, method or tool must provide the most accurate and comprehensive assessment of the patient. This is important because a key aspect of high dependency care is the ability to provide timely interventions and this requires accurate patient assessment.

Interventions can be delayed for a number of reasons, but one is when a member of staff does not feel confident in their clinical decision or judgement (i.e. if an individual is unsure), he or she is unlikely to pass on that information to someone who can orchestrate a therapeutic intervention. The common scenario is that individuals will wait until they feel there is sufficient evidence on which to base a clinical decision or judgement in which they are more confident and comfortable to escalate to other members of the team. Unfortunately, by that time, the patient may have exhausted physiological reserves and be requiring Level 2 or 3 care.

In many respects, this response is understandable; there are many factors involved in this complex subject but the concept of credibility is key (Kenward & Hodgetts 2002). It is easy, in terms of clinical decision-making, to wake a member of the medical staff at 3 am with news that 'my patient has a systolic blood pressure of 60 mmHg systolic with an unrecordable diastolic pressure, and a heart rate of 180 bpm'. Credibility is safe because the assessment is compelling and the clinical state of the patient would be universally regarded as one that requires immediate attention. However, it is more difficult with the patient who is slowly and discreetly deteriorating (often giving rise to the feeling that 'the patient is not quite right'), where vital signs are still within normal parameters, yet the nurse has concerns, often based on direct observation signs, such as colour, respirations, behaviour and the feel of the skin. In this case, the perceived potential loss of credibility is far greater.

The information used to make an assessment of the patient is important, as it relates directly to a judgement being made and that, in turn, drives the clinical decision (Dowding & Thompson 2003). Nurses who are caring for highly dependent patients need to be aware of which infor-

If a comprehensive assessment of the patient reveals nothing tangible yet that feeling of 'the patient not being quite right' prevails, it is important to still seek help or advice from a more senior member of the nursing team or a member of the medical staff.

mation is accurate or appropriate for each individual patient, and this element of patient assessment will be explored later in this chapter.

There are a number of strategies that may be used to enhance the speed and accuracy of clinical decision-making, which in turn will enable timely interventions, such as the use of trends, knowing the patient norms and baselines, and having a level of underpinning physiological knowledge, all of which will also be explored later in the chapter. The implementation of early warning scores can help to provide an objective measurement of change in the patient condition, and these can be used as an integral part of patient assessment prior to the patient requiring Level 2 care (see Chapter 1). Using underpinning knowledge can often help to articulate concerns in a way that preserves credibility and results in clinical action being taken. Box 2.1 provides an example of how the condition of a patient may be communicated. Method A is unlikely to result in prompt action, whereas Method B provides more information with rationale, and is more likely to prompt action and intervention.

> Patient assessment must allow a clinical decision to be made that results in a timely and appropriate intervention for the patient.

The importance of baseline observations

At some stage in their care, patients will have had their baseline observations performed. This is easier to achieve in elective surgical patients, as they are normally admitted 'well' (apart from their surgical complaint), either in hospital or as part of pre-operative assessment. Emergency surgical and medical patients are more difficult, as their observations are often deranged on admission and, of course, this may be one of the indications for admission. Where possible, it is vital to obtain a set of observations that reflect the norm for that patient and this is important for two reasons.

1. When a patient slowly deteriorates, one of the first signs to alert staff will be a slow deviation away from the baseline observations.

Box 2.1   Ways of communicating concern

Method A

'My patient feels cold and looks pale and I am not happy with him'

Method B

'Mr Smith, the 67-year-old gentleman who is now 6 hours post his abdominal aortic aneurysm repair, has been warm and well perfused since return from theatre. In the last 30 minutes, he has become peripherally vasoconstricted, and both arms and legs, and his face feel extremely cold to touch. I am concerned that he has peripherally vasoconstricted as a compensatory mechanism possibly as a response to haemorrhage. I would be grateful if you could come and review him with me.'

2. An individual patient's norms may not be 'textbook' norms. For example, a patient with chronic obstructive pulmonary disease (COPD) may be perfectly happy with a SpO_2 of 89%, whereas, in a patient without chronic lung disease, this level of saturation would be extremely worrying. Another example could be the physically fit individual who may have a resting heart rate of 40 bpm, which would be strictly defined as a bradycardia, and in other individuals would cause cardiovascular instability.

The reliance upon baseline observations means that they need to be accurate. Blood pressure must be taken with the correct sized cuff and the patient should be given the opportunity to 'settle down' first. Noting the peripheral perfusion of the patient prior to measuring the SpO_2 is important. If, for example, the patient is attending a pre-operative assessment clinic on a cold winter's morning, vasoconstriction will have occurred to conserve body temperature, and to measure the SpO_2, good peripheral perfusion is required. In this situation, it is important to have discussion first while the patient warms up and perform the observations later.

Where the person recording the baseline observations has any doubt in their accuracy (e.g. the SpO_2 in the patient who remains peripherally cold), there should be the facility to document these concerns to alert staff who may be caring for the patient at a later date. It may be several stages later that a problem becomes apparent, when the patient is highly dependent and those caring for the patient are unlikely to be the same as those who measured the baseline observations. The reliance is, therefore, on seamless documentation following the patient; this highlights the concept discussed in Chapter 1 that high dependency care is part of a continuum of care.

The patient's history in many ways provides a baseline for the patient, and it will also allow potential problems to be anticipated or, in the event of the patient's deterioration, may help to identify the more likely causes.

Direct patient observation

A vital element of patient assessment and ongoing monitoring is to look at, listen to and touch the patient. Observations gained from this activity can be valuable in isolation, but also in conjunction with other assessment and monitoring methods.

The following provide some examples of the information that can be gained through these activities.

Looking at the patient

- Skin condition: rashes resulting from the disease process or drug reaction; bruises may indicate a coagulopathy. Sweating, particularly on the forehead, may accompany respiratory distress.
- Patient behaviour: confusion, hallucinations or an altered mental state can be the result of a number of clinical states, such as hypoxia, electrolyte imbalance or sleep deprivation.
- Skin colour: pallor may reflect anaemia or vasoconstriction; a flushed appearance may be due to vasodilatation.

- Mouth opening and pursed lips: signs of respiratory distress.
- Patient movement: a lack of movement may indicate pain or the use of the accessory muscles of respiration may indicate respiratory distress.
- Mucous membrane colour: central cyanosis may present with a blue tinge.

Listening to the patient

- Respiratory signs: an inspiratory wheeze suggesting an obstructive airway problem or an expiratory wheeze in the presence of bronchospasm. A 'bubbly' sound may be due to pulmonary oedema.
- The way the patient speaks is also important: The breathless patient may only be able to speak two or three words before pausing to take a breath; sentences sound very interrupted. The patient may be confused, disorientated or describe feelings of anxiety.

Touching the patient

- Skin temperature: a cool skin can indicate vasoconstriction, which may be due to hypovolaemia, cardiac failure or an attempt to maintain core body temperature
- Skin condition: a lack of skin turgor may suggest dehydration, although caution should be exercised in the older patient where reduced skin turgor may naturally occur from reduced skin elasticity. Peripheral oedema may indicate fluid overload.

Physiological compensatory mechanisms

When a problem exists in a body system, the body system will attempt to maintain the function of that system by activating a compensatory mechanism, the aim being to maintain function until the problem is resolved.

For example, in hypoxia, the respiratory system will aim to maintain oxygenation and will initially activate two compensatory mechanisms to achieve this aim. One is to increase the respiratory rate and the second is to increase the tidal volume (depth) of each breath. If these measures work, and manage to maintain oxygenation, pulse oximetry will not initially detect a problem (i.e. it is still measuring good oxygenation and cannot detect whether this is being achieved with normal or excessive respiratory effort). Through direct patient observation, the signs of respiratory distress would be noted, such as tachypnoea, dyspnoea, increased work of breathing, colour changes, mouth breathing and sweating. If the cause of the hypoxia is not resolved, a point will be reached when the compensatory mechanisms can no longer maintain adequate oxygenation. Now the arterial saturation of oxygen will fall and the pulse oximeter will detect the change but, of course, now the patient is in an extremely vulnerable position, having exhausted the compensatory reserves.

This example not only describes the role of compensatory mechanisms, it also highlights the key role that direct patient observation has in the early detection of patient deterioration (i.e. when the patient is moving from Level 0 to Level 1 care). If there were to be a total reliance upon the pulse oximeter to alert staff to a problem, the patient would already be at Level 1 and possibly moving towards needing Level 2, if not Level 3 care.

Monitoring equipment is designed to monitor a function. Where the function is being maintained by a physiological compensatory mechanism, the monitoring equipment will not detect compensation, only that the function is within normal parameters.

The purpose of many items of commonly used monitoring equipment is to monitor a physiological function (e.g. pulse oximetry monitors oxygenation). The whole point of a compensatory mechanism is to maintain the function and, consequently, it is logical that, where the function is being maintained through compensation, the particular item of monitoring equipment will be unable to detect a problem until compensation is no longer possible.

Another example was described earlier in the chapter, where a young woman following a major gynaecological operation was haemorrhaging, yet her vital signs remained within 'normal' parameters. The aim is to maintain blood pressure in this clinical situation and the main compensatory mechanism that will achieve this is peripheral vasoconstriction. Two of the signs that alerted staff to a potential problem were pallor and cool peripheries, both suggesting peripheral vasoconstriction. As with all compensatory mechanisms, this is finite and a point will be reached where blood loss is so great that even maximum vasoconstriction is not able to maintain a blood pressure, and it will fall. It is at this point that the automated blood pressure machine will detect a problem but, again, the patient will have exhausted his or her physiological reserve and be in an extremely vulnerable position.

The fight and flight response

The so-called 'fight and flight response' is mediated by the sympathetic nervous system, which is part of the autonomic nervous system. Adrenaline (epinephrine) is released, which causes the signs and symptoms associated with this physiological response (Table 2.1). It is designed to be activated when the individual is in danger and the response should help the individual to 'survive' the danger or threat. The 'fight and flight response' is also activated during times of physiological stress, and the signs and symptoms associated with the response are important ones for the nurse to detect, as they can be early indicators of a change in the patient's condition.

Table 2.1 The flight and fight response

Physiological response	Effect of response	Assessment of response
Increased respiratory rate	To improve exchange of oxygen	Assessment of respiratory rate
Increased heart rate	To transport the oxygen more effectively	Assessment of heart rate
Peripheral vasoconstriction	To divert blood to essential organs	Cool and pale skin
Raised blood glucose	Via the breakdown of stored glycogen for increased energy	Blood sugar monitoring
Reduced renal perfusion	To divert blood to essential organs	Oliguria

The key signs and symptoms may include:

- an increase in heart rate and respiratory rate;
- oliguria;
- peripheral vasoconstriction;
- increased blood glucose;
- pupil dilation;
- a feeling of impending doom on the part of the patient.

The feeling of impending doom is caused by adrenaline and, if a patient expresses this level of anxiety, it should be regarded as a significant sign.

The peripheral vasoconstriction and oliguria are caused by the body diverting blood to 'more essential' organs; these are the heart, lungs and brain. In addition to the skin and kidneys being considered as 'non-essential', so too is the gut. A failure to detect activation of this response may lead to a prolonged period of time where there is reduced tissue perfusion, which endangers tissue viability, and reduced gut perfusion, leading to gut ischaemia and reduced renal perfusion, which could lead to acute renal failure.

There are clinical situations in which the full response may not be obvious. It is important for the nurse to appreciate these and to focus on other presenting signs:

- for the non-catheterized patient, it may be difficult to assess urine output;
- for the beta-blocked patient, tachycardia may not be present;
- for the patient receiving opiates, tachypnoea may not be present.

Trends and multianalysis

One of the reasons to observe a patient closely is to detect discreet slower changes in condition. Often the nurse will be alerted to a potential problem through direct observational signs, such as change in colour, behaviour or peripheral perfusion. Whilst the vital signs may remain within 'normal' parameters, they may be changing, albeit slowly, and will eventually become abnormal.

Before the patient arrives at this stage, the use of trends and multi-analysis can assist in determining that a potential problem exists. The trend of the vital signs will allow the nurse to track the direction in which they are moving. For example, four heart rate recordings made at 30 minute intervals over a 2-hour period in a post-operative patient are 60 bpm, 70 bpm, 80 bpm and 90 bpm. None of these recordings falls outside of a normal reading, yet there is a definite increasing trend, which, if continued, would soon rise outside of a normal parameter (i.e. greater than 100 bpm).

As previously stated, the more concern there is over a patient, the more frequently the patient is assessed. If the four heart rate recordings were made every 15 minutes, and not every 30 minutes, the increasing trend would be obvious in 1 hour and not 2. This would allow a faster decision to be made with a subsequent intervention.

> It can be easy to become absorbed by clinical values and the information being provided by monitors; but it is important to remember to ask the patient how they feel. That in itself can be valuable information.

It is rare that an isolated clinical value provides sufficient information on which to base a clinical judgement and decision. Combining a number of clinical values (multianalysis), such as heart rate, blood pressure, temperature and urine output, will provide a much clearer picture of the patient, particularly if they are combined with direct observation.

The previous example of an increasing heart rate in a post-operative patient could have many causes and, if this were the only clinical value assessed and no direct observation was undertaken, it would be extremely difficult to ascertain the cause accurately. However, if it were accompanied by a rising core temperature and the patient appeared flushed, then pyrexia would seem likely. If the core temperature were normal, yet the patient felt cold, looked pale and was oliguric, then hypovolaemia would seem more likely.

PATIENT MONITORING

Monitoring equipment versus direct patient assessment and observation

The importance of direct and indirect patient assessment and observation must never be underestimated, and the presence of monitoring equipment should not detract from this important nursing activity. It is highly dangerous and inappropriate to assume a sense of security because a patient is connected to numerous pieces of equipment and to rely on that equipment to 'sound the alarm' if and when the patient's condition deteriorates.

It is also false security to assume that what the equipment is telling you is always accurate (e.g. blood pressure), especially as equipment can give faulty or misleading readings. It is the accumulation of basic and comprehensive nursing observations and assessment, and the information gained from monitoring equipment that provide the mainstay of high dependency care. Technology must never be used as a replacement for comprehensive manual clinical assessment of the patient. Buckley et al (1997) and Beckman et al (1996) describe the ability of technology to replace direct observation by a trained professional as being flawed and how professionals, by using direct observations, had far higher success rates in detecting incidents than machines did.

> Be careful not to become overly dependent upon monitoring equipment. Remember to check the accuracy of the equipment frequently and compare equipment readings against manual recordings, for example, invasive blood pressure readings (arterial line) versus a manual blood pressure reading. Also, remember to allow and account for margins of error and the limitations of automated devices. These will be referred to in the respective manufacturer's guidelines.

Combining monitoring and direct patient observation information

As previously stated, it is a normal activity to assess, record and analyse the findings more frequently the sicker the patient becomes. The pulse may initially be assessed hourly, then half-hourly to every 15 minutes and, if the patient continues to cause concern, the inevitable choice will be to monitor the heart rate continuously, by attaching the patient to an ECG monitor (see Chapter 6). The same can apply to blood pressure, where even cycling the non-invasive blood pressure (NIBP) machine every 5 minutes may be insufficient and a continuous view is required; hence an arterial cannula is inserted, connected to a transducer and continuously displayed on a monitor screen (see Chapter 6).

Importantly, patient assessment is informed by a combination of information gained from monitoring equipment and that gained from direct patient observation. A reliance solely on the monitoring equipment may result in important information being missed and/or misinterpreted.

Example: continuous ECG monitoring

Heart rate, as displayed as a number on a monitor, will provide information regarding the heart rate, and the ECG tracing itself will indicate the rhythm. The radial pulse should still be checked as: (1) an ECG is only reflecting the electrical activity of the heart and not the mechanical response; and (2) the monitor cannot provide information regarding the volume of the pulse – weak and thready, or full and bounding.

It is possible to record the heart rate from a non-invasive blood pressure machine or a pulse oximeter. By recording it in this way, the feel of the pulse, an important assessment method, is omitted. Taking a radial pulse has three other key benefits, as follows.

1. In the conscious patient, it also allows the measurement of respiratory rate (i.e. the patient thinks that only the pulse is being counted and will remain unaware that the respiratory rate is also being counted).
2. It allows an assessment of peripheral perfusion.
3. The contact made by touching the patient's hand to record the radial pulse can be both comforting and reassuring for the patient.

Invasive versus non-invasive monitoring

Monitoring can be invasive or non-invasive. Any invasive technique, whether it be urinary catheterization, intubation of the trachea or cannulation of an artery to obtain arterial blood gas analysis and arterial blood pressure readings, will breach the body's normal defences against infection. The risks of infection posed to the highly dependent patient must be balanced against the benefits that can be gained. The balance may shift from minute to minute, or day to day and, therefore, requires continuous re-assessment.

Other deciding factors, particularly for invasive monitoring, may include the following.

- The expertise and competence of the nursing and medical staff, which is frequently related to the regularity of exposure to the specific item of monitoring. If a high dependency unit admits one patient per year who requires arterial cannulation for blood pressure monitoring, and the nursing or medical staff only gain their experience on this unit, then that level of exposure will not enable the acquisition of either expertise or competence.

- The availability of equipment will always be a deciding factor for obvious reasons. This can also be linked to the regularity of requiring the equipment, which can often be borrowed, if required infrequently, and may not be available at all times. A frequent use would suggest a need to purchase the equipment. Inevitably, cost becomes an influencing factor, and cost to benefit comparability should be made.

SEQUENTIAL PROBLEMS

High dependency care incorporates the current clinical situation, but it must also consider and identify potential sequential problems that may occur at a later date and implement preventative strategies.

Concurrent therapies

The highly dependent patient may have a number of concurrent therapeutic interventions, which can often exert deleterious effects on each other and on different body systems. This underlines the need for close observation to detect current changes but also an anticipatory role to prevent future problems. One of numerous possible examples is given below.

A 57-year-old gentleman is admitted to the surgical/trauma high dependency unit for post-operative care following fixation of a fractured femur and an exploratory laparotomy. He has a past medical history of two myocardial infarctions, hypertension, coronary artery bypass grafts and diabetes.

Twenty-four hours after being admitted, his urine output decreases to 15 ml/hour for 2 consecutive hours. He has also developed a cough with frothy sputum and has some sacral oedema. It is felt that he is overloaded and 40 mg of furosemide is prescribed to promote a diuresis. His serum potassium result from a blood sample taken 2 hours previously was 3.5 mmol/l (normal range 3.5–5.0 mmol/l). He is given the furosemide intravenously and, in the following hour, he passes 200 ml and in the hour following that he passes a further 250 ml.

In this example of a gentleman with a strong cardiac history, it is clearly important that the diagnosed fluid overload is treated, to relieve the additional strain being placed on his heart. The diuretic has an excellent effect and is fulfilling the rationale for prescription. However, in view of this patient's cardiac history, the maintenance of an adequate serum potassium level is also important for cardiac function. Prior to the diuresis, his potassium was at the lower end of the normal range and one of the key routes of potassium loss out of the body is via urine.

In addition to recording the volume of urine being passed, the nurse should also be considering the effect on the serum potassium levels and be taking proactive steps concurrently to replace his potassium to avoid any cardiac problems.

Potential problems associated with immobility

The highly dependent patient may be relatively immobile and is, therefore, at risk from the many complications of restricted mobility. Five of those are now discussed.

The highly dependent patient may have a number of risk factors for *deep vein thrombosis*. Hip or leg fractures, hip and knee replacements, major general surgery and major trauma are all strong risk factors (Anderson & Spencer 2003), and are common reasons for a patient to require high dependency care. Risk assessments should be performed and appropriate preventative measures taken, for example, early mobilization, anticoagulation, antiembolism stockings and intermittent pneumatic compression.

Chest infection can occur owing to reduced secretion clearance; basal collapse and ventilation to perfusion mismatches. Early involvement of the physiotherapist, attention to the patient's position, effective analgesia in the post-operative patient, early mobilization and the teaching of correct breathing techniques are important preventative measures.

There is a risk of *urinary infection* owing to urinary stasis, the presence of a urinary catheter or an increase in the urinary pH. Strict asepsis and infection control measures should be exercised from the catheterization procedure itself and throughout the period of time when the patient is catheterized. Ensuring a good urine output by maintaining renal perfusion and changing the patient's position on a regular basis should be integral to the plan of care for the patient.

A *loss of tissue viability* is a particular risk for the highly dependent patient. This is in part due to immobility but also can be due to factors such as vasoconstriction (caused by a reduced cardiac output or constrictor drugs such as noradrenaline). Chronic diseases, such as diabetes, may increase the risk of pressure sore formation. Therapeutic measures, such as epidural analgesia, may also limit sensory and motor function, rendering the patient unable to feel pressure or be able to move to relieve pressure. The maintenance of tissue viability can be enhanced by regular position changes, maintenance of tissue perfusion and the use of pressure-relieving mattresses and beds.

Healthcare-associated infections (HCAIs) are a potential risk to all hospital patients and the highly dependent patient has specific risk factors, perhaps the most obvious being that use of invasive devices and equipment is more likely in this category of patient. Despite advances being made in the control of HCAIs, the incidence of methicillin-resistant *Staphylococcus aureus* (MRSA) continues to increase (National Audit Office 2004) and, although there are a number of inter-related factors involved, the role of nurses and other healthcare professionals in basic infection control techniques and procedures is irrefutable. Another aspect that is particular to this group of patients is their relative immobility, which may restrict access to the bathroom for hand-washing. Therefore, in addition to ensuring education and facilities for staff, the same must be made available to patients.

CONCLUSION

The key requirements of the highly dependent patient are detailed observation and intervention. This chapter has explored a number of the many principles that underpin these requirements, and how the assessment skills of the nurse, an effective multidisciplinary team, the correct use of monitoring equipment and attention to both the current and potential problems can combine to produce a high standard of high dependency care.

Technology continues to advance, and certainly has its place in the diagnosis and management of patients. However, as has been discussed in the chapter, the more direct, non-technological methods have an equally important place in critical care, and every effort should be made to incorporate them into the portfolio of nursing assessment and observation skills.

References

Anderson F A, Spencer F A 2003 Risk factors for venous thromboembolism. Circulation 107(23, Suppl): 19–116

Beckman U, Baldwin I, Hart G K, Runciman W B 1996 An Australian incident monitoring study in intensive care: AIMS-ICU an analysis of the first year reporting. Anaesthesia and Intensive Care 24: 321–329

Buckley T, Short T, Rowbottom Y, Oh T 1997 Critical care incident reporting in the intensive care unit. Anaesthesia 52(5): 403–409

Department of Health 2000 Comprehensive critical care: a review of adult critical care services. Department of Health, London

Dowding D, Thompson C 2003 Using judgement to improve accuracy in decision-making. Nursing Times 100(22): 42–43

Kenward G, Hodgetts T J 2002 Nurse concern: a predictor of patient deterioration. Nursing Times 98(22): 38–39

National Audit Office 2004 Improving patient care by reducing the risk of hospital acquired infections: A progress report. The Stationery Office. London

Norman J, Cook A 2000 Medical emergencies. In: Sheppard M, Wright M (eds) Principles and practice of high dependency nursing. Baillière Tindall, London

Royal College of Nursing 2003 Guidance for nurse staffing in critical care. Royal College of Nursing, London

Smith G 2000 ALERT: Acute life-threatening events recognition and treatment, 1st edn. University of Portsmouth, Portsmouth

Chapter **3**

Interpersonal issues in high dependency care

John Allen Wilkinson and Chris Wilkinson

KEY LEARNING OBJECTIVES

- To understand that good communication practice is essential to good clinical practice
- To consider factors which influence the quality of communication that occurs within a healthcare setting
- To recognize that communication in critical care situations has the potential to be particularly effective when it is integrated into a therapeutic partnership
- To analyse the quality of communication in practice to ascertain the extent to which it is accessible, and understandable, attended to and perceived appropriately, remembered and motivating to be acted upon
- To explore the potential of different concepts of stress to guide the assessment and management of anxiety-provoking situations

INTRODUCTION

Almost 150 years ago, the most authoritative voice of professional nursing included the following advice:

I have often been surprised at the thoughtlessness (resulting in cruelty, quite unintentionally) of friends or of doctors who will hold a long conversation just in the room or the passage adjoining to the room of the patient, who . . . knows they are talking about him . . . [I]f friends and doctors did but watch, as nurses can and should watch, the features sharpening, and eyes glowing almost wild, of fever patients . . . these would never run the risk again of creating such expectation, or irritation of mind. Always sit within the patient's view . . . never speak to an invalid from behind, nor from the door, nor from any distance from him, nor when he is doing anything.

(Nightingale 1859: 34, 35, 37)

Florence Nightingale's legacy is her great emphasis upon core nursing skills, and her observations of interpersonal relationships with patients led her to a number of conclusions, which are summarized in Box 3.1.

Given the historical emphasis upon the importance of communication to good health care outcomes, it would be reasonable to assume the principles and practices of good communication are now well established within a modern health care provider such as the National Health Service (NHS). However, the findings of the regulatory authorities suggest otherwise. The Health Service Ombudsman (2002) and Commission for Health Improvement (2002) both report that much more needs to be done to improve communication with NHS patients and their families. Tingle (2003) comments that the devolvement in NHS governance puts great responsibility upon NHS staff working on the front line at ward and department level to implement policies and evidenced-based practice. He argues that the most effective NHS organizations are those that learn from critical incidents, have a commitment to lifelong learning and share good practice.

The central importance of identifying and valuing fundamental nursing skills to tackle the problems faced within contemporary health care continue to be championed by modern commentators such as Castledine (2003). In a refocus upon key practice priorities, the Department of Health (2001a) has launched the 'Essence of care programme' – a clinical benchmarking strategy designed to measure practice outcomes and disseminate recommended care delivery across a range of core practice fields. In 2003, the toolkit was republished and additionally included a new benchmark for communication (Department of Health 2003). 'Essence of care' is recommended as an appropriate toolkit to manage clinical effectiveness benchmarking across critical care networks by the Department of Health (2001b) in its strategic programme of action for the nursing contribution to the provision of comprehensive critical care for adults. In this blueprint for enhanced service provision, specific

---

Box 3.1 Communication advice offered by Florence Nightingale (summarized from Nightingale 1859)

- You should avoid talking about a patient, without including them, within their sight or hearing
- Nurses have skills in non-verbal communication to enable them to assess patient distress in response to poor communication
- Ensuring eye contact is an important aspect of good communication
- Physical proximity enhances human interaction
- Communication demands attention and should be practised in the absence of other activities to be most effective

attention is drawn to the central importance of the psychosocial care of patients and their visitors through periods of critical illness and beyond to the management of recovery or death.

This chapter will address a number of elementary topics that are relevant to interpersonal aspects of high dependency nursing. In doing so, there are recommendations of ways in which professionals, patients and their visitors may more effectively communicate to achieve better clinical outcomes.

COMMUNICATION WITH PATIENTS IN HIGH DEPENDENCY SETTINGS

Communication in intensive care settings has been the subject of much attention and ongoing research since the seminal work of Ashworth (1980). According to Lopez (2003), patient and family communication continues to be a research priority, suggesting the topic is still not fully understood nor adequately integrated into clinical practice. Rundell (1991) comments upon the wealth of literature that refers to both hospital wards and intensive care units, but draws attention to how little research had been conducted to investigate communication specifically within high dependency areas. Rundell makes the point that, while there are similarities between the needs of intensive care and high dependency unit patients in terms of critical illness, there is, however, a key difference in that patients in the former are generally unconscious, while in the latter they are more likely to be aware of their circumstances. It must be remembered that, irrespective of their state of consciousness, many people have a degree of awareness of their surroundings. A person with restricted mobility and unable to communicate may yet be able to hear perfectly and, in the absence of other stimuli, is likely to attend closely to what is said about them by others in close proximity.

Given the importance of effective communication to patient care and the identification of strategies to achieve this since the inception of professional nursing, it would perhaps be reasonable to expect that this is an aspect of care that requires little further attention. A review of the evidence suggests that this is not the case. Elliott & Wright (1999) reviewed the literature, and found that nurses do not provide enough verbal communication to meet the needs of unconscious or sedated patients within critical care settings. The authors report their own non-participant observational study undertaken in a general intensive care unit within a major teaching hospital and replicated the findings of previous work. Amazingly, nurses were observed to communicate with their patients for a mean of only 3 minutes and 15 seconds within a 4-hour episode, and this only increased to 5 minutes and 30 seconds when major clinical interventions were required. Positive messages to emerge from the findings of this work are that, in comparison with previous investigations, the participants in this research were found to communicate more and with enhanced variety to reflect perceived patient need. This finding suggests that the research participants knew how to communicate with their patients; however, they only did so infrequently.

It seems, therefore, that there is research evidence to suggest that the physical aspects of high dependency care can be complemented with attention to the development of a sense of partnership in practice related to skilled communication. To be able to communicate effectively, it is essential to be accessible to the other parties involved. In a setting that is likely to be dominated by extremely important attention to physical care needs, it is perhaps necessary to raise the profile of interpersonal care. Conducting her research in an intensive care setting, Leathart (1994a) found that, although many nurses were aware of the important contribution that good communication can make to patient recovery, it was often the case that this understanding was not acted upon in practice. An important way of implementing practice is through making interpersonal aspects of care a key component of a patient's care plan and including the needs of visitors as part of this area of care, the importance of which is stressed by Scullion (1994). Not only will this stress the importance of communication, but it will also demonstrate the value given to such care.

Fundamental processes in good communication are:

* being sensitive to the messages being conveyed by others (verbally and non-verbally); and
* responding in a way that is clear and understandable.

This is particularly relevant in high dependency settings where professionals, patients and their significant others are having to exchange information in a context that is potentially stressful for all parties.

In a high dependency care setting, there are likely to be fewer unconscious or sedated patients than within an intensive care setting; hence the literature will perhaps yield patient reports of better communication experiences. One anecdotal account suggests this is not the case. A patient's personal experience of high dependency care, which makes shocking reading, is offered by Barber (1997), who is a nurse himself. Some of Paul Barber's claims are controversial, but the conclusions he draws from his own perceptions of the care he received should provide food for thought for all high dependency care nurses. Barber found that:

* many nurses gave the impression of being focused upon technology rather than people;
* nursing notes reported a pain-free status although the patient was never directly asked about this;
* decisions about his own care were not encouraged and, when attempts were made to take control of some of his care, this was not welcomed;
* the patient – Paul Barber – felt that he should not complain through fear of being labelled as uncooperative;
* his own anxiety and that of his family about his transfer to a lower dependency area were poorly recognized and not addressed.

Patients are likely to enter into a high dependency setting by one of two sequences of events: as a planned elective event or, as was the case with Paul Barber, as the consequence of an emergency. The former is by definition predicted and is often associated with surgery. In these circumstances, the patient and his or her significant others, such as family or friends, can be prepared for what to expect. Read (1998) recommends that patients who have a planned elective admission are given opportunities to establish links with the team who will be caring for them and to discuss their post-therapy expectations. This is commonly achieved through a pre-intervention meeting, which may also include a visit to the critical care setting.

However, emergency admissions are almost certainly unexpected and, therefore, usually not planned. As can be seen from Paul Barber's experiences, this can lead to patient anxiety and confusion, which can be compounded by communication deficits. In addition to patients' needs, the high dependency clinical team is also frequently faced with the needs of those within the social network of the patients. It is, therefore, essential to include a patient's family, friends and significant others in a planned programme of communication.

COMMUNICATION WITH VISITORS IN HIGH DEPENDENCY SETTINGS AND DEALING WITH ENQUIRIES

In their review of the literature relating to families, nurses and critically ill patients, Holden et al (2002) found that, although nurses are often in a strong position to meet families' needs, these were frequently not adequately met. This they attribute to poor attention to the needs of patients' families within the literature, which is supported by research evidence that many nurses have difficulties within this area. The authors recommend better training to identify visitors' needs through questioning techniques and assessment of non-verbal cues. Also, some nurses are reported to need to be more aware of their own non-verbal presentation of self. Frequently, observed behaviour patterns of nurses at work in critical care settings point to an overemphasis upon technical efficiency to the detriment of human openness.

The theme of efficiency within high-tech care settings is highlighted within participant observation research conducted in Sweden reported by Wikstrom & Larsson (2003). Critical care nurses were observed to have well-developed roles and routines of behaviour, which were highly effective in coping with complex technological life-support apparatus and unpredictably unstable patients. Through the development of patterns of behaviour around care and patient management protocols, nurses and doctors were able to delineate areas of responsibility; this is very effective in promoting efficient teamwork. While there are clear advantages to working in a highly organized fashion, one of the disadvantages is that this can come across to visitors as threatening and make them feel excluded. Visitors are alienated by activities they do not comprehend and by language they do not understand.

It is clear, therefore, that methods to establish visitors' communication needs will be of great use to nurses in assessment stages of care planning. Reporting their research undertaken in Hong Kong, Lee et al (2000) collected data using the Critical Care Family Needs Inventory (CCFNI) developed by Leske (1991), demographic data and semistructured interviews. Findings from the study suggested that families' needs could be divided into three categories: cognitive, emotional and physical.

Cognitive needs can be best satisfied by providing specific information, which is clear, jargon-free and understandable. Hence it is important to avoid both overgeneralized responses, such as 'as well as can be expected' or 'comfortable', and on the other hand, to steer clear of technical jargon such as 'dysrhythmia' and 'catheterization'. As well as being understandable, information should be provided regularly by staff initiating contact at least once a day by telephone and explaining bedside procedures as they arise when visitors are in attendance. The value of consistency, that is, the same small team of nurses communicating with the same small group of visitors, is recommended as an important way to avoid confusion and the potential for misinterpretation or ambiguity. While written material has a useful function in the dissemination of information, it should not be used as a stand-alone tool, as it is poorly placed to meet emotional and physical needs.

Emotional needs are related to fear about the unknown and poor understanding, which can largely be addressed by attention to cognitive needs referred to above. However, the mode of information delivery was found to be strongly related to how well visitors are able to cope with the information they receive. In a UK critical care setting, the CCFNI is also reported as an effective assessment tool by Peel (2003), who argues the importance of fostering visitor empowerment through nurses assisting the patient and his or her family to set and reach goals so that all parties are effectively engaged in the plan of care, with which there is a real sense of ownership.

Physical needs are reported by Lee et al (2000) to be associated with family members sometimes requiring advice on their own health maintenance, so they retain sufficient stamina to support their loved one. There is an important role for nurses here in providing guidance on visiting that is sufficiently open to meet cognitive and emotional needs, and yet regulated in order to ensure adequate rest and recovery for patients and visitors alike. An important value of a patient- and visitor-centred access policy is highlighted by Damboise & Cardin (2003), who observed higher satisfaction levels from all stakeholders when visitors were afforded more open physical access regulated by service user rather than organizational needs. Usefully, for patients who have progressed to a more stable recovery phase, visitors were able to fill in forgotten details about the more acutely ill phase, which appeared to aid orientation and further physical and emotional recovery.

The importance of communication with patients and their relatives is well documented within the literature; so too is evidence that this is not always addressed effectively. The importance of utilizing communication skills has been emphasized and the challenges facing the use of these in high dependency settings has been explored. The processes involved in information exchange are analysed below in order to illustrate the application of skills as part of a process.

GETTING THE MESSAGE ACROSS

The process of interpersonal communication is dependent upon skilled use of communication skills to ensure that the message is accessible and understandable, attended to and perceived appropriately, remembered and motivated to be acted upon. It must be appreciated that the relationships between the components highlighted is complex, being idiosyncratic to each interaction and neither linear nor sequential. Consideration of each element in turn will indicate the contribution of each component to the whole process.

Ensuring that information is accessible and understandable

Nurses need to ensure that they are accessible to the patient and his or her visitors by overtly demonstrating their willingness to communicate. Detailed accounts of how to demonstrate an open posture and how to listen actively are well documented elsewhere (e.g. Betts 2002). As important as what is said is the accompanying behaviour of the skilled communicator. High dependency nursing demands time-consuming practical nursing skills, such as observation, assessment, physical care and the operation of complex equipment. Patient safety is clearly of utmost importance and, of course, should not be unnecessarily compromised. It has, however, been well documented by Menzies (1970) and, more recently, by Wilkinson (2002) that many nurses perceive the practical aspects of care to be less emotionally demanding upon themselves than interpersonal care. An implication of this is that attention can sometimes be directed away from the communication aspects of practice by overly rigorous attention to practical care.

Consider a situation where a nurse is paying great attention to technology, charts or notes. How accessible is this nurse being to patients and their visitors? The more insecure a nurse is with a piece of equipment, the more it is likely to dominate her attention. Equally, the less comfortable a particular nurse is with working in a high dependency setting, the less comfortable she may be working under the scrutiny of any visitors who are present. A nurse who appears underconfident will communicate this to patients and their visitors. In such circumstances, a coping mechanism may well be to 'cut off' from patients and their visitors, and to overly concern oneself with the technology. Junior staff have a responsibility to be sufficiently self-aware of any such tendency within themselves, and more senior staff need to take steps to provide education and support so that confidence through better understanding is facilitated.

In effective communication, the process is necessarily valued as much as the information being exchanged. It is, therefore, essential to make the time required to enable skills to be used effectively. It is accepted that practice that focuses upon unthinking adherence to routine often occurs without the conscious awareness of the individual (Stevens 1983). It is recommended by Barber (1993) that enhanced self-awareness is required in order to challenge such habitual practice. In professional nursing, this sort of critical enquiry into practice has achieved prominence in the context of reflective practice (Burns & Bulman 2000) often in combination with clinical supervision (Lindahl & Norberg 2002).

It is only possible to ensure the dissemination and hence accessibility of a nursing voice if nurses are confident of the positive outcomes of their practice, and of their ability to implement their recommendations. Confidence stems from training and experience, and Leathart (1994b), writing about intensive care nursing, argues that there is a need for improved training in the use of communication skills for critical care practitioners, which she recommends occurs in both classroom and work settings. In her investigation into the meaning of learning for critical care nurses, Little (1999) found that her research participants strongly valued the physical and technological aspects of practice. However, O'Riordan et al (2003), reporting a course for ward-based nurses designed to improve their skills in caring for highly dependent patients, found that, following completion of their course, participants became more confident. Consequently, better-educated nurses were more able to challenge staff appropriately and advocate assertively on behalf of patients, based upon their enhanced technical knowledge and communication skills.

Evidence of the existence of professional and lay theories in a range of domains, including healthcare, is presented by Furnham (1994), whose research demonstrates that there are differences in the way that health is interpreted between professionals and the laity. He comments that it is important to appreciate that, whatever view of health is held, it must be recognized that the view is valid for the holder. In high dependency care, nurses should be aware that their own values and understanding of a given issue or situation are likely to be different from those of a patient under their care. To enhance their understanding of a patient's perspective, nurses should have the resources and skills to assess their patients. Key messages should be conveyed in ways that are sensitive to the values held by patients and their significant others. According to research undertaken by Aitken (2003), expertise in critical care would appear to be characterized by the use of a wide range of information on which to base problem evaluation and the resulting decisions made. Thinking 'out of the box' and making themselves accessible to all the available information rather than jumping to conclusions seems to be the key to expert assessment in critical care nursing. Expert critical care nurses are able to focus upon those cues that are relevant and delineate these from the more peripheral distractions much more effectively than novice practitioners (Reischman & Yarandi 2002). One of the keys to enhancing expertise is, therefore, to better understand the processes involved in human attention and perception.

Attending to information and perceiving its meaning

Attention is a skill that can be learned and developed. It is an active process and you can choose how to allocate it. Attention is the ability to focus on different aspects of the flood of incoming information from the senses (Slack 1990). Attention is an active process that can be flexibly allocated, sometimes being divided between several tasks and sometimes focused on a single activity. The selectivity of human attention is sometimes illustrated in a high dependency unit, when a nurse may not be distracted by general background noise, but will be alert to the specific sounds of patient distress or monitoring alarms. The flexible nature of attention suggests that it is a skill that can be learned and developed. Expertise arises through knowledge, practice and experience. Hence a nurse who is experienced in a different specialty and moves into high dependency nursing will need time to regain the level of expertise enjoyed in a different field of practice.

Knowledge of attention is of relevance to nurses for two reasons. Firstly, the nurse needs to be aware of any personal sensory difficulties, as well as those of the patient and the patient's visitors. A number of authors have shown that sensory impairment or distortion can affect critically ill people (e.g. Kloosterman 1991). Secondly, it is important to remember that the mere provision of information by a nurse or a patient does not necessarily mean that it will be attended to by the intended recipient of that information. These issues are of extreme importance considering the significance of good communication skills to all fields of nursing. However, they are particularly relevant in high dependency care because of the attentional demands made upon nurses, patients and visitors, owing to the presence of monitoring equipment and the diversity of symptoms often accompanying critical illness.

Clarity of information substantially enhances human attention. Child (1996) categorizes factors that influence attention as external or internal. External factors include strategies such as the use of vibrant colours, novelty and humour, which have been used to good effect in health education literature, or in the design of complex comprehensive observation charts. Internal factors are associated with the disposition of the person attending to the stimuli; this is linked to their level of understanding, fatigue and motivation to attend.

'Perception is the process by which we organize and give meaning to sensory information by forming some mental representation of it' (Clark & Keeble 1990: 59). Perception is a complex information-processing activity, which is described by Gross (2001) as having two elements: the physiological functioning of the sensory organs (sight, smell, taste, hearing and touch), and a predisposition to conceptualize sensory stimuli in a particular way, which is likely to be influenced by personality, culture and experiences. These elements of perception combine to facilitate interactive processing. How a person perceives the world is reflected in attitudes and behaviour and this, in turn, shapes perceptions of the world. Hence perception is a dynamic and evaluative process, in which the individual is considered to make judgements based upon their sensory information and their way of making sense of the world (Gregory 1990).

Expectations are the product of life experiences, such as education, life events, gender and socialization. Many interpretations overlap with those of others, while some are highly individual. The influence of expectations helps to explain those situations when perception is distorted. From a nursing perspective, consider the administration of medicines and the similarity of the drug names *prednisolone* and *prednisone,* or *dipyridamole* and *disopyramide*. Consider also the abbreviation PID, which can represent both 'prolapsed intervertebral disc' and 'pelvic inflammatory disease', or MS, which can represent 'mitral stenosis' or 'multiple sclerosis'. It would be potentially disastrous if nurses relied on an automatic and passive mode of attention. In high dependency nursing, the unexpected can, and often does, occur, and it is necessary to actively pay attention to this. From a patient or client perspective, we may speculate what the use of technical jargon such as 'heart failure' or 'tumour' may mean. It is essential to anticipate that patients will not necessarily view healthcare, nor interpret its terminologies, in the same way as healthcare professionals.

The 'halo and horns' effects refer to a self-fulfilling prophecy characteristic of person perception. In the halo effect, a positive impression of a person leads to that person being consistently perceived in a favourable way. This, in turn, acts in a cyclical fashion, providing positive feedback that further promotes the original notion. The horns effect is the same process occurring with unfavourable impressions. In a classic study, Stockwell (1972) has drawn attention to the hazards of being labelled as an 'unpopular patient', which suggests that nurses have considerable influence upon the treatment and self-concept of those for whom they care. Despite communication being a feature of nursing curricula during the intervening years, Walsh (1995) has shown that some patients are still perceived by nurses to be less popular than others. In a high dependency setting, a patient may be perceived as unpopular because of poor response to treatment, which may provoke a sense of failure. The Code of Professional Conduct for nurses, midwives and health visitors (Nursing and Midwifery Council 2002) is very clear regarding the importance of nursing people without favour or prejudice, and it would be unprofessional to do otherwise knowingly. However, Mackellaig (1990) cautions that, in a critical care setting, unpopular long-term patients may be overly allocated to temporary agency nursing staff and this may convey an underlying message to patients or their visitors.

Attribution theory is considered by Davies (1996). There is experimental evidence that we tend to attribute our own actions to situational determinants and the actions of others to dispositional determinants. This has plausible application in nursing practice. For example, it may be perceived that a patient is angry because that is a feature of his or her personality (dispositional determinant), when in fact he is angry because a member of the nursing team has failed to keep a promise about something important to him (situational determinant). There are two important points to note from this. Firstly, it is important not to overlook situational determinants of behaviour, as they are frequently more addressable than dispositional elements. Secondly, it is often a mistake to draw conclusions about personality and its determinants from behaviour. Nursing observations inform assessment more accurately if a stream of behaviour is reported as it occurs, rather than the conclusions drawn. 'Reluctant to follow advice, poor attention span, expresses a pessimistic outlook and lack of interest in recovery' is likely to be more helpful than 'poorly motivated'.

Remembering information

Even clear information lucidly conveyed is inevitably reflected through the patients' own anxiety and distress, and that of their families. It is important to avoid the assumption that you only need give information once if you give it clearly. You may need to repeat and repeat again, in a variety of ways. Many nurses have experienced situations where a patient or visitor asks the same questions on several different occasions. A significant part of communication in nursing practice is that the information presented is remembered. In high dependency nursing, this is of particular importance for two reasons. First, when a patient is critically ill, there is frequently a great deal of information that patients and their significant others will request. Second, when a patient is highly dependent upon healthcare professionals, a key aspect of care is to give the information necessary to restore independence as quickly as is practicable to empower patient participation in recovery (Cahill 1996). These issues pose challenges upon memory and nurses need to understand this in order to assist the enhancement of the process. Memory is frequently conceptualized as a dynamic process, which involves encoding, storage and retrieval components (Eysenck & Keane 2000).

Encoding is the process by which memories are accessed from our experience and organized. Information that needs to be remembered must be attended to and perceived accurately. Remembering is easier if the new information can be related to existing memories and understanding, and it is helpful, therefore, if nurses can make use of their knowledge of this in communicating with others. A common way of doing this is by the use of analogies, for example, in likening the heart to a pump or the kidneys to filters, if it can be established that the recipient of the information can relate to these parallels. Cognitive learning theory suggests that encoding in memory will be enhanced if information is processed actively and deeply (McKenna 1995). This can be promoted if patients and their visitors are encouraged to link what is known with that which is new, and complex material is associated with that which is perceived to be simpler and already understood. Giving information in stages allows time for assimilation and hence this is a recommended approach.

Storage occurs when encoded memories are maintained as long-term files of information, often referred to as schemas. The storage of memories is not usually considered to be problematic in the absence of neurological damage. What is often blamed on failure of memory storage is frequently a problem associated with either ineffective encoding or ineffective retrieval.

The process by which information is accessed from memory is termed retrieval. When attempting to retrieve memories, it is important to make use of the same filing (i.e. schema) system as was used for encoding. It is important for nurses to appreciate that the schema used for encoding is likely to be idiosyncratic to the patient and hence may differ from the professional schema that they themselves have developed as a consequence of their expertise in high dependency care. To avoid interference between these two potentially different modes of memory storage, it is recommended that questions are posed that enable the patient to put the required information into context. For instance, it is often better to 'give patients examples of a good diet that they might follow?' than to outline the underpinning principles. If it is difficult for a patient or their visitors to remember important information, this can be a source of anxiety for them. In such circumstances, it is useful to consider that recognition is considerably easier than unprompted recall, and that the use of cues retains a degree of independence and achievement, which may be important to self-confidence.

Being motivated to act upon information

Motivation is concerned with the relationship between beliefs, values, attitudes and behaviour (Kent 1996). A belief is a representation of knowledge that is rightly or wrongly held by an individual, a value being a related judgement. It is the inter-linkage of beliefs and values that combine to form attitudes, which consequently may be a positive or negative predisposition towards an issue. This, in turn, contributes to choices about behaviour. For example, a patient may decide that he requires total rest to recover (a belief) and hence evaluate nursing insistence upon participation in a degree of contribution to his care as inappropriate (a value). In this instance, the patient's attitude towards contribution to his own care would be one of resistance to behaving cooperatively. The relationship between attitudes and behaviour is not one of simple causation, as it is a complex function of many variables. An understanding of this complexity is key to the motivation of self and others.

> Motivational theories can be divided into two types, push theories and pull theories. Under push theories we find such terms as drive, motive or even stimulus. Pull theories use such constructs as purpose, value or need. In terms of a well-known metaphor these are the pitchfork theories on one hand, and the carrot theories on the other. But our theory is neither of these. Since we prefer to look at the nature of the animal himself, ours is best described as a jackass theory.
>
> (Kelly 1958: 58)

Using Kelly's eloquent analogy, a number of strategies that nurses may utilize to motivate high dependency patients will be explored.

Push theories are associated with responding to some form of external drive to perform a given set of behaviours. Nurses or a patient's visitors may supply such stimuli in the form of verbal encouragement, which is often repeated regularly. Two issues arise from the use of this approach to motivation. Firstly, the importance of consistency in information provision. Asch (1952) has demonstrated the effect of the consistent opinions of others upon the promotion of compliance in individuals. Secondly, the message should be acceptable to the recipient. Lewin (1947) demonstrated experimentally that, if a message is perceived to be unacceptable, it will simply be ignored, even if the source of the message is accepted as being credible and trustworthy. However, if the same message is presented to a group in the form of a discussion topic, it was shown that the acceptability of the message increased and that this was accompanied by a tenfold increase in behaviour change. This research suggests that nurses should work closely with visitors to present a coordinated strategy of information provision so that the message is consistently reinforced. Asking visitors to nominate a link person through whom all information can be related is often a useful way of ensuring consistency of message between named nurse, patient and visitors.

Pull theories of motivation are centred on the notion of goal acquisition. Myles (1993) has used the hierarchy of needs model presented by Maslow (1970) to demonstrate how nursing care can be structured around this classic representation of human needs. It is important to acknowledge that the ascending sequential and linear presentation of Maslow's model is not an accurate reflection of the reality of human motivation, but is more a useful checklist of factors that may be motivational at a given time. It is, therefore, recommended that the taxonomy of needs (physiological needs; the need for safety, for love, esteem and a sense of belonging; cognitive needs; and the goal of self-actualization) is used as a basis for assessment rather than a prescription for care. In doing so, the model yields the potential to highlight factors that are important goals for an individual patient. If goals for nursing practice can be matched to patient-generated goals, there is an enhanced basis for the uptake of health promotion (Dines 1994).

'Jackass' or person-centred theories of motivation combine elements of push and pull theories in the context of the person's understanding of their experiences. This notion of the interaction between internal and external factors in influencing attitudes to health issues and their relationship to behaviour is exemplified by research into how individuals process information in the contexts of their social circumstances and emotions (Ogden 2000). The term social cognition model of health behaviour is used by Conner & Norman (1996) to identify a group of theories that seek to explain and predict health-related behaviour in order to indicate how a person might be motivated to select healthier options. The main recommendations to emerge from research into social cognition are summarized in Box 3.2.

In a high dependency setting, the potentially unstable nature of the patient's condition could result in changed attitudes as circumstances alter. This is, therefore, a challenge to nurses who need to reassess a patient's level of motivation frequently in order to respond with a range of motivating strategies.

STRESS AND HIGH DEPENDENCY SETTINGS

Foxall et al (1990) compared the frequency and sources of stress in a range of clinical settings, and came to the conclusion that nursing the critically ill is stressful. Specifically, Yam & Shui (2003) have reported the stressful nature of high dependency nursing and Cole et al (2001) demonstrate how this may be measured. From a patient perspective, Soehren (1995) has reviewed literature that suggests that critical illness is a stressful experience. A study by O'Malley et al (1991) identifies the significance of stress upon the relatives of the critically ill. It is clear from the literature that, for many of those involved, high dependency care settings are associated with stress.

The concept of stress is classically delineated and represented by three models, i.e. stimulus, response and cognitive–phenomenological–transactional (Baily & Clarke 1989). Each explanation will be considered in turn as issues relevant to high dependency nursing arise out of each approach.

The stimulus model of stress

In the stimulus model, stress is defined as something external to the individual in the environment, which impinges upon the person. Examples are factors that can be perceived by the senses, such as unpleasant sights, sounds, smells, temperatures and tastes. The dominance of environmental stressors, such as nursing acutely ill patients, nursing 'heavy'

> **Box 3.2   Summary of concepts considered to determine health behaviour (summarized from Connor & Norman 1996)**
>
> - Demographic variables, e.g. young males tend to be higher risk-takers and hence should be particularly targeted
> - Health promotion cues that are understandable and deemed relevant tend to alter behaviour, so every opportunity should be taken to offer advice about a healthier lifestyle
> - External locus of control in terms of powerful others is influential, and healthcare professionals should take advantage of the fact that many patients and their significant others will perceive them in this way
> - External locus of control in terms of luck, fate or religion may be influential to some patients, and so must be acknowledged or challenged as appropriate
> - Internal locus of control in terms of self-efficacy is influential through fostering a personal sense of self-efficacy
> - Intentions in terms of attitudes are likely to be shaped by significant others as well as rational argument and hence it is important to muster the support of those whom the patient values to reinforce health advice
> - In motivation, consider employing push, pull and person-focused factors
> - The perceived benefit of adopting a behaviour pattern should be stressed
> - The perceived cost of adopting a behaviour pattern should be stressed
> - Severity of threat evaluation related to continuing present behaviour should be stressed
> - Social support is important–get the relatives and all other significant others involved

long-term patients, prolongation of life in the critically ill, lack of time and inadequate patient–staff ratios were identified by White & Tonkin (1991) in their investigation of stressors in Australian intensive care units.

A number of high dependency units are being set up on general wards that may not be of an ideal design to facilitate both the technical and interpersonal aspects of care. In addition, a high dependency unit that is attached to a less acute practice setting may not have the appropriate nurse staffing establishment, in terms of numbers or levels of expertise, to satisfy the patient care demands of either specialty. Stressors imposed by such an environment have the potential to compromise communication because of inadequate time, unreasonable workloads and staff with an inadequate knowledge of the specialty in which they are working.

A strength of the stimulus explanation of stress is that it can direct attention to such stress-provoking factors. Nurses clearly have a responsibility to monitor the environment in which care is delivered to ensure that it is safe and conducive to recovery. The advice of Nightingale (1859) that hospitals should do patients no harm is as relevant in modern healthcare settings as it was when it was first suggested, according to contemporary commentators (Milligan & Robinson 2003). Stressful environmental stimuli that are generally accepted as undesirable, such as excessive noise, bright lights, heavy workloads and inadequate knowledge base, are measurable, and steps should be taken to address potential causes of patient, visitor or staff stress.

Some environmental factors, however, are less clearly identifiable as stressful. Ashbury (1984) argues that there is an increase in public awareness of the use of technological equipment in healthcare settings, such as a high dependency unit, although the consequences of this are unclear. Familiarization with technology may help to prepare patients and their visitors who witness its use mentally, although Clifford (1986) comments that exposure to 'life support' machinery on television may be entirely different from experiencing its use on oneself or a relative. Hence, for some individuals, the presence of equipment may be reassuring, while for others it may act as a source of stress. Clearly, the best way of ascertaining this is to assess people as individuals. The importance of this is exemplified by Bergbom-Engberg & Haljamäe (1993) who found that the same stressors are perceived differently by different nurses. From this research, it seems that the way that potentially stressful stimuli are interpreted is more important that the nature of the stimuli themselves.

Thus, an interpretation of stress as being attributable to stimuli alone is reductionist and static. This is a limitation, as it fails to acknowledge individual differences in the perception of what might be stressful. The assumption of linear and progressive causality of stress is additionally flawed because there is poor acknowledgement of human capacity to adapt and cope.

The response model of stress

The response model defines stress as the individual's physiological responses to perceived threat in an effort to maintain homeostasis. This is mediated principally through the release of catecholamines, which have been considered in other chapters, and is clearly highly relevant to the management of critical illness. The strength of this understanding of stress is that there is the establishment of a relationship between stress and disease, although the nature of this is unclear (Ogden 2000). Like the stimulus model, the response model can be criticized for being an overly deterministic explanation of stress, which fails to allow fully for individual interpretation and response to circumstances that might yield stress.

The cognitive–phenomenological–transactional model of stress

The cognitive–phenomenological–transactional model of stress is a consequence of the work of Lazarus and colleagues between the 1960s and the 1980s (Sarafino 1994). According to this approach, stress is defined as the result of an interaction between the individual and his or her understanding of his or her own situation. What can be stressful to one patient may not be stressful to another. Assumptions about a patient's state of stress are as invalid as any other assumptions a nurse can make without checking with reality. The key to the model is the idiosyncratic interpretation of threat and the perception of what can be done in response in the form of coping strategies. The model has three phases. Primary appraisal involves the initial assessment of challenge or demand. In this phase, the person may ask themselves questions such as 'what's happening?' or 'how will this affect me?' In other words, it is suggested that each individual makes an assessment, and evaluates whether he or she feels threatened or not. Secondary appraisal is an estimation of personal resources to counter, or coping resources to deal with, any perceived threat. In this phase, the person may ask questions such as 'what can I do?' or 'what help do I need?' Coping in response to appraisal may be to address a problem directly or to seek emotional release of tension (Clarke 1984). Finally, the reappraisal phase is an evaluation of the subsequent outcome in the light of the primary and secondary phases. Here the questions asked may be 'how am I coping?' or 'is the situation better or worse now?'

The strengths of this model lie in its highly individualistic and dynamic representation, which allows for differences and change both within and between people. It offers an explanation for stress in the absence of an apparent stressor, such as in the case of covert phobias or anxiety states. The model serves well to remind nurses that the way they interpret a given situation may differ from that of those they care for or their colleagues. Practice can be guided by the model, if the questions associated with each phase are used as a basis for assessment. A limitation in the application of the cognitive–phenomenological–transactional model of stress is that it requires a degree of articulacy to be able to voice the thought processes linked to each phase and not all individuals will be able to express this.

A composite explanation of stress

In summary, all representations of stress are relevant to high dependency nursing. Assessment of the environment will indicate avoidable stress-inducing factors. Assessment of the patient will indicate physiological responses that will potentially confound other physical pathology. It has been suggested that, at the heart of stress, however, are the interpretations and responses made by each individual linked to their perception of their situation. In this context, communication skills are as important as an environmental audit or physical examination. It is important to remember this in a care setting, which, for very good reasons, is likely to be dominated by environmental and physical demands upon human attention.

CONCLUSION

Good communication is part of therapy – just as much as drugs or interventions. An important aspect of high dependency care that should be borne in mind is its transient nature. This has substantial implications for communication, as patients rarely undergo all of their illness management exclusively within a high dependency setting. It is more usually the case that the rapid movement in and out of a high dependency unit leads to different teams of staff becoming involved in care and this is

> **Box 3.3 Summary of key interpersonal issues related to high dependency nursing**
>
> - Consider the context in which high dependency nursing is practised in relation to communication
> - Develop expertise in the use of a range of communication skills
> - Practise in a way that is conducive to partnership with each patient and his or her visitors
> - Understand that people are individuals with specific and idiosyncratic needs, and be rigorous in assessment to identify these
> - Plan care in the light of your assessment
> - Be aware that needs will be dynamic and will require frequent reassessment
> - Work collaboratively with other care workers and develop a consistent approach to care for each individual
> - Strive to make your message one that is accessible, understandable, attended to and perceived appropriately, memorable and motivating to be acted upon
> - Assess and manage stressful situations proactively using an eclectic interpretation

a potential source of deficits in the continuity of information. The management of severe illness often requires the contributions of a diverse range of healthcare professionals, both within and outside the high dependency care multidisciplinary team. The experience of being critically ill, and being at the centre of activity is likely to be extremely frightening for patients and their relatives. Good communication is the key to making sense of the complex activity that defines high dependency practice. A number of recommendations to this end emerge from the chapter and are summarized in Box 3.3.

References

Aitken L 2003 Critical care nurses' use of decision-making strategies. Journal of Clinical Nursing 12: 476–483

Asch S 1952 Effects of group pressure upon modification and distortion of judgements. In: Swanson G, Newcombe T, Hartley E (eds) Readings in social psychology. Holt, Rinehart & Winston, New York

Ashbury A 1984 Patients' memories and reactions to intensive care. Care of the Critically Ill 1(2): 12–13

Ashworth P 1980 Care to communicate. Royal College of Nursing, London

Baily R, Clarke M 1989 Stress and coping in nursing. Chapman & Hall, London

Barber P 1993 Who cares for the carers? Distance Learning Centre, South Bank University, London

Barber P 1997 Caring: the nature of the therapeutic relationship. In: Perry A, Jolly M (eds) Nursing: a knowledge base for practice, 2nd edn. Edward Arnold, London

Bergbom-Engberg I, Haljamäe H 1993 The communication process with ventilator patients in the ICU as perceived by the nursing staff. Intensive and Critical Care Nursing 9: 40–47

Betts A 2002 The nurse as communicator. In: Kenworthy N, Snowley G, Gilling C (eds) Common foundation studies in nursing, 3rd edn. Churchill Livingstone, Edinburgh

Burns S, Bulman C 2000 (eds) Reflective practice in nursing, 2nd edn. Blackwell Science, Oxford

Cahill J 1996 Patient participation: a concept analysis. Journal of Advanced Nursing 24: 561–571

Castledine G. 2003 Nurses must not integrate medical tasks into nursing. British Journal of Nursing 12: 67

Child D 1996 Psychology and the teacher, 5th edn. Cassell, London

Clark E, Keeble S 1990 Introduction to psychological knowledge. Distance Learning Centre, South Bank University, London

Clarke M 1984 Stress and coping: constructs for nursing. Journal of Advanced Nursing 9: 3–13

Clifford C 1986 Patients, relatives and nurses in a technological environment. Intensive Care Nursing 2: 67–72

Cole F, Slocumb E, Mastey J 2001 A measure of critical care nurses' post-code stress. Journal of Advanced Nursing 34: 281–288

Commission for Health Improvement 2002 South north divide in the NHS. Commission for Health Improvement, London

Connor M, Norman P (eds) 1996 Predicting health behaviour. Open University Press, Buckingham

Damboise C, Cardin S 2003 Family-centered critical care: how one unit implemented a plan. American Journal of Nursing 103(6): 56AA–56EE

Davies M 1996 Explaining people and events. In: Aitken V, Jellicoe H (eds) Behavioural sciences for health professionals. W B Saunders, London

Department of Health 2001a Essence of care toolkit. The Stationery Office, London

Department of Health 2001b The nursing contribution to the provision of comprehensive critical care for adults. The Stationery Office, London

Department of Health 2003 Essence of care: patient-focused benchmarks for clinical governance. NHS Modernisation Agency, London

Dines A 1994 A review of lay health beliefs research: insights for nursing practice in health promotion. Journal of Clinical Nursing 3: 329–338

Elliott R, Wright L 1999 Verbal communication: what do critical care nurses say to their unconscious or sedated patients? Journal of Advanced Nursing 29: 1412–1420

Eysenck M, Keane M 2000 Cognitive psychology: a student's handbook, 4th edn. Lawrence Erlbaum Associates, Hove

Foxall M, Zimmerman L, Standley R, Bene B 1990 A comparison of frequency and sources of nursing job stress perceived by intensive care, hospice and medical-surgical nurses. Journal of Advanced Nursing 15: 577–584

Furnham A 1994 Explaining health and illness: lay perceptions on current and future health, the causes of illness and the future of recovery. Social Science and Medicine 39: 715–725

Gregory R 1990 Eye and brain, 4th edn. Weidenfield & Nicholson, London

Gross R 2001 Psychology: the science of mind and behaviour, 3rd edn. Hodder & Stoughton, London

Health Service Ombudsman 2002 The Health Service Ombudsman, investigations completed April-July 2002 part 1. The Stationery Office, London

Holden J, Harrison L, Johnson M 2002 Families, nurses and intensive care patients: a review of the literature. Journal of Clinical Nursing 11: 140–148

Kelly G 1958 Man's construction of his alternatives. In: Lindzey G (ed) Assessment of human motives. Holt, Rinehart & Winston, New York

Kent V 1996 Attitudes. In: Aitken V, Jellicoe H (eds) Behavioural sciences for health professionals. W B Saunders, London

Kloosterman N 1991 Cultural care: the missing link in severe sensory alteration. Nursing Science Quarterly 4(3): 119–122

Leathart A 1994a Communication and socialisation (1): an exploratory study and explanation for nurse-patient communication in an ITU. Intensive and Critical Care Nursing 10: 93–104

Leathart A 1994b Communication and socialisation (2): perceptions of neophyte ITU nurses. Intensive and Critical Care Nursing 10: 142–154

Lee I, Chien W, Mackenzie A 2000 Needs of families with a relative in a critical care unit in Hong Kong. Journal of Clinical Nursing 9: 46–54

Leske S 1991 Internal psychometric properties of the critical care family needs inventory. Heart and Lung 20: 236–244

Lewin K 1947 Group decision and social change. In: Newcombe T, Hartley E (eds) Readings in social psychology. Holt, Rinehart & Winston, New York

Lindahl B, Norberg A 2002 Clinical group supervision in an intensive care unit: a space for relief, and for sharing emotions and experiences of care. Journal of Clinical Nursing 11: 809–818

Little C 1999 The meaning of learning in critical care nursing: a hermeneutic study. Journal of Advanced Nursing 30: 697–703

Lopez V 2003 Critical care nursing research priorities in Hong Kong. Journal of Advanced Nursing 43: 578–587

Mackellaig J 1990 A review of the psychological effects of intensive care on the isolated patient and his family. Care of the Critically Ill 6(3): 100–102

McKenna G 1995 Learning theories made easy: cognitivism. Nursing Standard 9: 29–31

Maslow A 1970 Motivation and personality. Harper & Row, New York

Menzies I 1970 The functioning of social systems as a defence mechanism against anxiety. Tavistock, London

Milligan F, Robinson K 2003 (eds) Limiting harm in health care: a nursing perspective. Blackwell Science, Oxford

Myles A 1993 Psychology and health care. In: Hinchliff S, Norman S, Schober J (eds) Nursing practice and health care, 2nd edn. Edward Arnold, London

Nightingale F 1859 Notes on nursing. Harrison & Sons, London (Republished 1980 by Churchill Livingstone, Edinburgh)

Nursing and Midwifery Council (2002) Code of professional conduct. Nursing and Midwifery Council, London

Ogden J 2000 Health psychology: a textbook, 2nd edn. Open University Press, Milton Keynes

O'Malley P, Favaloro R, Anderson B 1991 Critical nurse perception of family needs. Heart and Lung 20: 189–201

O'Riordan B, Gray K, McArthur-Rouse F 2003 Implementing a critical care course for ward nurses. Nursing Standard. 17(20): 41–44

Peel N 2003 The role of the critical care nurse in the delivery of bad news. British Journal of Nursing 12: 966–971

Read C 1998 Patients' information needs in intensive care and surgical wards. Nursing Standard 12(28): 37–39

Reischman R, Yarandi H 2002 Critical care cardiovascular nurse expert and novice diagnostic cue utilisation. Journal of Advanced Nursing 39: 24–34

Rundell S 1991 A study of nurse-patient interaction in a high dependency unit. Intensive Care Nursing 7: 171–178

Sarafino E 1994 Health psychology: biopsychosocial interactions, 2nd edn. Wiley, New York

Scullion P 1994 Personal cost, caring and communication: an analysis of communication between relatives and intensive care nurses. Intensive and Critical Care Nursing 10: 64–70

Slack J 1990 Attention. In: Roth I (ed.) Introduction to psychology, Vol. 2. Lawrence Erlbaum Associates, Hove

Soehren P 1995 Stressors perceived by cardiac surgical patients in the intensive care unit. American Journal of Critical Care 4(1): 71–76

Stevens R 1983 Freud and psychoanalysis. Open University Press, Milton Keynes

Stockwell F 1972 The unpopular patient. Royal College of Nursing, London

Tingle J 2003 Managing and improving health care delivery in 2003 (Editorial). British Journal of Nursing 12: 5

Tyler P, Ellison R 1994 Sources of stress and psychological well-being in high dependency nursing. Journal of Advanced Nursing 19: 469–476

Walsh M 1995 Why patients get the blame for being ill. Nursing Standard 9(37): 38–40

White D, Tonkin J 1991 Registered nurse stress in intensive care units – an Australian perspective. Intensive Care Nursing 7: 45–52

Wikstrom AC, Larsson U 2003 Patient on display – a study of everyday practice in intensive care. Journal of Advanced Nursing 43: 376–383

Wilkinson J 2002 The psychological basis of nursing. In: Kenworthy N, Snowley G, Gilling C (eds) Common foundation studies in nursing, 3rd edn. Churchill Livingstone, Edinburgh

Yam B, Shui A 2003 Perceived stress and sense of coherence among critical care nurses in Hong Kong: a pilot study. Journal of Clinical Nursing 12: 144–146

Chapter **4**

Social issues in high dependency care

Paul Mulligan

KEY LEARNING OBJECTIVES

- To be aware of the many social factors that influence the patient in high dependency care
- To explore through case example and reflection how an understanding of these factors may improve the quality of care

Prerequisite Knowledge

- Understanding of basic sociological terminology (e.g. race, ethnicity, gender and social class)
- Understanding of the concepts of interpersonal skills
- Understanding of the ethical principles of autonomy (freedom to choose and determine one's future), beneficence (doing good), non-maleficence (avoiding doing harm) and justice (fairness and equity) (Beauchamp & Childress 1994)

INTRODUCTION

We all have a medical history but, outside of a general practitioner's surgery or hospital ward, it is not something we often consider. Our personal histories are more important in our daily lives. It is only when we are admitted to a hospital ward or a high dependency unit that our medical histories come into play. For the nurse working in a hospital environment, dealing with patients every day, it is easy to lose sight of the fact that each patient is a person with his or her own unique history – an individual.

The fact that the patient might have been admitted urgently, with a severe life-threatening condition, means that the nurses tend to concentrate on dealing with medical priorities rather than anything else. They have to get the assessment, treatment, technology and the drugs right and, of course, there are other patients to care for, so there is a real danger that nurses could lose sight of each patient as an individual. So the patient may become a condition (e.g. the 'appendix' in bed 8), a chart, or a set of responses to monitors and machines. It is as though the patient as a person, with a social background, a family, an ethnic heritage and personal needs, is forgotten in the midst of what is happening to and around them. The length of time they will be in hospital care is often short. The aim within a busy unit is to reduce the patient's need for high dependency services and to 'step down' to less dependent care as quickly as is practical.

Yet the professional duty of registered nurses is much broader than that. The Nursing and Midwifery Council's (NMC) Code of Professional Conduct is clear about what a nurse's duty is: ' . . . to recognize and respect the uniqueness and dignity of each patient and client and respond to their need for care irrespective of their ethnicity, religious beliefs, personal attributes, nature of their health problem or any other factor' (NMC 2002: Clause 7).

The nurse is there to respond to the patient's need for care, and to coordinate and manage the delivery of that package of care. In the high dependency setting, that care is complex and directed by the medical condition of the patient. However, a professional nurse needs to be able to balance those aspects with insight, understanding and empathy for all the 'human' and individual needs of the patient. In other words, we have to take a 'holistic' approach to patients and their care. Understanding the patients' ethnicity or religion, for example, may have an effect on the way in which the programme of care is organized and delivered, their family/carers response to their illness, their need to interact with their family/carers' while in hospital and their attitude to life and death issues. Brykczynska (1992) says 'The most important and significant aspect of caring however is that delicate reintegration and synthesis of knowledge, skills, commitment, professional integrity and love, manifested each time a professional nurse consciously undertakes to nurse a patient or client. This is done because the nurse cares'. The Royal College of Nursing (RCN) has identified six defining characteristics of nursing – purpose, intervention, domain, focus, value base and partnership – and states that nursing is 'the use of clinical judgement in the provision of care to enable people to improve, maintain, or recover health, to cope with health problems, and to achieve the best possible quality of life, whatever their disease or disability, until death' (RCN 2003).

The aim of this chapter is to give the reader information and generate questions about some of the social factors that influence a patient's experience of high dependency care. Secondly, in order to help the reader integrate that knowledge, short case studies are presented in order to demonstrate how theory and practice integrate, and offer challenges to the ways in which care is delivered. Finally, nursing in high dependency care is an ethical activity for which we are personally and professionally accountable. Consideration should be made of how the ethical principles of autonomy, beneficence, non-maleficence and justice (Beauchamp

& Childress 1994) vie with each other so that balanced judgements can be made when delivering care.

THE FAMILY

Reflect on a family disaster/significant incident. How has that changed the dynamics in your family? What sort of social roles do you perform and how do they affect your relationship with other members of your family?
Have you had a personal experience of hospitals – either when you were a patient, or a member of your family? How has that influenced you?
What does you being a nurse mean within your family?

The patient in your care will be part of a social grouping; the most common of these is the family.

The family is a concept most people will be instantly familiar with. We are nearly all born into one and will probably die a member of one. Its influence is very powerful and yet it is vulnerable to the effects *of* social change as much as it is an agent *for* social change. It has been called variously an agent of social control and an agent of the state, and yet at no other time has the family undergone such radical and fundamental change as in the latter part of the 20th century and beginning of the 21st century. Understanding these changes will help to understand more about the patient.

The family has been described as being 'nuclear' or 'extended'. The classic distinction is that the nuclear family is the family of our current experience: it is small in number, self-reliant, economically self-fulfilling, geographically mobile, often with only one parent, possibly with both parents working. It is the creation of the industrial/technological age.

The extended family used to be the norm. It consists of wider 'kin' relationships living in close proximity, giving financial and social support. It undertook many of the caring, nurturing and healing roles that have subsequently been taken over by health professionals.

To some, the extended family may be an idealized construction. Nurses may make personal judgements about the value of the patient's family by the degree of their involvement in caring for the patient. You may have witnessed this happening; however, it is not the nurse's function to make a judgement about the role of the family, but it is their obligation to establish the level of family support that exists for each individual patient, and how the plan of care might best support and integrate with it. The important point is to try and understand the patients' own experience of family and how they live within their social grouping, what that means for them and who is important to them.

How is Danny's inability to choose (autonomy) to be balanced with the needs of the family (justice)?

Case example 4.1

Danny at 16 is the eldest son of a travelling family. He suffers a subarachnoid haemorrhage. His mother and twin elder sisters accompany him on admission. He comes to the high dependency unit (HDU) for stabilization prior to transfer to a neurosurgical unit. His condition deteriorates. He is ventilated and is making no respiratory effort. It seems that he is probably brain dead and the first set of brainstem tests confirm this. The father is unable to visit Danny but stays outside the unit. However, the 'family' have been informed. Over the next 2 days, nearly 100 'uncles', 'aunts' and 'cousins' visit Danny. The nurses are upset, as this appears to be a show of curiosity. The family are spoken to and his mother says that when someone is near to death the whole family must visit.

What is your idea of what constitutes the family? How do you project that idea on to the families of patients? What happens when your idealized view doesn't match the reality of the experience? It is not the role of nurses to impart their values on others, but to respect diversity. Just because their views may differ may not make their view the right or correct one.

Look at your ward/department/ environment from the perspective of a patient or a distressed relative. How would you view the actions and mannerisms of the staff if you were on the receiving end of their greeting, advice, comments or care? What standards would you expect if you or a member of your family were the patient?

Case example 4.1 – resolution

Relations between the nurses and the family come to a head, and the ward manager allows only the immediate family to visit. There is a great deal of shouting and arguing for a few hours. The visiting ceases except for close relatives, who are much happier with this arrangement but felt powerless to stop the traditional response of the extended family. The father asks for a priest and Danny is baptized. Removed from the scrutiny of the 'wider family', Danny's father is able to sit with his son and say his goodbye.

It can be stressful for the nurse dealing with the patient's family and relatives, especially where their values and norms differ. However, the care of the family is as much an integral part of the care of the patient and nurses must not use the excuse of level of care required for the patient as an excuse for not meeting the needs of the family. It might be that the nurse feels that the family should be coping and that they should be able to care for themselves, or that we don't understand the effects on the family that hospitalization causes.

Millar (1989) talks about the physical and biological crises that patients experience when admitted to intensive care (for 'intensive care', read also 'high dependency care' or 'general ward care'). The consequence is that their families are thrown into emotional turmoil owing to the real and perceived threats to the well-being of the patient and of themselves. This may put pressure on their abilities to cope.

The patient's choice (autonomy) to decide their treatment has to be balanced with the potential harm (non-maleficence) of the consequences.

Case example 4.2

Gordon aged 28 is a self-employed motorcycle courier. He is married to Sally and they have a 2-year-old daughter. Gordon is admitted following a road traffic accident (RTA) in which his left leg is badly crushed. He is admitted to the HDU and is told that surgical amputation is critical or he may die. He is denying the seriousness of his condition and refuses the operation. Sally is very upset and angry, and says 'well let him die then as at least I'll get the insurance', and keeps saying she knew something like this was going to happen. She talks about the financial consequences of his impending unemployability as a motorcycle courier and anticipates that she will have to give up her part-time work to care for him, as both their families live far away.

Who is providing social support? What can be done to alleviate fears, anxieties and worries? How can nursing care help all parties to cope (e.g. family, carers, friends, dependents, etc.)? How do you assess what support they need? Who do you discuss/organize this with? Who is included in the discussion?

Case example 4.2 – resolution

The nurses support Gordon in making his choice. He undergoes a below-knee amputation and is transferred to the surgical ward 24-hours post-op. The nurses encourage the wider family to visit and suggest ways in which they can help. Both Gordon and Sally's parents visit, and offer help and support. This enables Sally to work full time initially so that outstanding bills can be paid. The nurses contact the social service department, and a social worker is sought and takes up their case.

SOCIAL CLASS AND SOCIAL STRATIFICATION

Do you feel comfortable about the notion of class? How do you validate your answer? Do you believe social class differences exist? If so, what social class do you think you belong to?
Why do we generally feel uncomfortable talking about class?
Are there any moral or ethical issues around the judgements that we make in this regard?

An analysis of social grouping is provided by descriptions of social class and social stratification.

Although not necessarily explicitly, the patient requiring high dependency care will be categorized statistically within a social class. Understanding its broad outlines may help to understand specific individuals. When admitting a patient, we take note of their occupation. This is represented by the categories of social stratification (Box 4.1).

These are the categories used by *Social Trends* when analysing social data, and also by market researchers to imply or define a level of income, standard of living, and the individual's role and function in both employment and society. 'Social class' is a term that often creates strong feelings. It is sometimes used to categorize people in prejudicial stereotypes and high dependency care is not immune from this.

Box 4.1   Categories of social stratification (*Social Trends* 1996)

I	Professional	Higher managerial, administrative or professional
II	Intermediate	Intermediate management, administrative or professional
IIIn	Skilled non-manual	Supervisory or clerical and junior managerial, administrative or professional
IIIm	Skilled manual	Skilled manual workers
IV	Partly skilled manual	Semi-skilled and unskilled manual workers
V	Unskilled manual	State pensioners or widows (no other earners), or lowest grade workers or long-term unemployed.

Each unit will receive patients from across the so-called 'social' spectrum. The nursing and medical team will also reflect a wide variety of social, cultural and ethnic backgrounds. Both patients and staff will have their own prejudices. For example, patients who consider themselves traditionally working class may feel socially isolated in a unit where the staff are overtly 'middle class', since they may feel the staff are judgemental about their lifestyle, manner, pattern of speech and mode of understanding the world.

Case example 4.3

Colonel Grouse, 82, is admitted from the medical ward with bilateral pneumonia. He is to have continuous positive airway pressure (CPAP) for his respiratory failure. He is hypoxic, hypercarbic and pyrexial. He has moments of confusion. He is orientated to time and person, but insists he is in a different place. The patient in the bed opposite, Joe O'Reilly, is on total parenteral nutrition (TPN) following major abdominal surgery. Colonel Grouse becomes convinced Joe is in the IRA. He believes the TPN bag is Semtex explosive and that Joe's family is plotting a bombing or terrorist campaign. The Colonel talks to all nurses as if they are private soldiers and the doctors as junior officers. Despite explanation, his anxiety is not dissipated.

How does an understanding of class explain the Colonel's behaviour? What can be done to help him manage his misapprehensions? Is there anything in nursing behaviour that may exacerbate the scenario?

A particularly significant report in 1982 (The Black Report) considered health inequalities across the UK. It came to the conclusion that social class is a strong determinant of disease and ill health, and that the risk of death for those in groups IV and V was much greater than those in groups I and II at every stage of life. Poverty was declared to be a major determinant of ill health. There is evidence that those in poor health move down the social scale, since unemployment often follows, creating economic instability and loss of status. The idea of access to healthcare as determined by class suggests that some groups are disadvantaged by illiteracy, ignorance or lack of power to achieve the same health outcomes as those in higher socioeconomic groups.

Case example 4.3 – resolution

On such a small unit, it was not possible to separate the patients. The nurses tried to calm the Colonel down and tried to get Joe O'Reilly's family to pop over and talk to him. Nothing seemed to work. One nurse 'played the game' and acted like a deferential soldier. The Colonel responded and felt that at last someone was listening to him. The nurse defused the situation by distracting the Colonel during visiting time and by ignoring his most bizarre misapprehensions. A combination of antibiotics, good oxygenation and ventilation, and adapting responses to the situation helped return the patient to normal.

Is this action dishonest or untruthful?
Does it conflict with the patient's autonomy?

The authors of the report acknowledge there is no simple explanation but that:

> much of the evidence on social inequalities in health can be adequately understood in terms of specific features of the socioeconomic environment ... work accidents, overcrowding, cigarette smoking, which are strongly class related in Britain and also have clear causal significance.
> (Townsend & Davidson 1982, Whitehead 1992)

However, Hardey (1998) states that the term 'inequality' is nowhere to be found in 'The health of the nation' (Department of Health 1992) and that 'official' publications favour the term 'variations' in health.

In terms of ill health encountered in high dependency care, it would be very difficult to pinpoint specific factors of social inequality in many patients. The more vague the explanation, the more difficult it is to relate to practice. However, it appears that poverty, deprivation and ignorance are the most significant factors; these may be inferred from the patient's socioeconomic group and may be a result of ill health.

RACE

Reflect upon any personal experience of prejudice that you have had.
What do you honestly feel about the race of others?
Does this affect the way you care for others?

Another aspect of inequality is race. British society is multicultural, comprising many ethnic groups of people of both pure and mixed race.

Race is a biological concept whereby people may be categorized by physical criteria. Skin colour, for example, is the most obvious and widely used, but so are nasal shape, lip form, eye colour and hair type (Hardey 1998). Of course this categorization does not explain any of the real differences between people. The idea that inequality could be removed if the immigrant population was integrated into the host population is described as assimilation: the onus being on the immigrant to assimilate the host culture, to 'join the club' and succeed. However, this ignores differences, class divisions and prejudices within the host and immigrant populations. A criticism of this approach, which could be termed Marxist, suggests that there is a vested interest for the host culture not to achieve integration, as the immigrants provide the workforce for the national economies of Western society as cheap labour. This creates a climate of revolt where the host population believes 'they are taking over': this in turn may create an underclass where the indigenous (host) working class splits from the immigrant working class. This may create racism, which is discrimination solely on the grounds of race. Where discrimination enters the social structure of an organization, for example, then this is termed institutional racism. The health service, as part of society's social structure, is not immune from the effects of this and has been criticized as a mediator of racism through its employment practices. Most organizations, including the National Health Service (NHS), have antiracism policies such as equal opportunity practices. As a workable concept we talk about ethnicity, a description of people's experience and expression of common culture, language, diet, history, art, music. These groupings may contain cultural groups and subgroups.

Understanding cultural and ethnic variations will improve the care of patients and their families receiving high dependency care. However, it is dangerous to make assumptions about people based on knowledge received from books, previous experience or personal prejudices. The patient who calls himself a Muslim, Jew or Hindu may not behave in the way that textbooks suggest. The starting point must be the person's own experience and his or her individual needs.

How can we help patients and their relatives balance their own ethical principles (doing no harm – non-maleficence and beneficence, doing good)

Case example 4.4

Mr Aziz has been keeping a lonely vigil at his wife's bedside from early morning to late at night. By the second day, having refused food and drink, he begins to behave oddly. He appears to drop off to sleep over his wife's bed, but when roused he gets agitated after a nurse insists he leaves the unit for a break, or a drink and something to eat. On questioning, it becomes clear it is Ramadan and he is fasting, and he is going to do what he has to do, not what someone who is not a Muslim is telling him to do. Relations with the nursing staff are in a standoff position.

How could an assessment have prevented this? How can Mr Aziz be helped while still retaining his cultural and religious expression?

Case example 4.4 – resolution

The nurses consider it very odd that the children don't visit their mother. There are two adult daughters and a son who are seen in the hospital, but not in the high dependency unit. One nurse talks to them and discovers that Mr Aziz is feeling very guilty about his wife, is ignoring everything at home and is not looking after the youngest child, who is 10 years old. At the nurses' suggestion, the family decide to bring Mr Aziz's brother in to talk to him, and he realizes that he is ignoring the rest of the family and stopping them from caring. This seems to work during the patient's stay in the unit.

HEALTH BELIEFS

It may be easy to identify early on that some people will have a different way of looking at and experiencing the world. This will have a bearing on how the nurse cares for them; for example, with dietary requirements, gender issues when giving intimate nursing care and the variations on religious requirement when caring for a deceased patient. However, there are whole areas of belief that are not bound by cultural or racial expression, but all the same will influence the way that patients and their families make sense of their illness and their experience of high dependency care. These are the patient's own health beliefs.

These beliefs relate to how patients describe the illness in their own words, including the 'special' words that people use to describe medical conditions and, secondly, the cultural, social and emotional labels that they may attach to it. For example, when we consider the variety of words we use to describe pain – crushing, niggling, stabbing, aching, burning, searing and so on – we are making a judgement on the patients' pain by the words they use to describe it. If the words the patients use and the words the nurses use have different meanings, then effective communication has not taken place. Whenever we as nurses explain anything to patients or their families, we have to ensure that they understand what we are talking about. The discussion about social class and ethnicity has introduced some subtle concepts that may hinder understanding. The issue of lay health beliefs is, perhaps, even more subtle. People do not generally think about their health in universally similar ways. They may not have had a medical education, but they will have received ideas passed down through the generations and have particular experiences of health and ill health that will affect the way they think. Sayings, such as 'feed a cold and starve a fever', are an example of a lay health belief. In some cultures, this is more formalized: for example, the Hindu culture believes that some illnesses are hot and some are cold, and that they have to be treated in this 'hot' and 'cold' manner. The way that illness is explained is often mechanistic and this is a common belief within Western society. If the machine is broken, then there has to be a way of fixing it. It has a blockage, so it needs flushing out. If there is a leak, it needs plugging. The mechanistic model has its limitations, however.

> What remedies do you or your family rely upon in ill health? Are they 'scientific' (i.e. medically accepted remedies)? Have you ever been dissatisfied with an explanation regarding an illness or treatment from any health professional and, if so, why? Have you ever thought about what patients' perceptions of you might be like?

Case example 4.5

Sara is 7 years old, and is admitted following emergency bowel surgery and the creation of a temporary colostomy. Her parents are very protective, both spending as long as possible with Sara, apparently to the exclusion of the other children in the family. The parents are very quiet and do not relate to the nurses very well except to criticize the lateness of the doctor's round, the level of noise or the lack of clean sheets. The nurse caring for Sara discovers that she had diarrhoea for 2 weeks before admission and had been given large amounts of kaolin mixture to stop it. The side effect was to cause a blockage of nearly 'pure clay' as the surgeon wrote, which caused the bowel to become inflamed and rupture. As the relationship develops between the parents and the nurse, they say that they feel so guilty but they thought they were doing the right thing.

How can an understanding of 'lay' health beliefs help in understanding this situation? How can Sara's parents begin to overcome their guilt?

> The parents' ignorance of potential consequences seems to be the root cause. How is the education of the parents an ethical activity, and which principles are involved?

Case example 4.5 – resolution

Sara's parents remained very distant throughout her stay and, although the nurses had identified their feelings of guilt and shame, they were not able to address them in the HDU. However, communication between them and the paediatric surgical ward, and the use of family-centred care, meant that the problem was documented and a plan of care created to address the problem.

When something is explained to a patient, it is important that their understanding is checked. It is also very important to listen to the words that patients use, because words are often the key to the beliefs that patients express either consciously or unconsciously. The words that health professionals use are often taken for granted. Take the term 'high dependency care'. Patients may understand the term ICU but may not have heard of HDU. ICU implies or is often interpreted or perceived as meaning patients are sicker than HDU, whereas this may not be the case in reality. Dependency may mean something to do with alcohol or drug addiction, and the patient may think they are going to a 'drying out' clinic. If it is explained that high dependency is a little like intensive care, then it is important to find out what patients understand by intensive care. A similar consideration is that people perceive artificial ventilation (or 'being on a life support machine') as implying a certain level of severity or gravity, whereas this may not necessarily be the case within today's modern clinical practices. Many people experience hospital as a place of pain and suffering, and particularly believe that ICUs are places where people die. This belief has to be dealt with carefully and honestly. However, the challenge is to identify whether or not health beliefs are a significant factor in misunderstanding between patient and health professional.

IATROGENESIS

Patients' past experience of hospital may have been threatening, frightening, painful and distressing. Occasionally, the experience of hospital may have caused further pain on top of the admitting illness: patients may have contracted an infection in hospital, they may have undergone unnecessary treatments, and may have become more unwell as a direct result or failure of the treatment. The term used for this is 'iatrogenesis'; it comes from the Greek words *iatros* meaning doctor and *genesis* meaning origin, and is used to describe the harmful effects of medical and surgical treatments. Most treatments will have some degree of risk. This may be due to the side effects of the drugs used, the inexperience of the practitioner delivering the treatment, or as a consequence of the treatment being more painful and disfiguring than the disease itself. All these factors could apply to the patient requiring high dependency care.

The term iatrogenesis was coined by Ivan Illich (1977b) in his work *Medical Nemesis*. He criticized medicine and the healthcare system for creating three types of iatrogenesis:

- medical, where treatments cause actual harm to patients;
- social, where the power of medicine has so increased that it has 'medicalized' natural events such as birth and death;
- cultural, which is a consequence of the above, as complex urban industrialized communities give up caring for themselves and each other, and relinquish that care to the 'professional' carers.

It has long been recognized that hospitals are dangerous places: Florence Nightingale (1859) said 'It may seem a strange principle to enunciate as the very first requirement in a Hospital that it should do the sick no harm'. However, some of the sickest patients require high dependency care, and they often require some of the riskiest, most highly invasive interventions, such as chest drains, arterial lines, urinary catheters, intravenous catheters, central venous lines, biopsy and mechanical ventilation. Iatrogenic risks may be due to:

- the nature of the procedure;
- the inexperience of the operator;
- the appropriateness of the treatment.

A modern example of this could be where a patient contracts methicillin-resistant *Staphylococcus aureus* (MRSA) whilst undergoing elective surgery in a hospital setting. The care could be perceived as being due to poor professional standards/poor infection control practices.

> When patients are incapacitated how is their choice (autonomy) to be balanced with their needs and the needs of others requiring limited high dependency resources (justice)?

Case example 4.6

Gwen Teal, aged 83, is 24 hours post-op following total right hip replacement after a fall at home. She is underweight and appears a little malnourished. She lives alone and has some help from social services but has not been coping well. This is compounded by recently diagnosed mild dementia. She has developed a productive cough with green sputum. Her chest X-ray shows a consolidation in the right lung. She is admitted for high dependency care for chest physiotherapy, pulse oximetry and observation. The locum doctor says that the ward cannot cope with her.
On admission, her condition is very poor. The locum doctor insists on siting a central line. The first attempt is unsuccessful. On the second attempt, Gwen becomes very breathless and cyanosed. The doctor is again unsuccessful, and he leaves the unit saying he has to see another patient and will return later to put the line in again. The registrar is called, and a tension pneumothorax is diagnosed. A chest drain is inserted. The registrar reassesses Gwen's resuscitation status and decides she can return to the ward for palliative care. There are now no beds on the ward so she has to stay in the unit.

Which categories of iatrogenesis can be identified? How could the events have been predicted and prevented?

Case example 4.6 – resolution

Gwen remained very confused and repeatedly pulled out her i.v. cannula. Fortunately, she could not pull out the chest drain, despite repeated attempts. The feeling in the unit was that she was 'blocking a bed' and that she was just a nuisance making so much noise.

It is not just doctors who are responsible for iatrogenic incidents. Giraud et al (1993), in a study on incidents in French intensive care units, found that nurses committed twice as many errors as physicians. The main reasons cited were a heavy workload and a nurse–patient ratio of 1:4. This may also be true for high dependency units.

The power and influence of medicine in the Western world is widespread. Illich's (1977a) idea of social iatrogenesis is that birth and death

Think about the ways that, whilst caring for one of your patients , their condition has become worse, not better. Who and what were the factors involved?
How is society becoming more medicalized?

have been medicalized. More births occur in hospital than elsewhere and a higher percentage of these births are by caesarean section. The reasons for this are complex, but there is compelling evidence that the reduction in infant and maternal mortality and morbidity is a direct result of improvements in public health and greater medical intervention (Hicks & Allen 1999). Hardey (1998) suggests that death has moved out of the home and community into the hospital, away from a 'natural death' to one with a 'technological ending' (e.g. 'turning off' the ventilator and life support). How the process of death and dying is handled has immense significance for the patient and his family. The hospital environment can be a very alien place to some. High dependency care relies heavily upon technology, but such technology can be very frightening and alienating to the unprepared.

How can we 'demystify' the technology in high dependency care?

Case example 4.7

Mrs Black is dying. Her husband has been told her diagnosis and her prognosis, and appeared to take it in. She has a morphine intravenous infusion and seems pain-free but is only semiconscious. She has a cardiac monitor, central venous pressure monitor, temperature, blood pressure and oxygen saturation monitor recording her vital signs. Her husband is with her, but he seems to have lost sight of his wife, as his eyes are inexorably drawn to the machines. One alarms, the other bleeps. He reacts. He calls the nurse. The nurse resets the monitor. They alarm again. The nurse resets it again. There is an unusual trace, and Mr Black is becoming expert in observing the machines. He calls another nurse over.

The focus on technology can make our nursing care mechanistic. How can the needs of both husband and wife be met? (beneficence)

Case example 4.7 – resolution

The nurse sits down alongside Mr Black and asks him how he is feeling. He talks about his anxiety over all the monitoring. She again tells him the truth about his wife and says that his wife doesn't need the monitoring any more. When the monitoring is taken away, Mr Black is able to hold his wife's hand. This gives them the opportunity to talk and the possibility of eventually saying goodbye.

The hospice movement provides many good examples of how to respond to the specific needs of dying people and their families/carers. It attempts to demedicalize death, by giving greater choice and control back to patients and their families, and allowing patients to die at home. What can we learn from the values of the hospice movement in high dependency care?

Cultural iatrogenesis is perhaps more difficult to pin down. It has to do with the power and influence that the profession of medicine and, to some extent, that of nursing may have within society. The professions seem to have cornered a 'niche' market in terms of their knowledge and skills. This is reflected in the length and breadth of training, and the status that the individual members accrue within society (social groups I and II). Harrison et al (1990) argue that despite the various reorganizations of the NHS these have had a very limited effect on the dominance of the medical profession in society.

Illich (1977b) says that the only way forward is to 'demystify medical matters'. The laity, he argues, must be consulted on all decisions, and the individual must be assisted in developing autonomy, and be responsible for their coping ability. How far has the development within nursing moved towards meeting the above aims?

ADVOCACY

Think of an occasion when you have disagreed with a patient's medical or nursing treatment. What did you, or did you not do, do about it?

If you were not happy with what you did or did not do, why do you think that was, and what would you do differently next time?

One of the approaches that assist the individual is the concept of advocacy. The NMC's Code of Professional Conduct (2002) reflects the use of the concept of advocacy. The advocate is a 'voice for' – someone to take the place of, someone who will speak for you whether you are present, capable or not. This could present a picture of the nurse benignly 'standing' alongside the patient during their illness and hospitalization. The idea may be very appealing. Within the UK legal system, however, we have an understanding of advocacy based upon adversarial conflict. This image presupposes the nurse standing 'between' the patient and whoever he or she is in conflict with – the physician, the family, other nurses, hospital management or society at large. This presents a more complex picture of the role of the nurse. It can be argued that there are many things preventing nurses from executing their role, such as their own professionalism (or lack of it), their duty to the organization and their obligations to the other patients in their care, or their attitudes, their capability, prejudices, ignorance and lack of willingness or ability to embrace 'difference'.

One approach to care that has explored these avenues is primary nursing. Meutzel (1988) sees the relationship between the nurse and patient as a therapeutic relationship. It has three main elements:

- *reciprocity*, where the nurse may receive support and care;
- *intimacy*, a closeness which has meaning and value;
- *partnership*, which suggests a balance of power and an equality in the nurse–patient relationship.

The expression of the partnership of the nurse–patient relationship is, however, complex. Salvage (1991) says that it is not straightforward. as there is insufficient evidence that the patient explicitly wants this type of relationship. The situation where it appears to be most fruitful – but also most complex – is where patients are unable to speak for themselves. Patient who are unconscious or who are otherwise incapable of expressing their views could be without a voice. How is their autonomy and freedom to make choices respected? Nurses, with their skills, should anticipate, plan and deliver care to meet patients' needs, but what happens when there is disagreement between the patients' families/carers and the medical team?

> Is the success of PALS services a good thing or a bad thing? Does the success of PALS imply failure elsewhere in the NHS? Should the strategy be to reduce dependency/reliance on PALS?

The Kennedy Report (Learning from Bristol 2001) into the death of children following heart surgery at Bristol Royal Infirmary criticized the lack of openness and partnership between patients, carers and healthcare professionals. The response to the report from the Department of Health (2002) identifies the Patient Advocacy and Liaison Service (PALS) as a key method to respond to these criticisms, and bring about change locally and nationally. Does PALS represent a threat to the role of the nurse as advocate or an opportunity to expand the support and advocacy service to patients?

> How are the choices the patient makes (autonomy) balanced with the negative effects that the family may feel (non-maleficence)?

Case example 4.8

Brian Fuller is 72 years old. He has always spoken about 'living wills' and 'advanced directives', saying he 'didn't want to be a vegetable' and that he didn't want any Tom, Dick or Harry having any of his organs. His relatives have been persistent in trying to get him transferred to the local private hospital. Brian is none too fussed. He keeps asking about the patient in the next bed who is awaiting transfer to a specialist centre for transplantation. He is very moved by the plight of this patient and tells the nurse that he would give his organs if he died, saying that this has gone against everything that he has said before but that seeing the pain of a real situation has changed his mind. Later that day, Brian suffers a cardiac arrest in the high dependency unit and resuscitation is unsuccessful. His family are distraught. The doctors decide that it is not worth asking the family for organ donation because of the brittle relationship between them. The nurse knows, however, that Brian has changed his mind and broaches the subject. The family initially react badly, and one of the doctors is angry that the nurse has gone against their wishes.

How can you continue to be an advocate for the patient after their death? Where is your responsibility to maintain the partnership: with the patient, the family/carers or the doctors?

Case example 4.8 – resolution

The family can't believe that Brian has changed his mind so radically but, left with some literature and the opportunity to come back and ask questions, they give it some thought. The nurse stands by her principles and the doctor becomes more isolated in his opinions. The family agree to heart valves and corneal retrieval.

CONCLUSION

Nurses in the high dependency unit will often find themselves undertaking a number of activities using many complex aspects of their role. There is the patient's condition to treat and manage, the needs of the family/carer(s) to meet and their own personal needs to address. This may require that the nurse responds with technical skills at one moment and listening skills the next. When caring for patients, the nurse will require the insights of sociological theory and an understanding of how different cultural groups express themselves, in order to understand the patient in their care more fully.

A broad understanding of the issues that determine the medical imperatives of the situation, as well as its human aspects, will enable the nurse to reflect in the situation and on the situation. This may help in decision-making, by bringing to the fore the expertise needed to help and the ability to perform high-quality nursing care.

It is important to know what to do at a time of medical emergency, but it is also vital not to lose sight of the fact that nursing skills are being used in the care of a human being: a person with a unique history, a place in society, a family and a set of needs that transcend the purely clinical and the biases or preconceptions of individuals. The requirement of the NMC (2002: Clause 7) to provide holistic care may at times be daunting. Each patient is unique; no amount of tubes, wires, drugs and flashing screens should obscure that truth. The worried family/carers eager for news, reassurance or care in their own right will be a reminder that the person being cared for is not simply a patient.

The case examples in this chapter have highlighted some of the many factors that affect the patient who requires high dependency care. They have highlighted the ethical principles involved, and the personal and professional accountability demanded of each nurse. The patient, ill or injured, has a personality that was formed, in most cases, long before the illness or injury. Sometimes the condition affects the personality of the patient, and it also sometimes affects the reactions and opinions of the family/carers. The nurse may have to deal with the consequences of the interaction of such events and, as such, has a professional obligation to put aside any personal biases, prejudices or judgements.

Taking the time to consider the patients' needs, based on their social position, familial circumstances, ethnic background and traditions, their beliefs and personal opinions, will make the care better for the patients and families concerned and the responsibility of caring for the patient much more rewarding, within the context of high dependency care.

References

Beauchamp TL, Childress JF 1994 Principles of bioethics, 4th edn. Oxford University Press, New York

Brykczynska G 1992 Caring: a dying art? In: Jolley M, Brykczynska G (eds) Nursing care – the challenge to change. Edward Arnold, London, Ch 1

Department of Health 1992 The health of the nation: a strategy for health in England. HMSO, London

Department of Health 2002 Learning from Bristol: The Department of Health's response to the report of the Public Inquiry into children's heart surgery at the Bristol Royal Infirmary 1984–1995. Cmd5363. HMSO, London

Giraud T, Dhainaut J F, Vaxelaire J F et al 1993 Iatrogenic complications in adult intensive care units: a prospective two centre study. Critical Care Medicine 21(1): 40–51

Hardey M 1998 The social context of health. Open University Press, Buckingham

Harrison S, Hunter D J, Marnoch G, Pollit C 1990 The dynamics of British health policy. London, Unwin Hyman

Hicks J, Allen G 1999 A century of change: Trend in UK statistics since 1900. Research Paper 99/111 House of Commons Library. HMSO, London

Illich I 1977a Disabling professions. Marion Boyars, New York

Illich I 1977b Limits to medicine. Medical nemesis: the expropriation of health. Pelican Books, London

Learning from Bristol 2001 The Report from the Public Inquiry into children's heart surgery at the Bristol Royal Infirmary 1984–1995. Cmd5207(I). HMSO, London

Meutzel P 1988 Therapeutic nursing. In: Pearson A (ed.) Primary nursing: nursing in the Burford and Oxford nursing development units. Croom Helm, London

Millar B 1989 Critical support in critical care. Nursing Times 85(16): 31–32

Nightingale F 1859 Notes on nursing. (Reprinted 1980.) Churchill Livingstone, Edinburgh

Nursing and Midwifery Council 2002 Code of professional conduct. Nursing and Midwifery Council, London.

Royal College of Nursing (RCN) 2003 Defining nursing: Publication Code 001 998. RCN, London

Salvage J 1991 The new nursing: empowering patients or empowering nurses. In: Robinson J, Gray A, Elkin R (eds) Policy issues in nursing. Oxford University Press, Oxford

Social Trends 1996 HMSO, London

Townsend P, Davidson N (eds) 1982 The Black report. Pelican Books, London

Whitehead M 1992 The health divide in inequalities in health: The Black report. Harmondsworth, Penguin

Further reading

Bond J, Bond S 1995 Sociology and health care. Churchill Livingstone, Edinburgh

Kikuchi J F, Simmons H (eds) 1992 Philosophic inquiry in nursing. Sage, London

Porter R 1997 The greatest benefit to mankind. HarperCollins, London

Robinson K, Vaughan B 1992 Knowledge for nursing practice. Butterworth-Heinemann, London

SECTION 2

Clinical issues in high dependency care

SECTION CONTENTS

Chapter 5

Respiratory care

Debbie Field

KEY LEARNING OBJECTIVES

With Prerequisite knowledge of respiratory anatomy and physiology, readers of this chapter will be able:

- To better apply the concepts of respiratory physiology to their clinical practice in terms of patient assessment, evaluation, treatment options and care
- To identify the causes, signs and symptoms of respiratory failure
- To identify those patients who are at greater risk of developing respiratory distress/failure and who may require escalating levels of care
- To describe and give a rationale for patient assessment in relation to optimising and maintaining effective breathing
- To identify and give a rationale for the main principles of respiratory care, nursing interventions and prevention of complications
- To describe and give a rationale for adjuncts used to optimise respiratory function and care (e.g. oxygen therapy, non-invasive ventilation, tracheostomy)
- To identify and be aware of the usefulness and limitations of those technological interventions used in respiratory care and observation

INTRODUCTION

The purpose of this chapter is to demonstrate the importance of the nurse's role in relation to the delivery and effectiveness of respiratory care for those patients who are at risk of developing respiratory failure and require an increased level of care (Level 1/Level 2), whether within the ward environment or in a critical care environment. In both areas, nurses need to be able to apply their knowledge and skills in order to extrapolate, analyse and critically evaluate the data observed, the interventions and treatment being initiated and the nursing care implemented. This chapter is, therefore, designed to give nurses a greater understanding of the concepts of patient assessment, nursing care, therapeutic and technological intervention, treatment options and pharmacological agents in order to prevent complications and to optimize and maintain effective respiration for those patients who require a higher dependency of care in any setting. With greater understanding of respiratory care, nurses will ultimately effect a quality patient outcome by reducing morbidity and mortality in those patients who require Level 1 or Level 2 care.

Prerequisite knowledge

It is essential that the reader has an understanding of normal respiratory anatomy and physiology before studying this chapter (see 'Further reading'). This knowledge is summarized in Box 5.1. However, a brief overview of the basic physiological concepts will be presented in order to enhance the reader's application of these to patient assessment, intervention, treatment and care.

BASIC CONCEPTS OF RESPIRATORY PHYSIOLOGY

The primary function of the respiratory system is to supply adequate oxygen (O_2) to the tissues for the oxidation of respiratory substrates (carbohydrates, fats and proteins) in order to yield energy (cellular respiration) and to remove the waste product, carbon dioxide (CO_2). This is represented as:

Box 5.1   Prerequisite knowledge

Anatomy

- Major structures: mouth/nose, trachea, bronchi, lungs, diaphragm, pleura
- Blood supply
- Microstructures: alveoli, goblet cells
- Anatomical dead space

Physiology

- Lung volumes
- Carriage of gases
- Aerobic and anaerobic cellular respiration
- Oxyhaemoglobin dissociation curve
- Physiological dead space
- Ventilation–perfusion match ($\dot{V}/\dot{Q}$)
- Control of breathing
- Boyle's law
- Dalton's law

Acid–base balance
Determinants of work of breathing

$$O_2 + fuel = Energy + CO_2 + H_2O$$

This function is interdependent with the circulatory system's prime role of blood transport.

In order to achieve this primary function, there has to be:

- adequate airflow into and out of the lungs (pulmonary ventilation);
- exchange of O_2 and CO_2 at the alveolar level;
- effective transport of O_2 and CO_2 to the body and the pulmonary system (perfusion);
- normal cell function.

Adequate airflow into and out of the lungs

This is dependent upon:

- atmospheric pressure;
- chest wall compliance;
- respiratory muscle function;
- neural control;
- negative pressure gradient between mouth and alveoli;
- resistance of the airways to flow of air;
- elasticity of the lung tissue (lung compliance).

> This negative pressure also enhances venous return, which contributes to an adequate cardiac output.

Pulmonary ventilation happens in two phases: inspiration and expiration. The volume of the thoracic cavity is changed by muscle contraction and relaxation. During quiet inspiration, the diaphragm and external intercostal muscles contract, slightly enlarging the thoracic cavity (Figure 5.1). Increasing the volume decreases the pressure within the thoracic cavity and lungs (Boyle's law) and this creates a negative pressure within the lungs and thoracic cavity. Air then rushes down the pressure gradient through the mouth/nose from the atmosphere into the thoracic cavity, where the pressure then equalizes.

Figure 5.1 Inspiration.

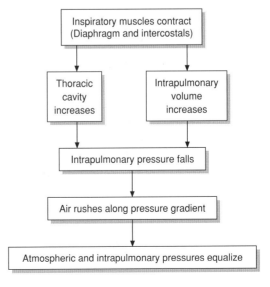

Inspiratory muscles contract
(Diaphragm and intercostals)

Thoracic cavity increases

Intrapulmonary volume increases

Intrapulmonary pressure falls

Air rushes along pressure gradient

Atmospheric and intrapulmonary pressures equalize

Expiration is normally a passive process (Figure 5.2) and only becomes active during exercise. In disease states, such as chronic obstructive pulmonary disease, expiration often becomes active most of the time owing to the patient's decreased lung compliance. Thus, the patient's work of breathing (WOB) increases.

Exchange of O_2 and CO_2 within the lungs

Gas exchange only takes place within the functioning units of the alveoli and where there is adequate alveolar capillary blood flow to allow movement of gases across the pulmonary capillary membrane by diffusion. Once there has been an exchange of gases at alveoli level, O_2 is transported to the tissues and CO_2 is excreted via the lungs during expiration.

Gas exchange is dependent upon:

- adequate surfactant production;
- matching of ventilation and perfusion ($\dot{V}/\dot{Q}$ match);
- alveolar ventilation.

Surfactant

Surfactant is a lipoprotein produced by the type II alveolar cells. Surfactant coats the outside of the alveoli and its function is to:

- reduce alveoli surface tension;
- aid diffusion of gases;
- contribute to the lungs' natural recoil during expiration;
- discourage alveolar collapse.

Reduction of surfactant directly affects gas diffusion and increases the work of breathing. The main causes of reduced surfactant production are:

- hypoxia;
- atelectasis;

Figure 5.2 Expiration.

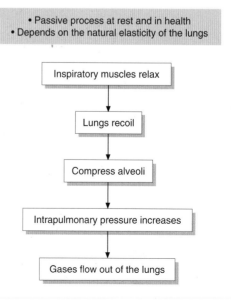

- Passive process at rest and in health
- Depends on the natural elasticity of the lungs

Inspiratory muscles relax

Lungs recoil

Compress alveoli

Intrapulmonary pressure increases

Gases flow out of the lungs

- positive pressure ventilation (continuous positive airway pressure, mechanical ventilation, etc.);
- acidosis;
- hyperoxygenation;
- starvation;
- pulmonary vascular congestion.

Ventilation–perfusion match

For gas exchange to be most efficient, there must be a close match between ventilation (the amount of gas reaching the alveoli) and perfusion (the blood flow in the pulmonary capillaries). Both ventilation and perfusion increase towards the lung base because of the effects of gravity; therefore, there will always be regional variations of ventilation and perfusion, which will vary according to body position. However, there are conditions that will make the $\dot{V}/\dot{Q}$ mismatch worse and lead to either acute or chronic hypoxaemia ($\dot{V}/\dot{Q}$ = ventilation/perfusion quotient, that is, the ratio between ventilation and perfusion within the lungs). These causes are:

- hypoventilation for any reason (e.g. excess sedation, pain, respiratory muscle weakness, etc.);
- atelectasis;
- alveoli consolidation;
- low cardiac output states;
- pulmonary oedema;
- obstructive lung disease;
- restrictive disease.

Alveolar ventilation

Although measuring minute ventilation will provide a rough and ready value for assessing respiratory efficiency, a much better and easily calculated index is the alveolar ventilation rate. This index takes into consideration the volume of air wasted in dead space areas (anatomical dead space) and measures the flow of fresh gases in and out of the alveoli during a particular time. Alveolar ventilation can be calculated as follows:

Alveolar ventilation (millilitres/minute) = Breaths per minute × tidal volume (ml/l) – dead space (ml/l)

Anatomical dead space in an average adult is often estimated as 150 ml; a more precise calculation of an individual's anatomical dead space is 1 ml per 1 lb body weight.

Example: A 150 lb adult with a respiratory rate of 12 breaths/minute (bpm) and tidal volume of 500 ml per breath will have an alveolar ventilation rate of 4200 ml/minute:

$$12 \times 500 - 150 = 4200 \text{ ml/minute}$$

Increasing the volume of each inspiration enhances alveolar ventilation and gas exchange more than raising the respiratory rate because anatomical space is constant in a particular individual. Alveolar ventilation drops dramatically during rapid shallow breathing because most of the inspired air never reaches the exchange sites.

Carriage of gases

A patient with a low haemoglobin will, therefore, carry less O_2 per 100 ml blood. This means that there is less available O_2 at tissue level for adequate cellular metabolism.

Figure 5.3 (a) The oxygen–haemoglobin dissociation curve. This curve applies when the pH is 7.4, blood temperature is 37°C and the PCO_2 is 5.3 kPa. It should also be assumed that haemoglobin concentration is 15 g/dl blood. (b) Factors influencing the position of the oxygen dissociation curve. (Reproduced from Hinchliff & Montague 1988 with kind permission.)

When demand exceeds supply (e.g. when a patient has an acute asthmatic attack), cellular metabolism changes from aerobic to anaerobic, which results in lactate production and metabolic acidosis, thus reducing the patient's O_2 reserve further.

Once haemoglobin is fully saturated, no further increase in PO_2 will increase the amount of O_2 carried by haemoglobin. Increasing patients' inspired O_2 will not increase their PO_2 if their haemoglobin is fully saturated. This is an important point to remember if you are caring for a patient who is anaemic.

This process is also dependent on an adequate cardiac output (see Chapter 6). The majority of O_2 is carried in combination with haemoglobin and only 0.3 ml of O_2 is carried dissolved in plasma. At a normal level of haemoglobin (15 g/dl), 20 ml of O_2 is carried per 100 ml of blood.

One important aspect in relation to the carriage of O_2 is the oxy-haemoglobin dissociation curve (see Figure 5.3), that is, the detachment

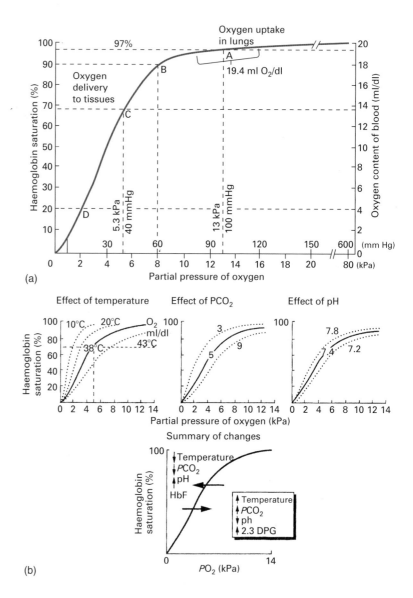

of O_2 from haemoglobin. The actual chemical structure of haemoglobin allows for varying affinity to O_2 molecules, which is dependent upon the partial pressure of O_2 (PO_2) within the capillary. A fit individual with normal lung function, therefore, who has a PO_2 of 13.3 kPa, will have used almost all of the O_2 binding capacity of haemoglobin and the haemoglobin is said to be approximately 98% saturated.

Where O_2 is extracted at tissue level, haemoglobin saturation is reduced to about 75% and O_2 is released to the tissues. This leaves about three-quarters of the haemoglobin oxygenated, which provides a reservoir for conditions when there is an increased demand for O_2 (e.g. during excerise or illness), in order to maintain aerobic metabolism.

Carbon dioxide

There are six different mechanisms involved in the carriage of CO_2:

Plasma
1. As dissolved CO_2 (10%)
2. Protein-bound
3. As bicarbonate (HCO_3)

Red blood cells
4. As dissolved CO_2 (10%)
5. Combined with haemoglobin
6. As bicarbonate (70%)

UNDERSTANDING CYANOSIS AND HYPOXIA

Cyanosis

When the haemoglobin (Hb) is oxygenated, it is bright red in colour, whereas deoxygenated Hb has a dark colour causing a dusky bluish coloration of the tissues. This is called *cyanosis* and occurs when there is more than 5 g/dl of reduced Hb in the blood, which equates to a Hb saturation of about 85–90%. It is most easily seen where the skin is thin and blood flows close to the surface, such as the mucous membranes.

There are two forms of cyanosis as outlined below.

• *Peripheral cyanosis*. This occurs when blood flow through the extremities is sluggish, which can be due to hypovolaemia, low cardiac output states, arteriovenous obstruction or cold weather. In this instance, the patient will appear pink centrally (i.e. mucous membranes within the mouth will be pink and glossy) but have cyanosed peripheries.
• *Central cyanosis*. The blood in the aorta leaving the heart has large amounts of deoxygenated Hb and the patient's mucous membranes will be dull, bluish in colour and dusky. This indicates a problem with oxygen transfer into the blood in the lungs, or mixing of oxygenated and deoxygenated blood. A patient who is centrally cyanosed needs immediate medical attention.

Hypoxia

When a patient is centrally cyanosed, the amount of oxygen being carried to the tissues is inadequate and this is called *hypoxia*. Hypoxia can be divided into the following four forms.

- *Hypoxic hypoxia* in which the PO_2 of the arterial blood is significantly reduced. This is the most common form of hypoxia seen clinically (see Figure 5.4).
- *Anaemic hypoxia* in which the PO_2 is adequate but the amount of Hb available to carry O_2 is reduced.
- *Stagnant hypoxia* in which the blood flow to the tissues is so low that adequate O_2 cannot be supplied to the tissues despite adequate PO_2 and Hb concentration.
- *Cytotoxic hypoxia,* in which the amount of O_2 supplied to the tissues is adequate but, because of the action of a toxic agent, the tissue cannot make use of the O_2 available.

The causes of hypoxic hypoxia are (Figure 5.4):

- gas exchange failure;
- ventilation mismatch within the lungs (pneumonia, atelectasis, asthma, pulmonary embolism);
- impaired gas transfer across the lungs (fibrotic lung disease, pulmonary oedema).

Arterial blood gases will show a low PaO_2 (8 kpa) with a normal or low $PaCO_2$, as the initial response to hypoxaemia is to increase ventilation by increasing respiratory rate. Pulse oximetry (SpO_2) will decrease below 90% on air. This is classified as *Type I respiratory failure*. First-line treatment for type I respiratory failure is oxygen therapy followed by investigation as to the cause of the failure.

When ventilation is inadequate, for whatever reason, the $PaCO_2$ will rise; if ventilation is halved, the $PaCO_2$ doubles. Blood gas analysis will demonstrate a low PaO_2 and a rising $PaCO_2$ (>7 kpa), known as hypercapnia. This is *Type II respiratory failure*, which can be caused by:

- ventilation failure (pump failure);
- respiratory depression (hypoventilation);
- respiratory muscle fatigue from whatever cause;
- mechanical defects (pneumothorax, bronchial obstruction).

Figure 5.4 Causes of hypoxia.

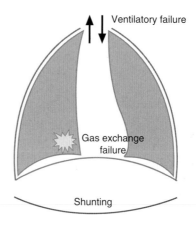

One of the most common conditions that manifests as type II respiratory failure is chronic obstructive pulmonary disease (COPD). Patients with COPD who require oxygen therapy need careful monitoring, as they are at risk of ventilatory depression if they are given high-concentration oxygen. Therefore it is recommended that these patients are initially treated with 35% oxygen and the oxygen level is increased incrementally to obtain saturations above 90%.

PRINCIPLES OF RESPIRATORY CARE

Nursing assessment, intervention and care must be based upon an individual and holistic approach to each patient for whom the nurse cares. It requires continuity of care if the nurse is to optimize and maintain effective respiration, with the ultimate aim of making the patient feel comfortable and cared for, and to prevent complications. Continuity of care is achieved through:

- effective communication throughout the team;
- proactive and creative nursing strategies, interventions and evaluation;
- an appropriate and effective framework of care;
- nursing audit;
- care reviews.

The patient at risk of developing respiratory failure needs continuous physiological and psychological observation and assessment, and well-planned nursing strategies. There is, therefore, an increased patient dependency on nursing care, nursing time and technology, such as non-invasive respiratory support, cardiac monitoring and oximetry.

The principle of respiratory care is to optimize and maintain ventilation and perfusion. This is achieved by:

- continuous observation and assessment of the patient;
- proactive patient-centred comfort care;
- positioning;
- assistance with physiotherapy techniques;
- oxygen therapy and non-invasive respiratory support;
- accurate fluid balance;
- adequate pain relief;
- temperature control;
- chest drain management;
- appropriate administration and evaluation of drug therapies in relation to respiratory function;
- continuity of care and review from the whole multidisciplinary team.

RESPIRATORY ASSESSMENT, OBSERVATION AND EVALUATION

The assessment of patients requires nurses to use their skills of observation, communication, monitoring, analysing and interpreting both objective and subjective data in order to deliver effective care. Observation skills, which include sight, hearing, touch and smell, should not be underestimated. They are important factors in assessing and collecting information about the patient's respiratory function. From such observations, nurses will often gain intuitive perceptions of how patients are reacting to hospital admission, the hospital environment, the course of treatment and care, and their whole sense of being. This intuitive knowledge is just as important as the meticulous collection of empirical data in relation to the patients' physiological status and it should never be trivialized. Respiratory assessment is an important part of holistic patient assessment and nurses should not regard it as a separate entity.

Normal respiratory work at rest consumes 2–3% of the total O_2 intake, but this increases to 40–50% in respiratory distress, leading to cardiovascular and neurological deterioration. Respiratory work may be increased, and ventilation and perfusion may be decreased well before the signs of hypercapnia and hypoxia are present.

Assessment for the signs and symptoms of potential respiratory failure demands that nurses look for subtle changes in patients' condition and vital signs. Remember, when assessing any patient, *look, listen and feel*, and all the time think of Airway, Breathing, Circulation, Disability and Environment.

With any good assessment, assessing a patient's respiratory status must begin with obtaining an in-depth history and should include the following.

- Relevant past medical history – to include asthma, chronic lung disease, etc.
- History of breathlessness – at rest or on exertion:
  - what makes the patient feel breathless?
  - what strategies do they use to alleviate their breathlessness?
- Patients exercise tolerance – how far can they walk?
- History of coughing – productive or dry?
  - If productive, what type of secretions, and their colour and consistency?
- Smoking history.
- Recent or chronic respiratory infections.
- Relevant drug history.
- How does the patient cope with stress?
- What is the patient's normal sleep pattern? In what position does he or she sleep?
- Nutritional history – has there been any recent weight loss or weight gain?

Once a thorough history has been obtained, it is important that the nurse assesses the patient's current respiratory function. This will include all of the general respiratory assessments and some of the adjuncts to a respiratory assessment (Box 5.2).

Risk factors

Whilst undertaking a general respiratory assessment, it is important to identify those patients who are commonly admitted to general clinical areas and who are most at risk of developing respiratory distress or fail-

Box 5.2   General respiratory assessment and adjuncts to respiratory assessment

General respiratory assessment

Overall appearance
Respiratory rate (RR: *remember* normal RR at rest is 10–14 bpm)
Respiratory rhythm and depth
Use of accessory muscles
Symmetry of chest wall movement
Position of trachea (middle or displaced)
Nose or mouth breathing (*remember* at rest we
breath through our nose; mouth breathing indicates
an increase in work of breathing)
Signs of peripheral or central cyanosis (*Remember* central
cynanosis means arterial desaturation and requires immediate
attention. Nurses should observe patients' mucous membranes
in their mouth, which will be dusky and dull on inspection if
central cyanosis is present)
Chest auscultation
Sputum and secretions
Cardiovascular status
Neurological status
Renal status (*remember* that any type of renal failure will affect
the body's ability to buffer an increase in hydrogen ions)
Pain assessment
Psychological status

Adjuncts to respiratory assessment

Pulse oximetry Chest X-ray

Blood profiles
Sputum culture and sensitivity
Bronchoscopy
Pulmonary lung function tests
Imaging: computed tomography
(CT) scan, magnetic resonance
imaging (MRI), ultrasound
Arterial blood gases/capillary blood
gases

Electrocardiogram

ure (Box 5.3). It is beyond the scope of this chapter to address the causes listed (see Further reading) and many are self-explanatory in their effect on respiratory function.

Identifying respiratory distress and failure

The clinical signs of respiratory distress signify a marked increase in *the work of breathing*, which will lead to hypoxaemia and eventually respiratory failure. One of the most significant and early signs of an increase in a patient's work of breathing is a rise in the patient's respiratory rate at rest from their normal rate (Box 5.4). This rise in respiratory rate initially minimizes the increase in respiratory work required as the patient's lung compliance falls. It may initially affect patients so little that they deny they are breathless. This is a result of the effect of compensatory factors, such as mouth opening and increased heart rate. It is, however, an extremely important sign and the nurse needs to look carefully at the trend of the patient's respiratory rate over time (Figure 5.5) It has been demonstrated by McGloin et al (1999) that these often subtle but important trends that predict a patient becoming critically ill often go unobserved

Box 5.3   Conditions that increase the risk of respiratory distress/failure

- Age of the patient (patients over the age of 65 years and who are going for surgery are at greater risk of post-operative pulmonary complications)
- Co-morbidity, e.g. asthma, chronic lung disease, cardiac disease
- General anaesthetic
- Type of surgery, e.g. cardiothoracic surgery, abdominal surgery
- Chest trauma
- Chest wall deformities
- Smoking
- Respiratory muscle weakness, e.g. myasthenia gravis, Guillain–Barré syndrome, poor nutritional status
- Immobilization
- Depression of respiratory centre, e.g. drugs, neurological injury
- Ventilation–perfusion mismatch, e.g pneumonia, hypoperfusion, pulmonary oedema, atelectasis

Box 5.4   Respiratory rate assessment

- Respiratory rate should always be assessed for a full 60 seconds
- Respiratory rate should not be taken from the pulse oximeter or dynomap
- Note the patient's use of any accessory muscles
- Record respiratory rate with SpO_2 and, if receiving oxygen, the percentage of oxygen
- Respiratory rates above or below normal must be reported to the nurse in charge

Figure 5.5 Respiratory rate over 3 days (4-hourly observations).

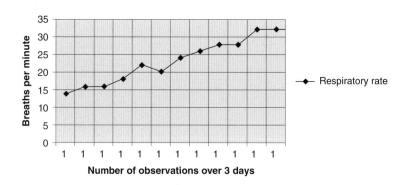

or are seen as insignificant. Consequently, there is an increase in patient mortality and morbidity at ward level, and an increase in patients requiring Level 2 and 3 care.

The most significant signs and symptoms of respiratory distress are manifested by the respiratory, cardiovascular and central nervous systems, and will include the following:

- increased respiratory rate above the patient's normal rate;
- tachypnoea (rate > 25 bpm);
- mouth opening;
- pursed lip breathing;
- cyanosis;
- feelings of breathlessness;
- increased use of accessory muscles;
- prominent sternocleidomastoid muscles;
- paradoxical breathing;
- diminishing breath sounds on chest auscultation;
- tachycardia;
- anxiety/fear;
- altered level of consciousness;
- confusion/agitation;
- sweating;
- fidgeting;
- furrowing of forehead.

A brief overview of some of the signs and symptoms will be given. However, some of the signs of respiratory distress are self-explanatory and two have already been addressed (respiratory rate and cyanosis).

> Patients whose respiratory rate has increased at rest will begin to talk in short sentences, pausing to take a breath during the sentence spoken. Eventually, they will not be able to speak at all as their respiratory distress increases.

> During severe exercise in fit individuals, they will use open-mouth panting in order to decrease respiratory work and anatomical dead space, as this is an autonomic response.

Mouth opening and pursed lip breathing

Commonly, the mouth opens at an early stage of respiratory distress. Initially, this is slight and variable, or occurring only during inspiration. It is often difficult to detect, but it becomes more and more obvious as the distress increases. *Even minor changes are significant.* There are two physiological benefits – a reduction in anatomical dead space and in respiratory work.

Pursed-lip breathing is often combined with open-mouth breathing, where the mouth opens with inspiration and the lips purse with expiration. Obstruction and prolongation of expiration by pursed lips is a natural positive end-expiratory pressure (PEEP) mechanism. It increases functional residual capacity and lung compliance, and benefits respiratory work and gas exchange.

> This manoeuvre is seen following severe exercise. When athletes finish running a race, for example, you will note that they often bend forward, open their mouths to breathe in, then purse their lips when breathing out.

Accessory muscles and breathing pattern

The use of accessory muscles will be observed in patients who develop moderate to severe respiratory distress. The use of these muscles indicates an increase in the work of breathing, with a consequent increase in oxygen demand. Accessory muscle action includes suprasternal retractions, intercostal retractions abdominal breathing and the use of the sternocleidomastoid muscles in the neck.

As respiratory distress increases, patients will demonstrate a pattern of rapid shallow breathing, reducing patients' tidal volume and consequently

Patients who have pre-existing lung disease may have chronic use of accessory muscle breathing but this will be further exaggerated if the patient has an exacerbation of chronic lung disease.

their alveolar ventilation. If respiratory distress worsens, breathing gradually becomes laboured and the use of accessory muscles will become even more prominent. Movement of the chest wall will change as the work of breathing increases. The rhythm of breathing will become dyssynchronous. Movement of the chest wall also relates to the anatomy of patients, and whether their movements are restricted by chest drains, wound site, dressings or chest wall trauma, causing a flail chest (see Box 5.5) or pain.

Confusion, agitation and altered levels of consciousness

Agitation and confusion must always be attributed to hypoxia and treated accordingly unless another cause for the patient's agitation and confusion can be directly identified. *If in any doubt, always* give supplemental oxygen and *never* give sedation!

Levels of consciousness decrease as respiratory distress increases. The patient often stares vacantly, seems drowsy and apathy is often noticeable. Although this is often attributed to hypercapnia, in the earlier stages of distress, there is a marked derangement of the blood gases. This may be due to decreased cerebral perfusion owing to the body's sympathetic response.

Tachycardia

In the response to an increase in the work of breathing and an increasing oxygen debt, there will be a corresponding increase in heart rate. This, in turn, will increase oxygen demand and a cycle of events is then established. If the patient has ischaemic heart disease, the increased heart rate may be enough to cause myocardial ischaemia and the patient may then complain of chest pain. A 12-lead electrocardiogram (ECG) may demonstrate ischaemic changes. As patients' hypoxaemia worsens and causes an acid–base imbalance, they could experience life-threatening arrhythmias. These may include atrial fibrillation, paroxysmal atrial tachycardia, ventricular tachycardia, ventricular fibrillation or severe bradycardia.

Box 5.5   Flail chest

- Injury to the chest wall produces instability of the thoracic cage and lung contusion
- When ribs are fractured in several places or combined with dislocations of the costochondral junctions or sternum, the negative intrapleural pressure generated on inspiration causes the isolated segment of the chest wall to collapse inwards (flail chest), compromising ventilation. This will be demonstrated by the patient in terms of *paradoxical breathing* (when the thoracic cage moves inward during inspiration, as opposed to normal inspiration when the rib cage expands in a symmetrical fashion)
- Chest wall injuries are *extremely painful*, which will further compromise the patient's respiratory function – the patient will hypoventilate

Feelings of breathlessness, anxiety and fear

As the work of breathing gets more and more difficult, patients express feelings that they cannot take a satisfactory breath, that they have 'air hunger', or feel like they are suffocating and breathless. This causes feelings of panic, anxiety and fear, and sets up a cycle of events (Figure 5.6). It is important to take into consideration these psychological manifestations when trying to establish certain treatments, such as trying to get patients to keep an oxygen mask on when they feel as if they are suffocating.

Diminished breath sounds

Listening to air entry is a difficult observation, as it requires experience to be able to interpret what is heard. It may take time to master the skill but, once mastered, it will be an important addition to a thorough respiratory assessment of the patient. It is important that nurses seek help and advice from colleagues within the multidisciplinary team (such as physiotherapists and doctors) in order to learn and master this observation.

There is a specific sequence of positions where you should place the stethoscope on the chest. This allows you to listen to all areas. The dome of the stethoscope should be used with the chest clear of clothing. Both anterior and posterior surfaces should be listened to, if possible.

Listening to air entry and breath sounds is a basic measure to ensure that there is flow of air to all areas of the lung. Common causes of decreased or non-existent air entry in self-ventilating patients are:

- hypoventilation;
- atelectasis;
- lobar collapse;
- sputum retention;
- pneumonia;
- pleural effusion;
- pneumothorax.

Breath sounds result from turbulent air passing over the larynx, and vary in loudness and rhythm depending on where the stethoscope is placed. There are three types of breath sounds:

- normal
- abnormal
- diminished.

Figure 5.6 A negative cycle of events.

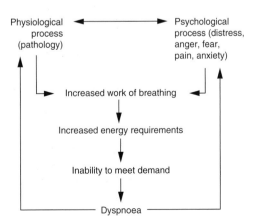

Normal breath sounds

- Vesicular – a gentle rustling noise, which is audible all over the periphery of the lungs. It is loudest on inspiration and fades away rapidly during the early part of expiration.
- Bronchial – high pitched and loud, with a pause between inspiration and expiration. Expiration equals inspiration and should only be heard over the trachea. If these bronchial sounds are heard over any other areas of the lung, it is indicative of lung pathology.
- Bronchovesicular – a combination of the above sounds, heard over major airways in most other parts of the lung.

Abnormal breath sounds

- *Wheezes* are characteristically an expiratory sound associated with forced airflow through abnormally collapsed or narrowed airways with residual trapping of air. Wheezes are commonly heard in patients suffering from chronic airway limitation or bronchial asthma, when the obstruction is due to secretions and bronchospasm.
- *Pleural friction rubs* – rough, grating and crackling sounds heard on inspiration and expiration. These are found in areas of pleural inflammation when the normally smooth surfaces of parietal and visceral pleura are roughened and rub on each other.
- *Crackles* are caused by excessive fluid within the airways. The fluid could be due to exudate, as in pneumonia or other infections of the lung, or transudate, as in congestive cardiac failure. They are typically inspiratory.

Other signs which may lead to respiratory distress

Sputum and secretions   If the patient is producing sputum, it is important to observe the colour, consistency and amount. This observation will also add to a better understanding of the patient's respiratory function. It is also important to note whether the patient is having increasing difficulty in expectorating his or her secretions. This could be due to:

- an increase in the tenacity and amount of secretions;
- the patient becoming more fatigued and unable to expectorate effectively.

Pain   Although there is a chapter in this book dedicated to the concept of pain, its importance cannot be overstressed here. If the patient at risk of developing respiratory failure is experiencing pain, whether physiological or psychological, and there is no nursing intervention to alleviate such discomfort, then that patient is put at further risk.

Significant conditions that will enhance pain and directly interfere with the patient's respiratory function are:

- chest trauma (including surgery);
- abdominal surgery;
- severe chest infections;
- pleural rub;
- pericarditis;

- psychological manifestations – feelings of insecurity, loneliness, isolation and depression, sleep deprivation.

Temperature   If the patient's core temperature is raised above normal on or during admission, or for 24 hours post-operatively, it is indicative of infection. A raised temperature will cause an increase in oxygen demand, which may lead to decreased respiratory function.

A decreased central temperature will also affect oxygen demand, as oxygen will not be so readily released to the tissues from the haemoglobin molecule. Therefore, there will be an increase in oxygen debt at tissue level with an increase in anaerobic respiration.

Peripheral temperature is an important but often overlooked observation, and a very important sign in patients who are at risk of developing respiratory failure. Cooling of the extremities with a gradient between the patient's core temperature and peripheral temperature is indicative of decreased perfusion. There will thus be anaerobic respiration at tissue level.

Measurable
respiratory signs

Peak expiratory flow rate (PEFR)   There will be a decreased PEFR in patients who develop respiratory failure. Those patients who already have asthma or chronic airway limitation will probably experience 'morning dips' in their PEFR as their respiratory failure worsens. These morning dips in PEFR are highly significant and should not be ignored.

Vital capacity   Observing a patient's vital capacity will demonstrate the strength of the respiratory muscles (directly proportional to the use of the muscle). This is especially important if patients have a history of neuromuscular disorder, such as multiple sclerosis, Guillain–Barré syndrome or myasthenia gravis. However, it relies on the patient to be able to cooperate with undertaking the manoeuvre consistently.

Pulse oximetry   Pulse oximetry has established itself as the most convenient non-invasive method of monitoring arterial saturation continuously. Its use is well established within all clinical areas. The normal range of SpO_2 for a patient breathing room air and with no significant lung disease is 95–99%.

Pulse oximetry is not foolproof and has its limitations. It requires those who use it to have an adequate understanding of respiratory physiology and basic principles of the management of acute respiratory dysfunction. The function of a pulse oximeter is affected by many variables, including ambient light, shivering, abnormal haemoglobins, pulse rate and rhythm, vasoconstriction and cardiac function. A pulse oximeter gives no indication of a patient's ventilation (i.e. the $PaCO_2$ level), only of their oxygenation and thus can give a false sense of security, if supplemental oxygen is being given. In addition, there may be a delay between the occurrence of a potentially hypoxic event, such as respiratory obstruction, and a pulse oximeter detecting low oxygen saturation. However, oximetry is a useful non-invasive monitor of a patient's cardiorespiratory system, which has undoubtedly improved patient safety in many circumstances.

> **Case example**
>
> An elderly woman post-operatively in the recovery room was receiving oxygen via a face mask. She became increasingly drowsy, despite having an oxygen saturation of 96%. The reason was that her respiratory rate and minute volume were low due to residual neuromuscular block and sedation, yet she was receiving high concentrations of inspired oxygen, so her oxygen saturation was maintained. She ended up with an arterial carbon dioxide concentration of 14.7 kpa (110 mmHg) and was ventilated for 24 hours on intensive care. Thus oximetry gives a good estimation of adequate oxygenation but no direct information about ventilation, particularly, as in this case, when supplemental oxygen is being administered.

Arterial blood gases   These will be taken as a final assessment of a patient's respiratory status once all other data have been extrapolated and analysed, and the doctor or senior nurse believes that they will add important and useful insight into the patient's condition, and consequent care and treatment. They are either taken using an arterial stab or via an arterial line. Arterial blood gases (ABGs) are taken for various reasons. In relation to respiratory assessment, the most common reason is to find out what is happening to the patient's pulmonary and ventilatory status.

Remember that:

- low PaO_2 levels (hypoxia) are bad;
- extremes of pH are bad;
- extremes of $PaCO_2$ are bad.

Normal values are as follows:

pH	7.35–7.45
$PaCO_2$	4.8–6.1 kPa (36–46 mmHg)
PaO_2	10–13 kPa (75–100 mmHg)
HCO_3	22–26 mmol/litre
SaO_2	95–100%
Acidosis	pH < 7.35
Alkalosis	pH > 7.45

Patients with hypoxaemia (respiratory failure type I) have:

- PaO_2 < 8 kPa (60 mmHg);
- $PaCO_2$ normal or low;
- pH normal or high.

Patients with respiratory failure Type II (acute) have:

- $PaCO_2$ > 7 kPa (50 mmHg);
- hypoxaemia (always);
- low pH [however, in chronic respiratory failure, the pH will be normalized, owing to compensation of the renal system and its excretion of bicarbonate ions (HCO_3)].

Case example

A 28-year-old lady has been admitted to the critical care environment following a laparotomy 5 hours ago. She has a morphine infusion *in situ* running at 5 mg/hour. She continues to be very sleepy, with a respiratory rate (RR) of 8 bpm. She is on supplemental oxygen of 40% via a Hudson mask, her pulse oximeter gives a saturation reading of 99%.

The doctor performs an arterial stab owing to her drowsiness and low RR. The results of her ABGs are:

- pH   7.16
- $PaCO_2$ 8.42 kPa (61.9 mmHg)
- PaO_2 15.6 kPa (115 mmHg)
- HCO_3 21.2 mmol/litre

Discussion

From the patient's pulse oximeter, it would appear that there is no respiratory problem. But one parameter should not be interpreted in isolation (and remember that pulse oximetry does not measure ventilation). What the nurse should feel worried about is the patient's low respiratory rate and that she remains drowsy 5 hours post-operatively. Her ABGs demonstrate a respiratory acidosis. This can be seen from her low pH of 7.1 and her high $PaCO_2$ of 8.42 kPa. Her PaO_2 is high because she is on supplemental oxygen. If the supplemental O_2 were removed, her ABGs would also show a hypoxaemia. The most probable cause for this patient's respiratory failure is oversedation with morphine infusion.

The nurse's responsibility in carrying out an in-depth and meticulous respiratory assessment on a patient who has been identified as at risk of developing respiratory failure cannot be overemphasized. A higher degree of care is required if the nurse is to observe, extrapolate and analyse such important and pertinent data and plan appropriate nursing care to optimize and maintain ventilation and perfusion.

NURSING INTERVENTIONS AND CARE

Nursing interventions and care can be viewed in two parts: general management and advanced management.

General management includes:

- positioning and comfort strategies;
- mobilizing;
- assistance with physiotherapy techniques
  - coughing and deep breathing exercises
  - rehabilitation;
- administering oxygen;
- drug therapy;
- chest drain management.

Advanced management includes:

- suctioning
  - nasopharyngeal;

- non-invasive ventilation
  - continuous positive airway pressure (CPAP)
  - non-invasive positive pressure ventilation (NIPPV);
- assistance with intubation;
- mechanical ventilation;
- tracheostomy care.

Positioning

Positioning may appear to be one of the most fundamental and essential of nursing care concepts, and not, therefore, worthy of in-depth discussion here. It is, however, a particularly important area of care in relation to optimising and maintaining ventilation and perfusion. Those patients who are at risk and need a higher intensity of care are usually bedfast, and will need frequent repositioning. However, those patients who have chronic lung disease need to be nursed in a position that they are used to and feel comfortable in. If they have not slept in a bed for a long time or find that their breathing is easier if they sit in a chair, then it is important to accommodate them. However, it must be remembered that these patients will also need repositioning. What must be remembered is that repositioning patients not only enhances respiratory function but is part of essential nursing care in order to prevent pressure sores. This is especially significant if the patients have poor perfusion because of their condition and are, therefore, more likely to develop pressure sores, thus increasing the risk of patient mortality.

The cardiopulmonary effects of turning or repositioning patients have been well documented (Gavigan et al 1990, Brooks-Brunn 1995, 2000). Frequent body repositioning can be effective in enhancing oxygen transport by changing the ventilation and perfusion of the lungs through gravitational effects. Changing the patient's position also enhances mobilization of secretions. Although frequent turning is important, it is also vital to monitor patients' responses, that is, their respiratory rate, respiratory effort and pulse oximetry, to different positions. This is because repositioning patients increases their oxygen demand.

Mobilization

Mobilization and ambulation are important aspects in the care of any patient who requires bedrest for whatever reason and who has been identified as at risk of developing respiratory failure. The physiological principles associated with early ambulation are extensions of the benefits of turning and repositioning the patient while in bed. Ambulation stimulates ventilation, increases perfusion and promotes secretion clearance and oxygenation. Further benefits of early ambulation can be seen in Box 5.6.

Deciding when and how the patient should be mobilized should be done on an individual basis in conjunction with the patient's nurse, doctor and physiotherapist. Some patients may worry about early mobilization, becoming anxious about pain and discomfort. It is, therefore, of paramount importance that the nurse explains to the patient the benefits of early mobilization. It is also important that the nurse monitors,

> **Box 5.6   Benefits of early ambulation**
>
> - Decreased venous pooling, thus reducing the risk of deep venous thrombosis and pulmonary emboli
> - Improved functional capacity
> - Decreased deconditioning related to bedrest, i.e. muscle weakness
> - Decreased physiological problems, such as depression and anxiety, in relation to bedrest

observes and provides optimal pain management as well as comfort strategies and interventions during this period.

Physiotherapy techniques

Chest physiotherapy reduces the risk of sputum retention, chest infection and consolidation. The physiotherapist and the nurse, therefore, play pivotal roles in implementing specific physiotherapy interventions related to respiratory care that ensure adequate ventilation and perfusion.

It is important that the nurse whose patient requires chest physiotherapy liaises with the physiotherapist as to what interventions are suitable for a particular patient and how to safely carry them out. Care needs to be truly collaborative and will include a plan of care and assessment tailored for those patients requiring chest physiotherapy. Physiotherapy care includes:

- effective positioning;
- deep breathing and coughing exercises;
- suctioning (oral and nasopharyngeal);
- postural drainage;
- saline nebulizers;
- mobilization.

It is not the intention of this chapter to explore all chest physiotherapy techniques, as this is primarily the domain of the physiotherapist. Certain physiotherapy interventions, however, may be facilitated equally by both nurse and physiotherapist.

Coughing and deep breathing exercises

If the patient is to undergo surgery, instruction on deep breathing and coughing exercises should ideally be given pre-operatively. This applies to all patients who are on bedrest and identified as at risk of developing pulmonary complications. These exercises are as important as frequent repositioning, early ambulation and pain management strategies.

The time-honoured tradition of 'cough and deep breath' is often thought of as the foundation of good pulmonary care. The concept can be attributed to Dripps & Waters (1941), who described three fundamental principles for patients who had or were at risk of developing pulmonary complications:

- the patient must be turned;
- the patient must cough;
- the patient must inflate his/her lungs adequately with deep breaths.

This should be encouraged every hour or every 30 minutes depending on the patient's physical and psychological condition. The limited human resources and complexity of today's nursing and medical care often mean a low priority for this procedure. If this essential nursing intervention is not valued, this puts patients further at risk of developing respiratory insufficiency.

Encouraging the patient to cough as a routine aspect of care is one method of facilitating clearance of airway secretions for those patients who have increased secretions or secretion management problems. Patients must be assessed on an individual basis in relation to whether they need to be encouraged to cough as a routine aspect of their care. The nurse must ask the following questions.

> It is important to remember that coughing is an expiratory manoeuvre that can cause pleural pressures to exceed airway pressure. This may result in alveoli collapse. Post-operative coughing is contraindicated in patients who have had ear surgery, eye surgery, neurosurgery or repair of large abdominal hernias because of this increase in pleural pressure.

- Does the patient have pre-existing lung disease?
- Does the patient have a history of secretion clearance problems?
- Is there evidence of increased secretions when listening to breath sounds?
- Will the patient benefit from coughing as an intervention?

If the nurse decides that the patient needs to be encouraged to cough, it is extremely important that effective coughing is taught, primarily by the physiotherapist. Once the patient understands the procedure, the nurse should continue to encourage and assist. The patient should be placed in an optimal position to reduce tension on the abdominal muscles. If the patient has a wound site (abdominal or chest), then splinting of the wound with a pillow, rolled-up towel or crossed arms should also be encouraged.

Deep breathing exercises

Normal ventilation occurs through pleural pressure changes caused by the contraction and relaxation of the diaphragm. Negative pleural pressure increases during inspiration and is decreased during expiration. Therefore, any disorder that interferes with the generation and maintenance of increased negative pleural pressure on inspiration will decrease the distending forces of the lung, and increase the risk of alveolar collapse and possible atelectasis.

In order to prevent pulmonary complications for those patients at risk of developing respiratory failure, it is imperative that the nurse encourages the patient to take regular effective deep breaths. The technique is:

- take a slow deep breath in;
- hold breath for at least 3 seconds in order to prevent alveolar collapse;
- repeat at least 3–6 times per hour.

As with coughing, patients should be assessed as to whether they are able to do deep breathing exercises. If they are, they should be placed in an optimal position that enables them to expand their lungs and in which they feel comfortable. Success in effective deep breathing exercises relies on five strategies:

- motivation of patient and staff;
- education of patient and staff;
- supervision of patient;
- comfort;
- assessment.

Oxygen therapy

It must be remembered that oxygen is a drug and should be prescribed by a doctor (unless in an emergency situation). As with any drug, the nurse must understand how to give it effectively and therapeutically, and know what positive and negative effects it may have on the patient. Remember, oxygen is a highly flammable substance.

The use of supplementary oxygen is the primary treatment for patients with respiratory failure (i.e. hypoxaemia) whether it is acute or chronic. Although giving supplementary oxygen to a patient with acute hypoxaemia may be of short-term benefit, it is important to find the cause of hypoxaemia and treat the underlying problem.

The benefits of oxygen therapy are as follows.

- It can correct hypoxaemia.
- Oxygen can reduce the work of breathing.
- It decreases myocardial workload.

Although the administration of oxygen may appear to be straightforward the nurse needs to have a full understanding of its hazards and of respiratory physiology (Box 5.7).

Box 5.7   Principles in the administration of oxygen

- Oxygen is a combustible gas and, therefore, a fire risk
- Compressed oxygen is very dry and must be humidified, if it is to be used for long periods, i.e. more than half an hour
- If hypoxaemia is not accompanied with carbon dioxide retention (hypercapnia), then high concentrations of oxygen up to 60% may be given
- In hypoxaemia associated with hypercapnia, the concentration of oxygen should not be more than 30%. Serial estimates of arterial carbon dioxide should be carried out before and during oxygen therapy to ensure that ventilation is not sufficiently depressed to cause significant carbon dioxide retention
- High concentration of oxygen (60% or more) over prolonged periods may cause severe lung damage. High concentrations of oxygen are toxic and damage the alveolar epithelium. Therefore, inspired oxygen concentrations should always be kept to a minimum while maintaining reasonable respiratory function. Meticulous assessment of the patient is essential

Methods of administration

A wide range of oxygen delivery systems are available that are capable of delivering 23% and 100% oxygen. Oxygen delivery systems are classified into two main categories: variable systems, which deliver a proportion of the ventilatory requirements, and fixed performance systems, which deliver the entire ventilatory requirements.

Oxygen delivery systems may be high-flow or low-flow systems, with a large range of masks and nasal cannulae. The choice of system will be dictated by what type of system the ward or unit has purchased; however, other factors that should be considered include the type of respiratory failure, how much inspired oxygen is required, and whether the flow needs to be high or low. *If high-flow oxygen (>3 litres/minute) is required for longer than 30 minutes, it should be humidified.*

Types of oxygen delivery systems used are:

- variable performance
  - nasal cannulae
  - Hudson mask
  - reservoir bags;
- fixed performance
  - Venturi systems.

Nasal cannulae (Figure 5.7)
Percentage of O_2 delivered:
2 litres/minute = 23–28%
3 litres/minute = 28–30%
4 litres/minute = 32–36%
5 litres/minute = 40%
6 litres/minute = Maximum 44%

Good points:

- generally comfortable;
- patient can eat and drink;
- no rebreathing of carbon dioxide.

Bad points:

- inaccurate delivery;
- if the patient is mouth breathing, then little O_2 will be inspired;

Figure 5.7 A nasal cannula.

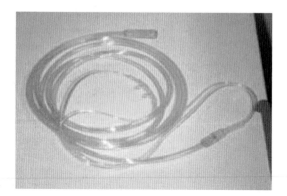

- dries the nasal passages;
- limited level of O_2 delivery.

Simple face masks (Figure 5.8)

Percentage of O_2 delivered:
4 litres/minute   = 35%
6 litres/minute   = 50%
8 litres/minute   = 55%
10 litres/minute = 60%
12 litres/minute = 65%

Good points:

- readily available on wards and all areas;
- nebulizers can be given.

Bad points:

- inaccurate delivery, particularly with high respiratory rates;
- eating and drinking is limited, especially if the patient is O_2 dependent;
- dries all the respiratory passages;
- rebreathing of CO_2 occurs.

Non-rebreather masks with reservoir bags   These are almost like simple facemasks but they have the addition of a reservoir bag attached. They also have either one or two valves over the exhalation port(s) of the mask. A non-rebreather mask achieves close to 100% oxygen by minimizing room air entrainment. It accomplishes this by attaching a reservoir bag to the mask filled with 100% oxygen. The reservoir bag has a flap valve to block exhaled gas from entering. Exhaled gas is directed out the side ports of the mask. These side ports have flap valves on the outside of the mask to block air entrainment on inspiration and instead draw gas from the 100% oxygen source in the reservoir bag. In actual

Figure 5.8 A simple face mask.

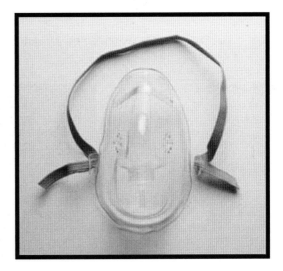

practice, one of the side port flap valves on the mask is removed as a safety precaution to allow room air entrainment, should the oxygen tubing become disconnected.

The non-rebreather mask is indicated for patients with acute severe hypoxemia (PaO_2 less than 60 mmHg on 50% oxygen). It is primarily designed to be a short-term device (less than 24 hours) because of the potential hazards of using 100% oxygen for prolonged periods

Good points:

- it can provide medium to high levels of oxygen;
- there is little rebreathing.

Bad points:

- high flows of O_2 without humidification are very drying and uncomfortable;
- the bag must be inflated prior to use to accommodate each breath;
- the mask must fit fairly tightly.

Fixed performance systems

Venturi system (colour-coded; Figure 5.9)
Percentage of O_2 delivered:

2 litres/minute = 24%
4 litres/minute = 28%
8 litres/minute = 35%
10 litres/minute = 40%
15 litres/minute = 60%

Each colour nozzle has different sized openings. The larger the opening, the higher the concentration of oxygen. Gas flow accelerates at a faster rate in the smaller port, causing a greater lateral pressure drop, which in turn causes a higher rate of room air entrainment. This results in the lower oxygen concentration in the 35% Venturi device.

Good points:

- accurate delivery of oxygen concentration in most circumstances;
- it can be humidified;
- the required flow rate and percentage of oxygen are marked on the valve.

Figure 5.9 The Venturi system.

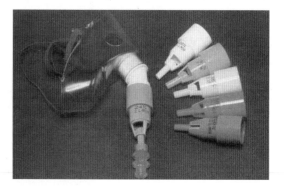

Bad points:

- patients with very high minute volumes may not receive accurate concentrations of oxygen;
- eating and drinking is limited;
- the oxygen flow rate must be altered if the percentage of oxygen is altered;
- coloured nozzles must be changed to alter the oxygen percentage;
- they must fit fairly tightly;
- the colour codes are not universal!

Caring for the patient requiring oxygen therapy

Finding out whether the treatment is effective is vital; therefore, frequent observation, assessment and monitoring of the patient's respiratory function during oxygen therapy are crucial, and will also include the following.

- Give a full explanation to the patient of what the treatment is for.
- If there is time, try to familiarize the patient with the oxygen mask or cannula.
- Ensure that the chosen system for the delivery of oxygen to the patient is set up correctly; if in any doubt, seek advice.
- Ensure that the patient is in the most effective and appropriate position to receive oxygen therapy.
- Nurses may need to stay with patients during the initial stages of treatment, especially if they are confused, agitated, anxious or frightened.
- Do not leave patients if they are hypoxic. Ensure that medical help has been summoned.
- Emphasize the importance of keeping the oxygen on.
- Check that the flow rate is correct for the percentage of oxygen that has been prescribed.
- Ensure that the doctor has set appropriate guidelines for the individual patient (i.e. limits to the patient's SpO_2 and RR against the inspired O_2 concentration that the patient is receiving).
- Always chart the patient's RR with their SpO_2 and the percentage or flow of oxygen that they are receiving, and whether they are mouth or nose breathing.

Non-invasive ventilation

The following explanation of non-invasive ventilation (NIV) is not intended to give the reader an in-depth understanding, but a brief overall description of what it is, its uses, the type of equipment used, contraindications, patient care and management. The reader is advised to seek further information from the books and papers listed under 'Further reading for NIV' at the end of the chapter.

The role of NIV has advanced rapidly over the last 7 years owing to advances in technology, increasing reports of success and the reconfiguration of critical care services within the UK (Department of Health 2000). Guidelines and recommendations for the use of NIV have been developed by two major agencies: the British Thoracic Society (BTS) and the NHS Modernisation Agency.

Definition   Non-invasive ventilation refers to the provision of ventilatory support through the patient's upper airway using a full facial mask or nasal mask. It therefore does not require the patient to be intubated with a tracheal tube, laryngeal mask or tracheostomy.

There is some confusion between continuous positive airway pressure ventilation and NIV in relation to whether the use of non-invasive CPAP in acute respiratory failure constitutes ventilatory support. CPAP does not provide ventilatory support and, therefore, should not be considered as a form of NIV. However, non-invasive CPAP will be discussed simultaneously with NIV because of the associated issues.

Non-invasive CPAP   CPAP is a system that provides continuous positive pressure within the lungs throughout the respiratory cycle but does not provide any mechanical breaths. For this reason, the work of breathing is entirely assumed by the patient. Therefore, the patient must be able sustain effective spontaneous breathing. Consequently, close observation of the patient's respiratory function during the treatment is vital.

The physiological effects of CPAP are as follows.

- It will expand alveoli that have poor air entry and thus increase the functional capacity of the lungs.
- It will increase the area of the lung available for gas exchange, which will improve the patient's oxygenation.
- There will be a decrease in the patient's work of breathing.
- Owing to the continuous positive pressure applied to the lungs, venous return will be impaired
  - This may cause the patient to have a reduced cardiac output in the first stages of the treatment.
  - Reduction in venous return is advantageous when CPAP is being used to treat left ventricular failure with pulmonary oedema

It is used for the following:

- Type I respiratory failure with a normal or low $PaCO_2$;
- left ventricular failure with pulmonary oedema;
- reduced air entry to lung bases (atelectasis);
- obstructive sleep apnoea without significant hypercapnia.

Specific contraindications for non-invasive CPAP are:

- apnoea;
- respiratory muscle fatigue;
- progressive hypoventilation;
- hypercapnia.

Non-invasive CPAP is easier and cheaper to deliver, and has been shown to be successful in a variety of studies (Brett & Sinclair 1993, Gachot et al 1992). However, CPAP needs to be used with caution in patients with hypoxaemic respiratory failure, as a recent prospective randomized trial demonstrated that non-invasive CPAP delayed intubation and had a higher number of adverse events compared with patients who underwent standard treatment (Delclaux et al 2000).

The basic equipment required is:

- piped oxygen supply;
- high-flow generator (Figure 5.10);
- oxygen analyser pressure relief valve (20 cm H_2O valve);
- CPAP mask;
- CPAP mask headstraps or cap;
- CPAP valve (Figure 5.11);
- elephant tubing;
- bacterial filter;
- humidification;
- pulse oximeter;
- wall suction.

The CPAP circuit set-up will vary between hospitals depending on the equipment they hold; however, the principles of care and management of the patient remain the same. It is imperative that the nurse caring for the patient undergoing CPAP knows how the equipment works.

Non-invasive ventilation provides positive airway pressure to the patient using a mask via a variety of ventilatory machines that have been specifically designed for NIV. It provides mechanical breaths to the patient by setting the ventilator's inspiratory positive airway pressure (IPAP) and an expiratory positive airway pressure (EPAP) level that functions as positive end-expiratory pressure.

NIV is an alternative method to support ventilation in selected patients with acute respiratory failure that may prevent intensive care admissions. However, NIV is not suitable for all patients with respiratory failure.

Figure 5.10 A high-flow generator.

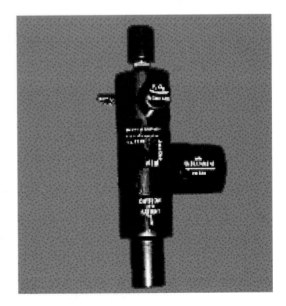

Figure 5.11 CPAP valves.

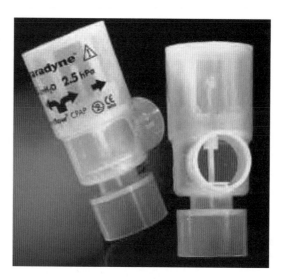

Key points   The BTS Standards of Care Committee (2002) has set out key points to using NIV, which are listed below. For details of the full BTS recommendations on NIV, see the BTS website (www.brit-thoracic.org.uk).

- Non-invasive ventilation works – an evidence-based verdict.
- NIV can be used in any hospital given the following minimum facilities:
  – a consultant committed to developing an NIV service;
  – nurses on a respiratory ward, high dependency unit or intensive care unit who are keen to be involved in NIV
  – an intensive care unit to provide back-up for patients who do not improve on NIV;
  – non-invasive ventilator and a selection of masks.
- NIV is particularly indicated in:
  – COPD with a respiratory acidosis pH 7.25–7.35 (H^+ 45–56 nmol/l);
  – hypercapnic respiratory failure secondary to chest wall deformity (scoliosis, thoracoplasty) or neuromuscular diseases;
  – cardiogenic pulmonary oedema unresponsive to CPAP;
  – weaning from tracheal intubation.
- NIV is not indicated in:
  – impaired consciousness;
  – severe hypoxaemia;
  – patients with copious respiratory secretions.
- The benefits of an acute NIV service are likely to be:
  – fewer patients referred to intensive care for intubation;
  – shorter stays on intensive care;
  – fewer deaths of patients with acute respiratory failure.

The BTS Standards of Care Committee (2002) describe three goals of NIV:

1. as a holding measure to assist ventilation in patients at an earlier stage than that at which tracheal intubation would be considered;

2. as a trial with a view to intubation if NIV fails;
3. as the ceiling of treatment in patients who are not candidates for intubation.

A very important issue that needs to be discussed with the patient, family and multidisciplinary team is the decision about intubation if NIV fails. This decision should be made early in each patient, taking into consideration the severity of the underlying disease and previous level of disability, and the decision made should *always* be documented in the patient's notes.

NIV in COPD   Many studies have demonstrated that NIV has been successful in certain patients with an acute exacerbation of COPD (Kramer et al 1995, Brochard et al 1995, Nava et al 1998, Plant et al 2001, Ram et al 2004). These studies show that successful NIV is possible and that prevention of endotracheal intubation is advantageous. A reduction in the incidence of nosocomial infection is a consistent and important advantage of NIV compared with mechanical ventilation. NIV is now being regarded as a new standard of care in the management of acute exacerbations of COPD.

The equipment required for NIV is as follows:

- an appropriate non-invasive ventilator – refer to BTS Guidelines (2002);
- oxygen supply (piped or cylinder);
- suitable patient–ventilator interfaces
  - nasal masks
  - full facial masks
  - nasal plugs
  - headstraps;
- humidification;
- pulse oximeter;
- wall suction;
- Ambu bag (manual resuscitation bag).

Starting NIV (inclusive of non-invasive CPAP)   This is a brief guide to starting NIV and non-invasive CPAP. There are no absolute methods for success, but the key to an effective outcome lies in the following:

- the selection of appropriate patients;
- the availability of suitable equipment;
- familiarity with the equipment;
- adequate staffing levels;
- adequate ongoing staff training in the concepts and use of NIV/CPAP;
- development of local guidelines and protocols by the multidisciplinary team responsible for initiating a NIV/CPAP service.

Individuals suitable for an acute trial of NIV or non-invasive CPAP should fulfil the following criteria:

- acute respiratory failure
  - Type I – CPAP
  - Type II – NIV;
- normal or near-normal bulbar function;

- ability to clear bronchial secretions;
- haemodynamic stability;
- functioning gastrointestinal tract;
- able to cooperate with treatment;

  Contraindications for NIV/CPAP:

- immediate need for intubation;
- unconscious patients;*
- severe haemodynamic instability;*
- severe bulbar weakness;*
- extensive facial trauma;
- upper airway obstruction;
- absent cough reflex;*
- evolving myocardial infarction;
- highly confused or uncooperative patient;
- undrained pneumothorax;*
- recent oesophageal or gastric surgery;*
- copious respiratory secretions;*
- vomiting;
- bowel obstruction;*
- confusion/agitation;*
- severe co-morbidity;*
- life-threatening hypoxaemia.*

Getting started

The practical aspects of using NIV and non-invasive CPAP

- Call the appropriate clinical team who set up NIV/CPAP.
- Is the patient suitable for either treatment?
  - Refer to national and/or local guidelines.
- Have all conventional medical therapies been explored and optimized?
- Is conventional intubation and mechanical ventilation more suitable?
- Remember that NIV/CPAP is not universally successful.
- What decisions have been made if NIV/CPAP fails?
- Where should treatment be carried out?
  - Remember that the patient's dependency will move to level 2; therefore, there will be an increase in nurse–patient ratio (1:2–1:4).
  - Commencing NIV/CPAP in the first stages of treatment is labour-intensive if it is to be successful.
- What equipment is available to set up the treatment?
  - Is it suitable for the job in hand?
  - Are the staff familiar with the equipment being used?
- It is advisable to set up the equipment and check that it is working correctly *before* introducing it to the patient
- Inform the critical care outreach team.

Establishing NIV/CPAP The first few hours of treatment are extremely important and will establish whether the treatment will have any chance of success or not. Time spent fitting the mask and building the patient's

---

*NIV may be used despite the presence of these contraindications, if it is to be the 'ceiling' of treatment.

confidence in the first few hours will be well invested. Patients are often very frightened and anxious, which will add to their feelings of breathlessness. They need your time, comfort and care.

- Explain to the patient what you are going to do and why, and the sensations the patient is likely to experience.
- Allow the patient to handle the mask and equipment, if there is time.
- Initial settings of the equipment should have already been decided by the clinical team or with the use of a local protocol.
    - The settings will be based upon the equipment being used.
    - Titration of the settings will depend upon the patient's response to treatment.
- The fitting of the mask is crucial to the success of the technique.
    - Often this is where many problems arise, as the patient–ventilator/CPAP circuit interface may not be adequate with only a very limited choice of masks for use.
    - If the patient wears dentures, they should keep them in as they may help with producing an adequate seal. However, if the dentures are ill fitting, they should be removed.
    - Use the mask the patient prefers. However, patients who are mouth-breathing, who are slightly confused or very dyspnoeic should be fitted with a full-face mask.
    - It is best to let patients hold the mask firmly to their face first. Once happy, – secure the mask using the headstraps.
    - Full-face masks can make some patients feel very claustrophobic and they will not tolerate the treatment no matter how hard you try. If using a nasal mask, remind them that they should breath through their nose and keep their mouth closed.
- Ensure the patient is in a comfortable position before commencing treatment.
- Ensure pulse oximeter is attached to the patient.
- Encourage and stay with the patient until treatment is established.
- Initially, some patients may only be able to tolerate NIV/CPAP for short periods. These may be increased with encouragement and care from the nurse. However, it is important to explore why they cannot tolerate it for longer periods:
    - Is ventilation adequate?
    - Are patient and ventilator synchronized?
    - Is the mask comfortable?
    - Is the patient confused?
    - Have other medical problems developed?
    - However, short periods of use are better than nothing!
- Give the patient a call bell.
- Breaks from NIV/CPAP should be made for drugs, physiotherapy, meals, nebulizers and overall patient comfort.

Monitoring the patient   Close observation of patients and their response to the treatment is paramount. Monitoring will vary depending on the location in which the patient is receiving treatment.

- All patients should be continuously monitored with oximetry, especially for the first 24 hours of treatment.
  - Remember oximetry *does not* measure ventilation.
  - Ensure that limits of SpO_2 are set for the patient by the clinician *or* that there is a protocol in use to guide practice.
- In severely ill patients, continuous ECG monitoring and insertion of an arterial line will be required.
- Arterial blood gas tensions should be checked 30–60 minutes following the establishment of treatment unless the patient's condition is rapidly deteriorating.
  - Frequency of subsequent measurements will depend upon the patient's progress.
- Clinical reassessment must routinely take place 1 hour after the patient has been established on NIV/CPAP.
- Physiological monitoring is not a substitute for clinical assessment and observation of the patient. Clinical features that should be assessed are described earlier in 'Identifying respiratory failure distress and'.
  - Improvement in breathlessness is usually seen within 1–2 hours, if the treatment is effective. There is usually an improvement in the patient's neurological state at the same time.

Defining failure

Assessment and definition of treatment failure will depend upon the role of NIV/CPAP in each individual patient, and should be stated prior to treatment. However, the following factors should be taken into account:

- deterioration in the patient's condition;
- failure to improve or deterioration of arterial blood gas tensions;
- development of new symptoms or complications, such as
  - pneumothorax
  - sputum retention
  - nasal bridge erosion;
- intolerance or failure of coordination with the ventilator in relation to NIV;
- failure to alleviate symptoms;
- deteriorating conscious level;
- patient and carer wish to withdraw treatment.

Practical problems

Side effects and complications do not always cause NIV/CPAP to be discontinued but do limit the efficacy of the treatment. The most common problems are:

- mask discomfort;
- dry nose;
- air leaks around the mask;
- eye irritation from air leaks;
- gastric distension;
- pressure sores from tightness of mask/headstraps, especially on the bridge of the nose and around the back of the ears. Pressure-relieving dressings, such as Granuflex, should be applied on initiating therapy (Callaghan & Trapp 1998).

Weaning   Clinical improvement and stability of the patient's condition are the most important factors in determining when NIV/CPAP may be safely withdrawn. Protocols have also been shown to improve the efficacy of weaning. Therefore, local weaning protocols should be developed with the multidisciplinary team.

The use of NIV brings new opportunities in the management of patients with ventilatory failure, particularly with regard to location and the timing of intervention.

Tracheostomy

The following brief description about caring for patients with tracheostomies will only refer to those patients who have cuffed tracheostomy tubes and who will eventually be decannulated prior to leaving hospital.

A tracheostomy is an opening in the anterior wall of the trachea that provides airway access into the trachea.

Indications for tracheostomy

- To maintain a patent airway
  - after total laryngectomy
  - upper airway oedema
  - upper airway stenosis
  - traumatic injuries;
- To protect the airway
  - altered conscious state
  - uncoordinated swallowing
  - vocal cord paralysis
  - removal of protective structures;
- Assistance in secretion clearance
  - respiratory muscle weakness
  - neuromuscular disease;
- Prolonged airway protection
  - prolonged coma
  - high lesion spinal cord injury
  - neuromuscular disease
  - respiratory failure;
- Assistance in artificial ventilation
  - prolonged mechanical ventilation
  - home mechanical ventilatory support.

Types of tracheostomy

- Surgical:
  - performed in an operating theatre;
  - does not require neck extension, therefore, suitable for patients with unstable spines;
  - for more difficult procedures;
  - performed for patients requiring permanent tracheotomies.
- Percutaneous:
  - can be performed in an ITU environment;
  - requires neck extension;
  - non-permanent tracheostomy.

Complications

Immediate

- Haemorrhage
- Pneumothorax
- Subcutaneous and mediastinal emphysema
- Respiratory and cardiovascular collapse
- Dislodged tube

Late

- Airway obstruction
  - secretions
  - improper tube placement
  - overinflated cuff
- Infection
- Aspiration
  - secretions
  - gastric contents
- Tracheal damage
  - progressive fistula
- Dislodged tube

Tracheostomy tubes
(Figure 5.12)

- Single lumen tubes:
  - outer tube only, no inner;
  - non-fenestrated.
- Double lumen tubes:
  - inner and outer cannula;
  - used in longer term care;
  - may or may not be fenestrated.
- Non-fenestrated tubes:
  - no holes in the cannula.
- Fenestrated tubes:
  - an opening or hole in the posterior wall of the inner cannula;
  - when cuff deflated, assists airflow up into the larynx for speech;
  - cannot suction with fenestrated cannula *in situ*, therefore, has to be changed to non-fenestrated cannula.
- Cuffed tubes:
  - cuff maintains a seal against the tracheal wall and, therefore, stops air leaks;
  - minimizes the movement of the tube, reducing risk of tracheal trauma;
  - minimizes but does not necessarily prevent aspiration;
  - requires effective tracheal cuff management.
- Non-cuffed tubes:
  - allow patients to speak;
  - useful in the weaning process.

Emergency equipment

This equipment must be kept at the patient's bedside at all times, and should be taken with the patient when transported off the unit or ward area:

- suctioning equipment;
- 10 ml syringe for cuff inflation/deflation;

Figure 5.12 Types of
tracheostomy tube. (a) Cuffed
tracheostomy tube.
(b) Tracheostomy tube with
inner cannula. (c) Fenestrated
tracheostomy tube.

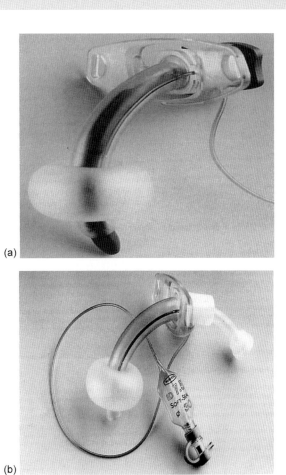

(a)

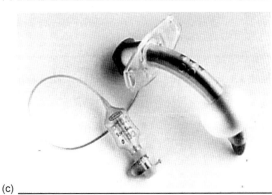

(b)

(c) _____

- tracheal dilator;
- replacement tracheostomy tubes
  - one a size smaller than that *in situ*
  - one the same size;
- Ambu bag (manual resuscitation bag);
- oxygen supply and equipment.

Essential equipment   Essential equipment comprises:

- humidification equipment;
- tracheal masks;
- sterile water;
- cuff pressure monitor;
- stoma dressings;
- securing tape;
- communication aids;
- call bell.

Caring for the patient   There are five major factors that must be considered in caring for a
with a tracheostomy   patient with a tracheostomy:

1. humidification;
2. mobilization of secretions;
3. airway patency;
4. cuff management and swallowing;
5. psychological impact and comfort care.

Caring for patients with a tracheostomy in whatever setting must involve the multidisciplinary team, and should include:

- an anaesthetist;
- a nurse;
- a physiotherapist;
- a speech therapist;
- a dietician.

The patient's nasopharynx, which provides the natural humidification mechanism for the airway, has been bypassed by the tracheostomy. It is, therefore, extremely important that some form of humidification is used.

- Ensure that the patient is well hydrated: This will permit the mucosal surface to remain moist and ensure that the viscid secretions remain on top of the cilia. Effective hydration will also ensure that the secretions remain thin and mobile.
- Use a condenser humidifier (e.g. ThermoVent). This makes use of the patient's own moisture breathed out through the tracheostomy tube. As patients exhale, the water vapour with the patient's breath condenses on a pleated paper filter and is revaporized on inhalation

If the patient requires oxygen, this should be supplied via an Aquapac system and tracheostomy mask.

Mobilization of secretions   This is extremely important in order to maintain a patent airway and reduce the risk of infection. This can be achieved by:

- effective position of the patient when in bed;
- regular chest physiotherapy;
- encouraging the patient to mobilize as soon as possible;
- deep breathing exercises;

- effective humidification;
- effective hydration;
- using saline nebulizers.

NB The practice of instilling normal saline directly into the tracheostomy tube in order to loosen and mobilize secretions has *no* research-based evidence. The author, therefore, does not advocate its use and does not see it as best practice.

Suctioning (maintaining airway patency) Suctioning is an invasive procedure; it is uncomfortable and often frightening for the patient. It must, therefore, be performed by an experienced and competent practitioner. An individual assessment must also be carried out as to whether a patient requires suctioning and it should not be given as 'routine'.

Studies carried out to explore nurses' knowledge and competence in performing tracheal suctioning have demonstrated a poor level of knowledge, which was also been reflected in practice, as suctioning was performed against many research recommendations (Tanser et al 1997, Celik & Elbas 2000, Day et al 2001, 2002).

Tracheal suctioning is an essential aspects of airway management but carries with it risks and complications. It is imperative that nurses are familiar with current research recommendations on all aspects of tracheal suctioning (Box 5.8).

Suctioning aims to stimulate a cough and remove excess secretions. The following complications can occur:

- mucosal damage;
- atelectasis;
- hypoxia;
- cardiac arrhythmias;
- hypotension;
- bronchospasm;
- trachebronchial infection;
- pain;
- anxiety/fear;
- feelings of breathlessness;
- feelings of suffocation.

A procedural synopsis is given below. The nurse should be wearing gloves, apron and goggles during the suctioning procedure. Remember that it is an aseptic technique.

- Set the suction pressure appropriately (80–120 mmHg occluded).
- Ensure catheters of the correct size are used.
- Ensure that emergency equipment is at hand and that it is working.
- Explain the procedure fully to the patient.
- Pre-oxygenate the patient using either tracheal mask oxygen or a rebreath bag.
- Insert the catheter gently and slowly into the tracheostomy to just above the carina or when the patient begins to cough.

Box 5.8   Recommended practice for tracheal suctioning

Action	Recommended practice
Assessment	In order to determine the need for suctioning and the effectiveness of the suctioning procedure, a thorough assessment of the patient should be made including chest auscultation (Glass & Grap 1995, Day 2000)
Patient preparation	Reassurance and explanation should always be given before and after suctioning, as it is a frightening and unpleasant experience (Fiorentini 1992, Griggs 1998)
Pre-oxygenation	Suctioning may frequently lead to hypoxaemia, which can cause cardiac arrhythmias, hypotension, cardiac arrest and even death. In order to prevent these complications, pre-oxygenation is recommended prior to suctioning (Wainwright & Gould 1996)
Infection control	Suctioning is an invasive procedure; therefore, there is an increased risk of infection (Pierce 1995). Hands should be washed before and after suctioning, and suctioning should be treated as an aseptic technique. Aprons, gloves and goggles should be worn (Wood 1998, Parker 1999, Pratt et al 2001)
Catheter selection	The external diameter of the suction catheter should not exceed one-half of the internal diameter of the tube (Wood 1998). Larger catheters have been shown to cause trauma and hypoxia
Applied negative pressure	The correct suctioning pressure should be set between 80 and 120 mmHg occluded for an adult. Higher pressures have been shown to cause trauma, hypoxia and atelectasis (Czarnik et al 1991, Luce et al 1993). Too little pressure will be ineffective. Pressure should only be applied during withdrawal of the catheter and this should be applied continuously as opposed to intermittently
Duration of suction	The procedure should take no more than 10–15 seconds (Boggs 1993)
Number of suction passes	The number of suction passes may contribute to the occurrence of complications. Therefore, no more than three suction passes should be made during any one suction episode (Glass & Grap 1995)

- Only apply suction when withdrawing the catheter (suction must be continuous rather than intermittent during withdrawal).
- Insertion and withdrawal of the suction catheter should not take any longer than 10–15 seconds.
- A new catheter should always be used for any further insertions.
- No more than three catheters should be passed in one suction episode.
- Observe the patient throughout and post-procedure for signs of respiratory distress, hypoxia, cardiac instability or any other complications.
- Observe the secretions obtained and report the findings.
- *Do not suction the patient's mouth to clear any secretions coughed up with the catheter that has just been down the patient's trachea!*

Tracheostomy cuff management   Tracheal injury has been lessened to some extent owing to the fact that tracheostomy tubes use low-pressure cuffs and many modifications have been made to make them safer. However, complications still exist and increase the longer the tracheostomy tube has to stay *in situ* with the cuff inflated. Proper management of the tracheostomy cuff is essential, if the nurse is to lessen the risk of tracheal and laryngeal damage.

Laryngeal trauma
- Pressure necrosis: pressure of the tracheostomy tube against the fragile laryngeal mucosa can potentially create tissue necrosis. The degree of irritation varies proportionally with the size of the tracheostomy tube.
- Movement of the tracheostomy tube against the laryngeal mucosa is an additional source of tissue irritation, and potential tissue abrasion and possible necrosis.
- Granulomas or polyps can also occur during the healing of abraded tissue, which may create obstruction.
- Glottic incompetence: long-term intubation can interfere with the normal protective responses of the larynx. These include laryngeal closure and the ability to clear aspirated material from the airway.

Tracheal trauma   The major cause of tracheal trauma is cuff overinflation. Although the incidence of injury has been significantly reduced, owing to the use of high-volume low-pressure cuffs, damage still occurs as a result of healthcare professionals' lack of understanding of upper airway anatomy and physiology, and appropriate management of the tracheostomy tube.

The soft 'floppy' characteristics of the low-pressure cuff are lost when air even slightly exceeds 20 mmHg. The low-pressure cuff then acts as a high-pressure cuff. A high-pressure cuff is associated with a much greater incidence of trauma, with the subsequent development of tracheal stenosis or tracheal malacia.

Healthcare professionals who are not aware of the risks of adding additional air to low-pressure cuffs without using an appropriate measuring tool (cuff manometer) place their patients at risk for these complications. A cycle of events emerges where the tracheal walls around the overinflated cuff soften and break down. The cuff to tracheal wall seal then becomes inadequate. As the space around the cuff is eroded, an air leak develops. The practitioner attempts to obtain a seal by injecting more air into the cuff and so the process continues. Therefore, careful cuff management is paramount.

Cuff management
- Tracheostomy cuff pressures should not exceed 20 mmHg.
- Cuff pressures should be checked at least every 8 hours using a cuff manometer.
- Minimal occlusion volume is advocated when caring for patients with a tracheostomy (Box 5.9).

Benefits of cuff deflation
- Normalized airflow through the upper airway for the preservation of airway protection reflexes – thus improved muscle tone.
- Reduced risk of trauma to the mucosal tissue – potential for oral communication.
- Decreased interference with laryngeal elevation during swallowing.
- More complete access to the upper airway during suctioning.

Pilot protocol for cuff deflation
- Discuss with the multidisciplinary team the appropriateness of the patient for a trial of cuff deflation.
- Suction the patient using the established suctioning procedure, through the tracheostomy tube. The cuff is inflated.
- Allow the patient to rest. Reinsert the suction catheter carefully into tracheostomy tube. Insert the syringe into the cuff valve. Apply suction while *slowly* removing air from the cuff with the syringe. Suction as required.
- Reinflate the cuff to baseline. Allow the patient to rest. Suction orally, if needed.
- Insert the syringe into the cuff valve and *slowly* withdraw air until the cuff is fully deflated, 2 cm^3 at a time. *NB Rapid cuff deflation can cause laryngeal spasm.* Slow deflation allows the patient to get used to airflow passing through their upper airway.
- Continually assess the patient's respiratory and haemodynamic status and psychological well-being.
- A speech therapist should assess the patient's ability to voice with the newly created leak by encouraging vocalization, initially during inspiration. Re-establish use of the upper airway by having the patient vocalize an extended 'ah' or blow gently.

Box 5.9   Minimal occlusion volume

- Inflate the tracheostomy cuff to the point where air can no longer be heard escaping from around the cuff into the upper airway
- This is achieved through auscultation of the trachea with a stethoscope
- Cuff pressure *must not* exceed 20 mmHg

- A speech therapist should assess the patient's swallowing.
- Keep reassuring the patient.
- A speech therapist should trial a speaking valve, if appropriate.
- Plan periods of cuff deflation with the team and the patient.

Psychological support   The psychological impact of having a tracheostomy, although it may not be permanent, should not be underestimated. There are two main areas that affect the patient: communication and altered body image.

Cuffed tracheostomy tubes do not allow airflow through the larynx and over the vocal cords; the patient, therefore, is unable to speak or show emotion. It is imperative that an effective system of communication is set up between the patient, multidisciplinary team and their family. Involving the speech therapist is paramount.

Aids to communication
- If the ratio of nurse to patient is less than 1:1, give the patient a call bell:
  - Make sure that it works!
  - Make sure that the patient can use it!
  - Make sure that it is accessible
  - Answer the call bell promptly.
- Paper and pencil.
- Magic board.
- Alphabet board.
- Picture board.
- Common phrase board.
- Computer aids.
- Cuff deflation.
- Speaking valves.
- Lip reading.

CHEST DRAIN MANAGEMENT

Indications for insertion of chest drain

- Pneumothorax;
- Following thoracic and/or cardiac surgery;
- Chest trauma (e.g. haemothorax);
- Empyema (uses open drainage system).

Principles of chest drains (Figure 5.13)

- A chest drain is a conduit to remove air or fluid from the pleural cavity.
- The fluid can be blood, pus or a pleural effusion.
- Chest drains allow re-expansion of the underlying lung.
- Entry of air or drained fluid back into the chest cavity must be prevented.

Essential components of a chest drain

- The drain must be unobstructed (no clamping or kinking of tubes).
- The collection chamber *must* be below chest level.
- A one-way mechanism, such as a water seal.

Figure 5.13 Basic principles of chest drainage.

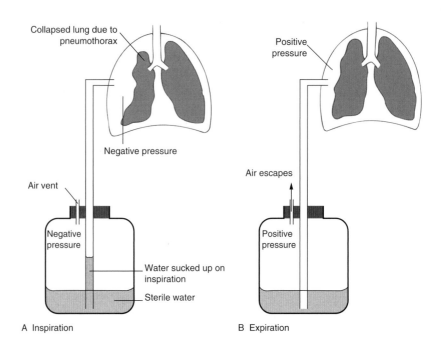

Collapsed lung due to pneumothorax

Negative pressure

Positive pressure

Air vent

Air escapes

Negative pressure

Positive pressure

Water sucked up on inspiration

Sterile water

A Inspiration

B Expiration

Mechanism of action

- Drainage occurs during expiration when pleural pressure is positive.
- Fluid or air within pleural cavity drains into a water seal.
- Air bubbles through a water seal to the outside world.
- The length of the drain below the fluid level is important; if greater than 2–3 cm, it increases resistance to air drainage.

Assessment

Fluid level and type of fluid within the chest drain bottle

This should be recorded regularly. Any signs of fresh bleeding into the drain must be reported immediately. If the fluid looks cloudy or infected, a specimen must be sent for culture and sensitivity.

Fluid swing

There should always be a 'swing' of fluid in the tube of the chest drainage bottle during inspiration and expiration, if the system is patent. This should also be recorded.

Bubble/air leak

If the chest drain is *in situ* for the treatment of a pneumothorax, then there should be a visible bubbling within the chest drain until the pneumothorax has resolved. It is important when assessing for such an air leak that the patient is sitting upright, and is asked to take a deep breath in and out and to cough.

Pain and discomfort

Chest drain tubes can be extremely painful and cause discomfort, especially if they are not secured correctly and are accidentally pulled.

Infection   The longer a chest drain is *in situ*, the more likely the risk of infection around the site of insertion. The patient will often complain of increased pain and discomfort around this area. Careful observation of the site is needed. If the infection goes unchecked, it can translocate into the pleural cavity and cause an empyema.

Respiratory function   Continuous assessment of a patient's respiratory function during chest drain therapy is essential in order to prevent complications (Box 5.10). Complications arising from chest drains can include:

- infection;
- surgical emphysema;
- pain;
- blocked drain;
- broken seal;
- tension pneumothorax;
- air leak from insertion site.

Box 5.10   Troubleshooting chest drains

If the bubbling suddenly stops

- Check there are no kinks in the tubing system
- Check the level of fluid. Is there an adequate seal? Is the level too high and does the drainage bottle need changing?
- Ask the patient to cough
- If unresolved, inform the medical staff
- Observe for tension pneumothorax

If the drain is blocked

- Check that there are no kinks in the tubing
- Check level of fluid is not too high, as this may stop drainage
- If the drain is on low-flow suction, increase this slightly
- Milk the tubing (This is the only time that tubes should be milked, as it may dislodge the blockage)

If unresolved, inform medical staff

- Continue to observe patient's respiratory function and signs of tension pneumothorax

If there is a broken underwater seal

- Sit the patient down
- Re-connect drain and/or re-establish underwater seal

- Ask the patient to take a deep breath in and out
- Ask the patient to cough
- Assess the patient's respiratory function
- Inform medical staff

If there is an air leak around the insertion site

- Assess the insertion site for infection
- Does the drain site need further suturing?
- Ensure adequate dressing around the site, **Do not use Sleek**
- Look for signs of surgical emphysema

If the chest drain falls out

- Put the patient into bed
- Inform medical staff
- Put a gauze dressing over the insertion site
- Assess the patient's respiratory function

Signs of tension pneumothorax

- Bubbling ceases within the chest drain
- No fluid swing
- Respiratory rate rapidly increases
- Heart rate increases
- Patient exhibits signs of shock
- Displaced mediastinum
- Respiratory arrest

Dos and don'ts of chest drains

- Avoid clamping of the drain, as it can result in a tension pneumothorax.
- Avoid milking chest drains, as this causes an increase in intrapleural pressure and may lead to further pneumothoracies and cardiac instability.
- A drain should only be clamped when changing the bottle.
- Always keep the drain below the level of the patient.
- If lifted above the chest level, the contents of the drain can siphon back into chest.
- If disconnection occurs, reconnect and ask the patient to cough.
- If there is a persistent air leak, consider low-pressure suction.
- Observe for post-expansion pulmonary oedema.
- Secure the chest drain to the patient's skin with a non-bulky dressing.
- Do not pin tubing to the patient's nightwear or bedding.
- Encourage the patient to mobilize as soon as possible and when appropriate.

Removal of the chest drain

- Remove the drain as soon as it has served its purpose.
- For a simple pneumothorax it can often be removed within 24 hours.
- Give appropriate analgesia prior to drain removal.
- To remove the drain, ask the patient to perform a Valsalva manoeuvre.
- Remove the drain at the height of expiration or inspiration.
- Tie pre-inserted purse string or Z stitch.
- Perform a post-procedure chest X-ray to exclude a pneumothorax.
- Observe the patient's respiratory function.

CONCLUSION

This chapter has given nurses a greater understanding of the concepts of patient assessment, nursing care and therapeutic interventions in order to optimize and maintain effective respiration for those patients who require higher levels of care (Level 1 and Level 2 care) in any setting. Nurses caring for such patients must realize that they are the pivot for effective respiratory care and prevention of complications. To achieve this, the nurse caring for the high dependency patient must be knowledgeable, proactive, dynamic and creative in all aspects of nursing care and intervention.

By using their clinical wisdom and demonstrating an understanding of both the physiological and psychological response to breathing, nurses will realize that they are not just instruments of other professionals in curing the patient but rather are uniquely significant in the patient's recovery.

The definitive outcome of such good nursing care will be improvement in the quality of patient care and comfort, especially in terms of reducing patient morbidity and mortality.

References

Boggs R L 1993 Airway management. In: Boggs R L, Woodridge-King M (eds) AACN procedure manual for critical care, 3rd edn. W B Saunders, Philadelphia

Brett A, Sinclair D G 1993 Use of continuous positive airway pressure in the management of community acquired pneumonia. Thorax 48:1280–1281

British Thoracic Society Standards of Care Committee 2002 Non-invasive ventilation in acute respiratory failure. Thorax 57: 192–211

Brooks-Brunn J A 1995 Postoperative atelectasis and pneumonia. Heart and Lung 24: 94–115

Brooks-Brunn J A 2000 Risk factors associated with postoperative pulmonary complications following total abdominal hysterectomy. Clinical Nursing Research 9:27–46

Brouchard L, Mancebo J, Wysocki M et al 1995 Non-invasive ventilation for acute exacerbation of chronic obstructive pulmonary disease. New England Journal of Medicine 333: 817–822

Callaghan S, Trapp M 1998 Evaluating two dressings for the prevention of nasal bridge pressure sores. Professional Nurse 13:361–364

Celik S, Elbas N 2000 The standard of suction for patients undergoing endotracheal intubation. Intensive Critical Care Nursing 16: 191–198

Czarnik R E, Stone K S, Everhart C C 1991 Differential effects of continuous versus intermittent suction on tracheal tissue. Heart and Lung 20: 144–151

Day T 2000 Tracheal suctioning: when, why and how? Nursing Times 96: 13–15

Day T, Wainwright S, Wilson-Barnett J 2001 An evaluation of a teaching intervention to improve the practice of endotracheal suctioning in intensive care units. Journal of Clinical Nursing 10: 682–696

Day T, Farnell S, Haynes S et al 2002 Tracheal suctioning: an exploration of nurses' knowledge and competence in acute and high dependency ward areas. Journal of Advanced Nursing 39: 35–45

Declaux C, L'Her E, Alberti C et al 2000 Treatment of acute hypoxemic nonhypercapnic respiratory insufficiency with continuous positive airway pressure delivered by a face mask: A randomized controlled trial. Journal of the American Medical Association 284: 2352–2360

Department of Health 2000 Comprehensive critical care. A review of adult critical care services. May. HMSO, London

Dripps R D Waters R M 1941 Nursing care of surgical patients 1: the 'stir up'. American Journal of Nursing 41: 534–537

Fiorentini A 1992 Potential hazards of tracheobronchial suctioning. Intensive and Critical Care Nursing 8: 217–226

Gachot B, Clair B, Wolff M et al 1992 Continuous positive airway pressure by face mask or mechanical ventilation in patients with human immunodeficiency virus infection and severe *Pneumocystis carinii* pneumonia. Intensive Care Medicine 18: 155–159

Gavigan M, Kline-O'Sullivan C, Klumpp-Lybrand B 1990 The effect of regular turning on CABG patients. Critical Care Nursing Quarterly 12: 69–76

Glass C, Grap M 1995 Ten tips for safer suctioning. American Journal of Nursing 95: 51–53

Griggs A 1998 Tracheostomy: suctioning and humidification. Nursing Standard 13(2): 49–53

Hinchliff S, Montague S 1988 Physiology for nursing practice. Baillière Tindall, London

Kramer N, Meyer T J, Meharg J et al 1995 Randomized, prospective trial of noninvasive positive pressure ventilation in acute respiratory failure. American Journal of Respiratory and Critical Care Medicine 151: 1799–1806

Luce J M, Pierson D J, Tyler M L 1993 Intensive respiratory care, 2nd edn. WB Saunders Company, Philadelphia

McGloin H, Adams S K, Singer M 1999 Unexpected deaths and referrals to intensive care of patients on general wards. Are some cases potentially avoidable? Journal of the Royal College of Physicians of London 33: 255–259

Nava S, Ambrosino N, Clini E et al 1998 Noninvasive mechanical ventilation in the weaning of patients with respiratory failure due to chronic obstructive pulmonary disease. A randomized, controlled trial. Annals of Internal Medicine 128: 721–728

Parker L J 1999 Importance of handwashing in the prevention of cross-infection. British Journal of Nursing 8(11): 716–720

Pierce L 1995 Guide to mechanical ventilation and respiratory care. WB Saunders, Philadelphia: 92–143

Plant P K, Owen J L, Elliott M W 2001 Non-invasive ventilation in acute exacerbations of chronic obstructive pulmonary disease: long term survival and predictors of in-hospital outcome. Thorax 56: 708–712

Pratt R J, Pellowe C, Loveday H P et al 2001 The epic project: developing national evidence-based guidelines for preventing healthcare associated infections. Phase I: Guidelines for preventing hospital-acquired infections. Department of Health (England). Journal of Hospital Infection 47(Suppl): S3–82

Ram F, Picot J, Lightwater J et al 2004 Non-invasive positive pressure ventilation for treatment of respiratory failure due to exacerbations of chronic obstructive pulmonary disease. Cochrane Database System Review 3:CD004104

Tanser S, Walker M, Macnaughton P 1997 Tracheostomy care on the wards – an audit of nursing knowledge. Clinical Intensive Care 8: 105(Abstract)

Wainwright S, Gould D 1996 Endotracheal suctioning: an example of the problems of relevance and rigour in clinical research. Journal of Clinical Nursing 5: 389–398

Wood C J 1998 Endotracheal suctioning: a literature review. Intensive Critical Care Nursing 14: 124–136

Further reading

Pre-requisite knowledge

Nunn J F 1993 Nunn's applied respiratory physiology, 4th edn. Butterworth Heinemann, Oxford

Riley M E 2003 Removing chest drains – a critical reflection of a complex clinical decision. Nursing in Critical Care 8: 212–221

West J B 1995 Pulmonary pathophysiology, 5th edn. Williams & Wilkins, Philadelphia

Non-invasive ventilation

Layfield C 2002 Non-invasive BiPAP – implementation of a new service. Intensive and Critical Care Nursing 18: 310–319

NHS Modernisation Agency 2002 Critical care programme, weaning and long term ventilation. www.criticalcare.nhs.uk

Plant PK, Owen JL, Parrott S et al 2003 Cost effectiveness of ward based non-invasive ventilation for acute exacerbations of chronic obstructive pulmonary disease: economic analysis of randomised controlled trial. British Medical Journal 326: 956

Ram F, Picot J, Lightwater J et al 2004 Non-invasive positive pressure ventilation for treatment of respiratory failure due to exacerbations of chronic obstructive pulmonary disease. Cochrane Database System Review 3: CD004104

Serra A 2000 Tracheostomy care. Nursing Standard 14(42): 45–52

Simonds AK (ed.) 2001 Non-invasive respiratory support, 2nd edn. Arnold, London

Chapter **6**

Cardiac care

Susan Laight, Mary Currie and Nigel Davies

KEY LEARNING OBJECTIVES

- To relate the structure and function of the cardiovascular system with specific reference to the knowledge required for providing care to high dependency patients
- To undertake a comprehensive cardiovascular nursing assessment and plan appropriate care
- To make best use of monitoring equipment and other devices commonly used to assess cardiovascular status in high dependency patients
- To understand the rationale for care in a patient with low cardiac output and relate this to the concept of shock
- To recognize common conduction defects and care for a patient with a temporary pacing system
- To consider the nurse's role in advanced life support
- To explore advances in the care of clients with acute myocardial infarction and recognize ECG changes manifested by clients with chest pain
- To demonstrate a greater awareness of the cardiac drugs most commonly used for high dependency patients and the nurse's role in the maintenance of the patient's stability

INTRODUCTION

This chapter will discuss the cardiovascular aspects of high dependency care, commonly needed either for patients with a primary cardiac condition (e.g. acute myocardial infarction or cardiac surgery) or for patients with underlying ischaemic heart disease who are admitted to hospital for other reasons (e.g. elective surgery).

Around 11% of male and 7% of female admissions to National Health Service (NHS) hospitals in England are due to cardiovascular disease (Petersen et al 2004: 67). It is estimated that there are about 1.5 million men and about 1.15 million women living in the UK who have coronary heart disease (CHD). Additionally, cardiovascular disease (heart disease, stroke and other diseases of the circulatory system) has been shown to be the second most commonly reported longstanding illness in Great Britain (Petersen et al 2004: 42). To address this problem, the National Service Framework for coronary heart disease was published as part of a strategy to reduce mortality rates and ensure equity of health care (Department of Health 2000). The progress of this action plan has resulted in a reduction of deaths from cardiovascular disease (Department of Health 2004).

Despite excellent progress with reducing deaths, there is still a high underlying prevalence of heart disease. Nurses need to be equipped with an appreciation of the principles of cardiac care, not only in designated cardiac or coronary care units, but also by those caring for patients in other medical and surgical high dependency areas.

BACKGROUND PHYSIOLOGY

In this section, an overview will be given of the control mechanisms that can affect cardiac output. These may be manipulated by medical and nursing interventions for patients requiring high dependency care.

An introduction to the knowledge required by nurses caring for high dependency patients is also given. You may wish to explore cardiovascular physiology in greater depth by consulting one of the textbooks and electrocardiography (ECG) sources suggested at the end of this chapter.

Cardiac output

In health, the normal cardiac output (CO) is around 5 litres/minute at rest increasing to 25 litres/minute during exercise. It represents the amount of blood ejected by the heart in a minute and is calculated by multiplying the stroke volume (SV) by the heart rate (HR):

$$CO = SV \times HR$$

Heart rate and stroke volume are both controlled by, and dependent upon, a number of factors (summarized in Box 6.1) including the action of the conduction system, and the effectiveness of the heart muscle and the peripheral vasculature.

The cardiac cycle

The cardiac cycle is the period from the end of one heartbeat to the end of the next. The heart contracts (systole) and then relaxes (diastole). At an average heart rate of 72 beats/minute, each cardiac cycle lasts 0.8 seconds, with the relaxation phase (0.5 seconds) being slightly longer.

Box 6.1   Factors affecting the cardiac output

Factors controlling the heart rate

Conducting system
- Inherent 'pacemaker' cells

Nervous control
- Sympathetic nervous system increases heart rate
- Parasympathetic nerves (vagus) decrease heart rate

Hormonal control
- Adrenaline (epinephrine) from the adrenal medulla

Stretch
- Increased venous return can stretch the right atrial wall and result in an increase in heart rate by 10–15% (Bainbridge reflex)

Temperature
- Affects the sinoatrial (SA) and atrioventricular (AV) nodes. Raised temperatures increase heart rate; low temperatures decrease heart rate, e.g. in hypothermia and following cardiac surgery

Drugs
- Drugs that affect heart rate are known as chronotropes. Examples of positive chronotropes which increase heart rate are atropine and adrenaline; negative chronotropes include beta-adrenergic blocking agents

Other factors
- Electrolyte concentration
- Hormones (other than adrenaline)

Factors affecting stroke volume

Pre-load
- Volume of blood returning to the heart

Contractility
- 'Elasticity' of the myocardium

Afterload
- Resistance to ventricular ejection, e.g. aortic valve, peripheral vascular resistance

The terms 'systole' and 'diastole' are usually used to refer to the contraction and relaxation of the ventricles, respectively. The sequence of events happens in both the right and left sides of the heart; however, the pressure exerted by the right side is less owing to the resistance to flow being less in the pulmonary circulation than in the systemic circulation. This difference is reflected in the comparative size of the muscular walls of the left and right sides of the heart. Despite the lower pressure exerted by the right side of the heart, the same amount of blood is ejected with each contraction.

In late diastole, the atria and ventricles are relaxed and blood enters the atria. When enough blood has entered the atria, the pressure causes the mitral and tricuspid valves to open, for blood to pass into the ventricles. Towards the end of diastole, the atria contract and pump some more blood into the ventricles. The ventricles receive 80% of their blood passively before the atria contract; the last 20% is sometimes referred to as the 'atrial kick' and its absence (e.g. in people with atrial fibrillation) can sometimes lead to symptoms of dyspnoea and fatigue secondary to reduced left ventricular function. Confusion and 'light-headedness' may also occur with faster heart rates. The amount of blood remaining in the ventricles at the end of diastole is called the ventricular end-diastolic volume (EDV).

As the ventricles begin to contract, the pressure in them begins to rise. This causes the mitral and tricuspid valves to close and so prevent backflow of blood into the atria. This can be heard as the first heart sound. When the pressure in the ventricles exceeds the pressure in the great arteries, the aortic and pulmonary valves open, causing rapid ejection of blood at first. The amount of blood ejected is called the stroke volume. The ejection fraction is the ratio between stroke volume and end-diastolic volume, and is normally between 60% and 70%.

Almost as soon as the ventricular muscle relaxes, the pulmonary and aortic valves close. This can be heard as the second heart sound. As ventricular pressure falls below atrial pressure, the mitral and tricuspid valves open, and ventricular filling occurs fairly rapidly.

The conduction system and the normal ECG

The conduction system within the heart consists of the sinoatrial (SA) node, the atrioventricular (AV) node, the atrioventricular bundle (also known as the bundle of His), the left and right bundle branches, and the Purkinje fibres (Figure 6.1). The electrical activity that occurs when an impulse passes along this system can be observed on an ECG. Figure 6.2 shows a normal ECG complex.

The impulse is initiated in the SA node, which has the ability to self-generate an impulse (automaticity). The impulse spreads through the atria and is represented on the ECG by the P wave. The SA node controls the pace of the heart and is known as the heart's normal pacemaker. Although its inherent rate is about 100 per minute, the actual heart rate is slowed to an average of 70–80 per minute by the effects of the parasympathetic nervous system, exerted through the vagus nerve. Other parts of the conducting system also have 'pacemaker' ability, although at slower rates. For example, the AV node has an inherent rate of 40–60 per minute, and the Purkinje fibres about 20–40 per minute.

The atria and ventricles are separated by connective tissue, which does not permit the spread of impulses. Therefore, the AV node and AV bundle provide the only connection. Conduction through the AV node is delayed for approximately 0.1 seconds, which allows the atria to contract and empty into the ventricles before the ventricles are depolarized and subsequently contract. This pause can be seen on the ECG during the PR interval, when the wave returns to the isoelectric (zero amplitude) line for a short period.

Figure 6.1 Conduction system. (Reproduced from Jowett & Thompson 1995, p 22, by kind permission of Baillière Tindall.)

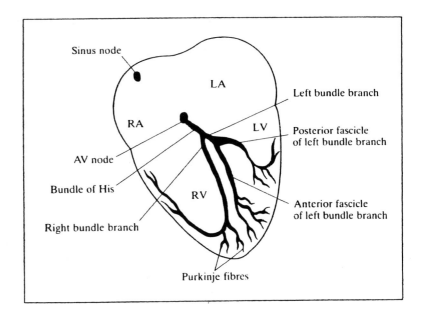

Figure 6.2 The normal ECG complex.

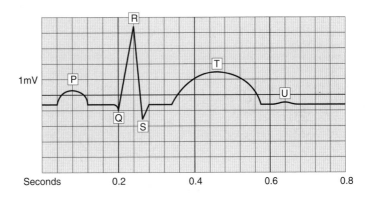

When the impulse leaves the AV node, it is conducted rapidly, which results in both ventricles contracting more or less simultaneously. The speed of depolarization through the ventricles is shown by the narrow QRS complex.

An impulse generated by the conduction system leads to depolarization (or electrical activity) in the heart, which then causes the heart muscle to contract. The ECG waveform is, therefore, a representation of the electrical activity of the heart rather than actual contraction.

Chemical changes: the role of potassium, sodium and calcium

Electricity is the movement of electrons along a conductor. Within the heart, electrical activity is made possible by a wave of chemical changes that pass along the cardiac cells (Box 6.2). The interlacing structures of cardiac cells facilitate this wave transmission throughout the heart. Key to this process is the permeability of the cell membrane in cardiac

Box 6.2   Changes during a heartbeat

Resting phase (termed 'polarized' because there is a difference in electrical charge of −90 mV across the membrane)	Active transport of potassium into cell	Intracellular potassium concentration is higher than extracellular	Isoelectric line on ECG
	Active transport of sodium out of cell	Extracellular sodium concentration higher than intracellular	
Depolarization	Sodium ion 'fast' channels open	Sodium floods into the cell	PQRS on ECG
Repolarization	Sodium and calcium 'slow' channels open	Sodium and calcium continue to move into the cell	ECG returns to resting potential T wave on ECG
	Electrostatic and concentration gradient affects potassium ions	Potassium leaves the cell	
	Sodium exchanged for potassium by enzyme action	Potassium and sodium ions return to their resting states	

tissue. This permeability can vary in response to two forces (concentration gradient and electrostatic forces) at work across the cell membrane. The complex checks and balances of these forces determine the movement of potassium, sodium and calcium ions across the cell wall.

At rest, the intracellular potassium is maintained at a higher concentration than outside the cell, whilst the intracellular sodium is kept lower than the extracellular concentration. These ions are not, however, in balance, and a charge of −90 mV inside the cell can be measured. This means the cell is, therefore, polarized. When the cell is excited, sodium ion channels open in the cell membrane, allowing sodium to flood into the cell making it positively charged. This sudden movement of ions forms the basis of the electric current and 'depolarization'. This translates into the PQRS complex on the ECG. Potassium now moves out of the cell in response to this change in electrostatic charge, coupled with the concentration gradient. In addition, calcium channels open and calcium flows into the cell at this time, helping to maintain the positive charge despite the reduction of potassium inside the cell. Ultimately, the sodium is removed from the cell by enzyme action that actively exchanges it for potassium and the cell returns to its resting 'polarized' state. This is the process of 'repolarization' and forms the T and U waves of the ECG.

Effectiveness of the heart muscle

The Frank–Starling mechanism (Guyton & Hall 1996: 115–116) explains that the greater the amount of stretch of the myocardial fibres at the end of diastole, the greater the force of the ensuing contraction. Up to a certain point, with healthy myocardium, the more filling that takes place, the greater the contractility and the greater the stroke volume (i.e. more fluid entering is followed by more fluid being pumped out).

In practice, with patients who have impaired left ventricular function (i.e. heart failure) cardiac output becomes compromised when pre-load is increased. This can also occur, for example, following a blood transfusion or fluid administration, where the heart muscle does not have the capacity (or elasticity) to increase stroke volume. More fluid enters the circulation but is not pumped adequately, resulting in pooling in the pulmonary or peripheral vasculature, leading to oedema.

Positive inotropes are frequently administered in acute settings to patients with the aim of improving the effectiveness of the heart muscle's action. An inotrope is a substance that affects the contractility of the heart. The term is often used incorrectly in practice to refer only to positive inotropic drugs that increase contractility (Box 6.3). Strictly speaking, positive inotropes increase contractility, for example adrenaline (epinephrine), dopamine, whereas negative inotropes decrease contractility, for example calcium antagonists (nifedipine, verapamil) and beta-adrenergic blocking agents (atenolol, propranolol).

ASSESSMENT

In order to make a comprehensive assessment of a patient's cardiovascular status, the following approaches may be adopted:

- interpretation of vital signs;
- physical examination;
- interview with patient and any close family/friends;
- review of previous health information;
- review of cardiac risk factors;
- analysis of laboratory findings.

> The stress caused to the patient by multiple assessments should be avoided. In evaluating the patient's condition, the multidisciplinary team should work as a whole.

For patients needing high dependency care, this assessment needs to be undertaken collaboratively with other members of the healthcare team, including doctors, physiotherapists, cardiac technicians and support workers. Repeated assessments by these different health professionals should be avoided, particularly in acutely ill patients, and assessment should be ongoing and synonymous with evaluation. Communication and coordination of activities between the multidisciplinary healthcare team are vital to reduce the amount of disruption and disturbance for the patient.

Box 6.3   Positive inotropes

Adrenaline (epinephrine)
Dopamine   } naturally occurring catecholamines
Noradrenaline (norepinephrine)
Dobutamine   synthetic substance
All act directly on adrenergic receptors:

- Alpha-1 effects: vasoconstriction of most peripheral vessels; some increased myocardial contractility
- Beta-1 effects: increased heart rate, rate of AV conduction and myocardial contractility
- Beta-2 effects: peripheral vasodilatation of some vascular beds, e.g. some skeletal muscle, bronchodilatation

Adrenaline (epinephrine)

Has beta effects at lower doses. At higher doses, e.g. during resuscitation, alpha effects produce a higher blood pressure leading to increased coronary and cerebral perfusion.

Dopamine

Increases stroke volume but has less effect on heart rate. Causes peripheral vasoconstriction but may have a selective renal arterial vasodilatation effect, which is most marked at low doses. Can cause localized peripheral tissue ischaemia and should, therefore, always be given via a central line.

Noradrenaline (norepinephrine)

Generally only given under full monitoring conditions in intensive care environments. Useful in septic shock.

Dobutamine

Increases force of myocardial contraction with only a small increase in heart rate. Used predominantly for cardiogenic shock and heart failure.

All catecholamines have very short biological half-lives (1–2 minutes) due largely to reuptake into tissues and to degradation in the liver and lungs. A steady-state plasma concentration is achieved within 5–10 minutes after the start of a continuous infusion. Discontinuation of the infusion even for only a short time (e.g. reloading syringes) can have a marked effect on the patient.
Adrenaline (epinephrine) and noradrenaline (norepinephrine) have 100 times greater potency than dopamine and dobutamine.

Interpretation of vital signs

Observation of a patient's vital signs often constitutes a large proportion of a high dependency nurse's time. The interpretation of alterations in vital signs gives an insight into changes occurring within the patient's internal environment and the homeostatic mechanisms being used to counter any problems. Changes can act as triggers to other aspects of the patient's care. For example, an increase in heart rate and blood pressure may be a result of pain, while emotions such as anxiety can also affect vital signs. Therefore, vital signs must be interpreted correctly and not in isolation from other factors. Furthermore, baseline observations, preferably obtained before the acute event, can be useful for comparison.

Pulse and heart rate

Arterial pulses should be examined for rate, rhythm and volume. The radial artery is usually used but may be difficult to palpate if there is peripheral shutdown, in which case the femoral or carotid arteries should be palpated. The pulse should be counted for 1 minute to assess heart rate and rhythm; however, it is more usual in high dependency or cardiac units to rely upon continuous ECG monitoring to obtain these details. In this case, care should be taken to assess whether there is a peripheral pulse deficit by recording any difference between the apical rate and the peripheral pulse. Normal heart rate in the resting adult is around 70 beats/minute, but can be between 60 and 100 beats/minute, and should be regular.

The volume of the pulse depends on the pulse pressure, which is the difference between the systolic and diastolic blood pressure. A small volume pulse is often seen following a myocardial infarction, whereas large volumes can be found in patients with anaemia or aortic regurgitation.

ECG monitoring

Monitoring the ECG gives a continuous picture of the heart's electrical activity, which includes the heart rate. There are different situations in which continuous ECG monitoring may be performed (Box 6.4) but the overall aim is to identify or anticipate potentially life-threatening disturbances as early as possible. However, it should be remembered that the monitor trace is just an additional tool for assessment and that observing the patient's general condition and status is essential.

> The ECG monitor trace is just an additional tool for assessment. Don't lose sight of the patient and what *all* the vital signs are telling you.

The reason for continuous ECG monitoring needs to be explained to the patient and family, together with the explanation that being attached to the monitor does not necessarily imply that they are critically ill.

The ECG tracing should be observed for the following features:

- rate;
- rhythm;
- PR interval;
- narrow or broad QRS complex;
- ectopic beats.

A regular heart rate between 60 and 100 per minute is known as sinus rhythm. (A slight slowing and quickening with respiration, known as sinus arrhythmia, is quite normal.) Slower rates (less than 60 per minute) are referred to as sinus bradycardia. Rates faster than 100 are known as

Box 6.4   Indications for continuous cardiac monitoring

- Surveillance of heart rate and rhythm
- Dysrhythmia identification and evaluation
- Acute myocardial infarction
- Undiagnosed chest pain
- Unstable angina
- Atrial–ventricular block (third-degree/complete heart block and some patients with second-degree, depending on symptoms)
- Evaluation of temporary pacing
- Evaluation of response to drug therapy
- Peri-operatively and post-operatively (length of time will depend on procedure and other factors, e.g. effect of drug therapy)
- Emergency and life-threatening conditions, e.g. trauma, overdose, poisoning
- Patients with a history of syncope or blackout

sinus tachycardia, if the rhythm remains regular and controlled by the sinoatrial node (Figure 6.3 and Box 6.5).

Nurses working in areas where ECG monitoring takes places should be familiar with the operation of the monitor, including setting alarm limits appropriately and dealing with common problems (Table 6.1).

Blood pressure   Arterial blood pressure is an important clinical observation that is used extensively to assess and monitor patient progress. For high dependency patients, it may be recorded in three ways:

Figure 6.3 ECG tracings. Cardiac arrhythmias (Reproduced from Hinchliff et al 1996, p. 393, by kind permission of Baillière Tindall.)

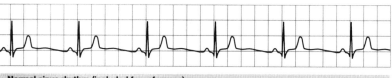

Normal sinus rhythm (included for reference)

Description
Each P wave is followed by a QRS complex
Rate 60-100 beats/min – in this
example the rate is 63 beats/min

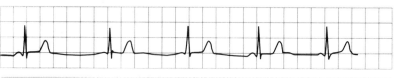

Sinus bradycardia

Description	Causes	Treatment
Sinus rhythm (i.e. each P wave is followed by a QRS complex); however, the heart rate at rest is less than 60 beats/min – in this example the rate is 50 beats/min	May be normal in athletes Hypothermia Increased vagal tone due to bowel straining, vomiting, intubation, mechanical ventilation, pain β-blocking drugs	Atropine, isoprenaline If unresponsive to these, may require temporary ventricular pacemaker

Figure 6.3—*continued*

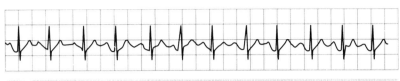

Sinus tachycardia

Description
Sinus rhythm (i.e. each P wave is followed by a QRS complex); however, the heart rate at rest is greater than 100 beats/min – in this example the rate is 125 beats/min

Causes
Physiological response to fever, exercise, anxiety, pain
May accompany shock, left ventricular failure, cardiac tamponade, hyperthyroidism, pulmonary embolism
Sympathetic stimulating drugs

Treatment
Correction of the underlying cause

Box 6.5   ECG electrode skin preparation

Although self-adhesive ECG electrodes usually require minimal skin preparation, the following steps can help if the signal is poor:

- Rub the skin lightly with dry gauze or a proprietary 'skin prep' tape to remove loose dry skin
- Shave the skin, if the patient is particularly hirsute, to improve electrode contact (and make removal painless)
- Excess body oil and perspiration should be removed by washing with soap and water. Wiping the skin with alcohol-impregnated swabs is no longer recommended, as the alcohol dries the skin excessively

The electrode site should be observed daily for allergic reaction

---

- using a stethoscope and sphygmomanometer;
- using an automatic device with cuff that measures non-invasively;
- direct and continuous intra-arterial measurement.

The decision concerning which method is to be adopted will depend on the acuity of the patient, the resources available in the ward or unit and whether rapid changes in blood pressure are likely to occur. Arterial measurement follows the insertion of a catheter into an artery, often the radial, which is then connected to a transducer. The advantages of this method (i.e. continuous measurement and observation of a wave form) need to be weighed against the potential disadvantages (e.g. risk of accidental dislodgement and subsequent bleeding, potential infection, peripheral artery damage and embolism; see Figure 6.4).

When using a non-invasive device, the cuff should be an appropriate size for the patient, otherwise an inaccurate recording can be made. The bladder of the cuff should be at least 80% of the arm circumference in length and 40% of the arm circumference in width.

Homeostatic mechanisms may initially mask the effect of compromised cardiac output. Arterial vasodilation may give rise to a low diastolic blood pressure. When the difference between the systolic and

Table 6.1 Troubleshooting ECG monitors

Problem	Cause	Solution
Interference (regular pattern)	Electrical interference from other mains sources	Avoid crossing wires. During 12-lead recordings, briefly disconnect non-essential mains-powered equipment (e.g. electrical mattresses)
	Broken lead	Replace lead
Interference (irregular pattern)	Patient movement or muscle tension	Keep the patient warm and comfortable. During 12-lead recordings explain to the patient that they need to relax and lie still. Explore any anxieties that the procedure evokes
Wandering baseline	Relates to chest movement, exacerbated by poor electrode contact	Reposition electrodes
False heart rate count	The numerical heart rate display is calculated electronically by the height of the R wave; if the T waves are of equivalent height the displayed rate may be doubled	Select a lead that has smaller T waves, adjust the trigger level (see monitor instructions)
	The numerical heart rate display may be low if the amplitude (height) of the ECG is very small	Increase the gain on the monitor, check the electrodes have good contact, try a different lead selection
Skin excoriation under electrode	Patient allergic to electrode	Wash skin under electrodes at least daily and vary electrode position; consider alternative brand

diastolic blood pressures is narrowed, it is the result of arterial vasoconstriction (Smith 2000).

Central venous pressure

The central venous pressure (CVP) is measured following insertion of a line into either the subclavian or internal jugular vein, which is then advanced along the vein until its tip is near the right atrium. The CVP is, therefore, reflective of the pressure in the right atrium.

Measurement of the CVP will:

• assist with establishing the pressure in the right atrium (filling pressure or pre-load);
• assist the evaluation of circulatory failure;
• act as a guide in fluid replacement;
• reflect response to treatment.

Figure 6.4 Arterial pressure monitoring. (Reproduced from Hartshorn et al 1997, p. 94.)

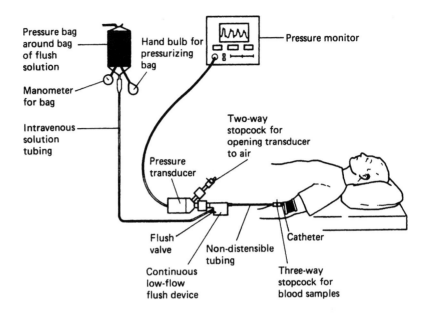

The normal CVP range is 3–10 mmHg (5–12 cmH$_2$O), although considerable variation exists in what is considered a normal value. The trend of the readings is considered more important in its association with other signs. For example, if the CVP begins to rise while urine output drops, a decreased cardiac output may be indicated with circulatory overload. The CVP can be measured as follows.

- Electronically using a transducer system similar to that used for measuring arterial blood pressure (see Figure 6.4). Continuous measurements can then be obtained.
- Manually using a hard plastic water manometer that is placed on an intravenous infusion set. Measurements are obtained intermittently (Figure 6.5).

The recording should be made with the patient in the same 'baseline' position with the zero point of the manometer level with the patient's right atrium.

Manual methods measure the pressure in centimetres of water (cmH$_2$O), whereas electronic systems usually use millimetres of mercury (mmHg). Care should be taken when interpreting changes in CVP to check if the method used has been changed; for example, soon after a patient has been transferred from a ward, where the CVP has been recorded manually, to a high dependency area, where the pressure is transduced electronically, or if the patient's position has changed (1 mmHg is equal to 1.36 cmH$_2$O). Situations that commonly produce an elevated CVP include congestive heart failure, cardiac tamponade, vasoconstrictive states where the blood volume has remained the same but the vascular bed has become smaller, and increased blood volume as a result, for example, of overtransfusion. A low CVP is usually seen with

From giving set
Manometer
O-point of manometer at
level of midaxillary line
Right atrium
Catheter inserted via
subclavian vein
Three-way tap

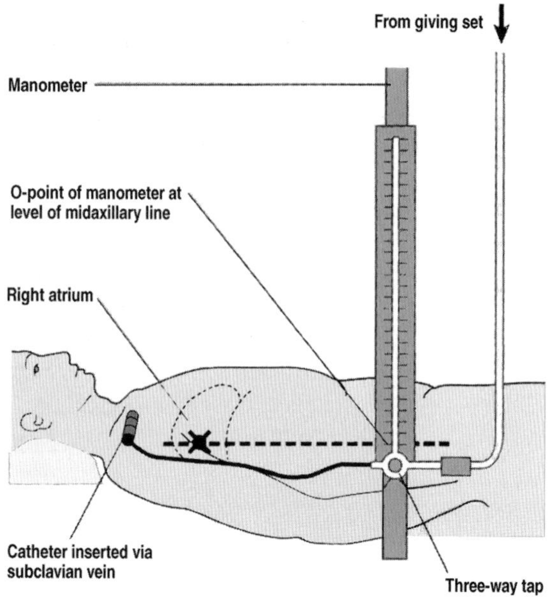

Figure 6.5 Measuring central venous pressure using a fluid manometer. (Reproduced from Hinchliff et al 1996, p.432, by kind permission of Baillière Tindall.)

20
15
10
5
0
–5
CVP ↑
Congestive cardiac failure
Cardiac tamponade
Vasoconstruction e.g.
noradrenaline
Normal CVP ~
3-10mm Hg or
5-12cm H_2O
CVP ↓
Dehydration e.g. vomiting
Vasodilation e.g. nifedipine

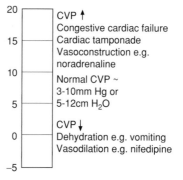

Figure 6.6 Factors affecting central venous pressure readings.

hypovolaemia owing to blood or fluid loss, or through drug-induced vasodilatation (Figure 6.6).

Measuring cardiac output indirectly is often adequate for many clinical situations. This can be done by reviewing blood pressure, heart rate and CVP measurements and relating this to information obtained during a physical examination of the patient (e.g. skin colour, peripheral temperature and changes in urine output). Occasionally it may be necessary to measure cardiac output invasively and there are a variety of techniques for assessing this, including a pulmonary artery flotation catheter (Swan et al 1970), and continuous real time monitoring via a specialized arterial line or oesophageal Doppler (Singer 1996). Echocardiography is a non-invasive alternative for estimating cardiac output.

> Indirect measurement of cardiac output may be adequate for most clinical situations. Review blood pressure, heart rate and CVP. Relate this to skin colour, urine output and peripheral temperature in the patient.

Physical examination

Observation of a patient's physical state can aid the assessment of their cardiovascular status greatly. Nurses are increasingly developing the skills required to perform a comprehensive physical assessment, and the information obtained by using this approach can be invaluable. Aspects of a physical examination particularly pertinent to the cardiovascular assessment include skin colour and temperature, level of consciousness and urine output.

Skin colour and temperature

Any signs of pallor or cyanosis should be noted together with hypothermia or hyperthermia, and of peripheral 'shutdown'. Simply squeezing the fingertip for 5 seconds can test peripheral refill: once the pressure is released, the original fingertip colour should return in less than 2 seconds (Figure 6.7). A prolonged peripheral refill time indicates poor peripheral circulation (Smith 2000). Peripheral symptoms of atheroma include intermittent claudication. This induces cramp-like pain in muscles during exercise owing to narrowing or blockage of the arteries reducing oxygen delivery to the tissues. The pain should resolve with rest (British Vascular Foundation 2003).

Level of consciousness

A swift assessment of neurological deficit may be attained by reference to the AVPU scale as advocated by Smith (2000). This scale directs health professionals to consider whether the patient is (A) *a*wake, (V) responding to *v*erbal stimuli, (P) only responding to *p*ain or (U) fully *u*nconscious (Box 6.6). If a deficit is found, then a fuller neurological assessment (i.e. Glasgow coma score) should be performed. Neurological deficit in a patient with underlying cardiovascular disease may be due to thromboembolic events (e.g. stroke or transient ischaemic attack; TIA) or to hypoxia as a result of heart failure.

Urine output

The urine output is a fundamental indicator of physiological function. The mechanism of kidney function requires and seeks to maintain a large blood flow (25% of the cardiac output). If this cannot be achieved, the urine output falls below 0.5 ml/kg per hour and should be investigated promptly. Hypovolaemia is the commonest reason for a low urine output and may only require increased fluid intake; however, in the presence of heart failure, inotropic support and diuretic therapy may also be required. If there is no response to fluid administration, renal and post-renal causes of the low urine output will require investigation (Park & Roe 2000).

Fluid balance monitoring is essential for meaningful analysis of urine output. All fluids received should be measured and documented along

Figure 6.7 Assessing peripheral refill.

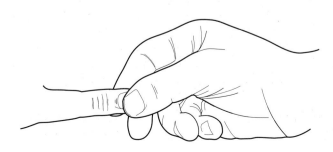

Box 6.6 AVPU scale for assessing conscious level

A	Alert
V	Responds to voice
	Airway at risk below this line
P	Responds to pain
U	Unresponsive

with all outputs. Generally, where urine output is inadequate, catheterization will be required in order to assess response to treatment.

Interview

Nurses can gain a wealth of information from the patient and any accompanying family or close friend, which may be pertinent to the cardiovascular assessment. The information may be collected in a structured interview or over a period of time. In acute situations, information may be obtained from patients about their experience of the situation. For example, the patient may have a sensation of palpitations to accompany the tachycardia noted on the ECG monitor or their pain may be associated with inspiration.

Review of previous health information

Valuable details that may contribute to the current assessment of patients may be culled from previous information recorded. Information that may be readily available can be found in 'old' notes relating to previous hospital admissions, recent notes recorded before the current acute episode or from 'patient-held' details (e.g. current medications or anticoagulation clinic results). Medical notes may contain information about longstanding conditions (e.g. hypertension) or previous treatments (e.g. the response to nitrates). Nursing notes may give an indication of the patients' perception of their illness or their social situation, which they may not be able to communicate because of their current acuity. Furthermore, they may contain information relating to patients' normal coping strategies and previous experiences of aspects of high dependency care. Charts (e.g. vital signs, fluid balance), previous ECGs, echocardiogram and angiogram reports along with laboratory results will provide 'baseline' information to compare with current assessments.

Review of cardiac risk factors

An assessment of the patient's risk factors is useful in developing the management plan. There are two groups of risk factors: non-modifiable (those we cannot change), for example, age, gender and a family history of heart disease. Then there are the modifiable risk factors (those that can be prevented or controlled), for example, hypertension, high blood cholesterol, diabetes mellitus, smoking, obesity, lack of exercise and poor diet (high in saturated fats, and low in fresh fruit and vegetable intake). Identifying cardiac risk factors can assist the nurse with educating both patient and carers, and reduce the chance of future cardiac events (Department of Health 2000).

Analysis of laboratory findings

Results obtained primarily from blood samples will aid the assessment (Lab Test Online website). This will include the interpretation of results obtained from equipment located within many high dependency units. Information that is frequently of use in acute settings to the cardiovascular assessment includes the following.

Serum potassium (K+) levels

In healthy individuals, the normal level is 3.6–4.6 mmol/l; however, a higher level (4.5–5.0 mmol/l) may need to be maintained in some cases where the cardiac muscle is particularly irritable (e.g. after cardiac surgery). Variation from the norm (both higher and lower levels) can lead to cardiac arrest.

Renal function

Patients with cardiac disease (typically those with heart failure) require close monitoring of their renal function, especially for those on angiotensin-converting enzyme (ACE) inhibitors or spironolactone, as both these drugs can have a detrimental effect on renal function.

Coagulation times

Clotting times will be needed for both hypovolaemic patients and those with a primary cardiac condition requiring anticoagulation. Laboratory analysis of activated partial thromboplastin time (APTT) and the international normalized ratio (INR) for prothrombin time should be assessed for patients who have been anticoagulated with heparin or warfarin, respectively.

Red blood cell status

Haemoglobin and haematocrit or packed cell volume (PCV) will be needed for hypovolaemic patients or those where fluid replacement is anticipated.

Arterial blood gases

The metabolic status is derived from the partial pressures of oxygen and carbon dioxide (see Chapter 5 for a full account of the interpretation of arterial blood gases).

Typical normal values from blood samples are shown in Table 6.2.

Table 6.2 Typical normal values

Hb	13.5–17.5 g/dl (male)
	11.5–15.5 g/dl (female)
Hct/PCV	0.4–0.45 (M)
	0.36–0.44 (F)
Platelet count	150–400 (10^9 litres)
APTT	25–37 seconds
ACT	< 150 seconds
K+	3.6–4.6 mmol/l
Na	135–146 mmol/l
INR	0.8–1.2
	2.0–3.5* (warfarin therapeutic range)

* The therapeutic goal for INR will vary according to each patient's diagnosis and condition. The precise therapeutic goal must always be confirmed by the Haematology Department.

> **Case example 6.1**
>
> Christine Stevens was a 32-year-old lady admitted to the gynaecology ward with hyperemesis. She was 14 weeks pregnant and had been vomiting since the second week of pregnancy. On admission, her heart rate was 110 with a thready pulse, her blood pressure was 88/53, she had a delayed peripheral refill time (> 2 seconds) and she was actively vomiting.
>
> As rehydration was a priority, Ms Stevens was cannulated. At this time, blood samples for electrolytes, urea and full blood count were obtained. Normal saline 500 ml was administered intravenously over 10 minutes.
>
> The blood samples showed that her potassium level was 1.5 mmol/l and her sodium was 119 mmol/l. As hypokalaemia can be immediately life threatening, the assistance of the intensive care outreach team was requested. ECG monitoring was commenced and intravenous potassium was administered via a central venous line using a volumetric pump.

LOW CARDIAC OUTPUT

The distinctions between the terms low cardiac output state, acute circulatory collapse and the various types of 'shock' are largely arbitrary. The terms can be used to denote a clinical picture in which there is inadequate perfusion of oxygen and other essential substances in the tissues caused by:

- heart muscle pump failure;
- hypovolaemia;
- abnormalities in peripheral resistance;
- a combination of one or more of the above.

The different types and typical manifestations of shock are listed in Boxes 6.7 and 6.8.

Pathophysiological changes

Cardiac changes

Cardiac output may be either absent or reduced owing to disruption of electrical activity, impaired contractility or inadequate filling. In the early stages, as shock begins to develop, there is more sympathetic activity, which increases the heart rate and force of contraction. This is accompanied by vasoconstriction, increasing the venous return to the heart. This compensatory mechanism ceases to work when the circulating volume is reduced by more than 15%.

The increased heart rate causes a decreased diastolic filling time that reduces coronary perfusion. Dysrhythmias can further reduce the diastolic filling time and also lead to inefficient ventricular contractions, decreasing cardiac output.

Bleeding into the pericardial sac (cardiac tamponade) can precipitate cardiogenic shock, particularly following cardiac surgery or chest injuries. This impairs effective emptying or filling of the heart.

In the later stages of shock, a number of vasoactive kinins (e.g. bradykinin, histamine) are released that have potent vasodilator effects, further decreasing the circulating volume.

Box 6.7   Types of shock

Hypovolaemic

This is not manifested until between 15% and 25% of the circulating volume is lost.

- Haemorrhage
- Dehydration
- Burns

Cardiogenic

- Acute myocardial infarction
- Arrhythmias
- Tamponade
- Pulmonary embolism (caused by an inadequate cardiac output)

Neurogenic

- Spinal cord injury
- Spinal and epidural analgesia
- Severe pain
- Extreme fright (autonomic nervous system activity causes reflex vasodilatation and loss of arteriolar tone, resulting in pooling of blood and loss of venous return)

Septic

The following are examples of patients who are particularly susceptible to septic shock.

- Older patients in hospital
- Following invasive procedure, particularly genitourinary instrumentation
- Where there is an underlying disease that limits the use of compensatory mechanisms (caused by an overwhelming infection that results in peripheral vasodilatation leading to inadequate circulating volume)

Anaphylactic

- Antigen–antibody reaction (the release of toxic substances, e.g. histamine, produces vasodilatation and pooling of blood)

Peripheral vessel changes

Initially, vasoconstriction diverts blood to the vital organs, and blood pressure, particularly diastolic pressure, may be maintained. Blood flow to the skin and renal circulation are reduced. Prolonged vasoconstriction causes tissue hypoxia and acidosis, which eventually leads to microcirculatory failure if not reversed or treated. Accumulating metabolites and the local acidosis cause relaxation of the pre-capillary sphincters, which results in the pooling of blood.

> **Box 6.8   Typical manifestations of shock**
>
> - Systolic blood pressure < 90 mmHg or reduction of > 25% of its normal reading
> - Weak, rapid and thready pulse
> - Cold and clammy skin, prolonged peripheral refill time (> 2 seconds)
> - Oliguria – urine output less than 0.5 ml/kg body weight per hour
> - Mental confusion or other signs of altered orientation, such as agitation
>
> The classic picture may show some variations, e.g. in septic shock the patient's skin may be warm and dry, and the pulse bounding.

Fluid shifts

Early in hypovolaemic and cardiogenic shock, fluid moves from the interstitial spaces into capillaries, thus increasing the circulating volume. However, this fluid shift is later reversed and fluid leaves the vascular space. This reversal is caused by the effects of hypoxia on cellular metabolism. Ion-pumping mechanisms fail owing to lack of 'energy', potassium leaves the cell and sodium enters. Water follows sodium, leaving the vasculature and extending the hypovolaemia.

In septic shock, toxins result in increased permeability of capillaries with small proteins and fluid leaving the circulation. Fluid can leave the circulation at a rate of 200 ml/hour with the patient developing severe oedema and hypovolaemia.

Renal changes

In the initial stages of shock, the kidneys promote conservation of water through activation of antidiuretic hormone (ADH) from the posterior pituitary gland, and through the renin–angiotensin–aldosterone response (Guyton & Hall 1996: 227–229). Prolonged renal ischaemia may lead to acute renal failure with the onset of oliguria or anuria.

Coagulation changes

Microcirculatory changes can lead to pooling and stasis of blood, which predisposes to platelet aggregation. Disseminated intravascular coagulation is often seen in patients with septic shock with very rapid consumption of clotting factors, leading to bleeding, particularly from mucosal surfaces.

Acid–base disequilibrium

Initially, owing to hyperventilation, respiratory alkalosis can develop. However, once tissue hypoxia occurs, anaerobic metabolism is induced and lactic acid accumulates, producing a metabolic acidosis (see Chapter 5).

Intestine and liver

Prolonged vasoconstriction is thought to cause intestinal ischaemia and necrosis, which permits intestinal bacteria to gain access to the bloodstream leading to sepsis. If the liver has sustained ischaemic damage, it is unable to undertake its metabolic and detoxification functions or produce clotting factors.

Pulmonary changes   Extensive left ventricular damage (in cardiogenic shock) will result in vascular congestion and pulmonary oedema. Ventilation:perfusion ratios are disturbed and hypoxaemia results.

CARE OF THE PATIENT WITH A LOW CARDIAC OUTPUT

The aim of nursing and medical interventions is to preserve oxygen and nutrient transport to the vital organs, and to elicit the cause (if not known) of the low output state. Aspects of the initial management of a patient displaying signs of shock are shown in Figure 6.8. Depending on the response to initial treatment, the patient may be stabilized quickly and able to remain in a lower dependency care setting, or may require transfer to another critical care or intensive therapy unit where more comprehensive care is available. Advanced life support may be necessary (see page 148)

With all patients, continuous monitoring of heart rate and blood pressure is necessary. Oxygen should generally be administered as appropriate in relation to assessment of oxygen saturation or blood gas analysis. Pulse oximetry may only be useful if the patient is not peripherally 'shut down'. Skin colour and temperature, together with an assessment of the patient's conscious level, also need to be considered. The insertion of

Figure 6.8 The management of shock.

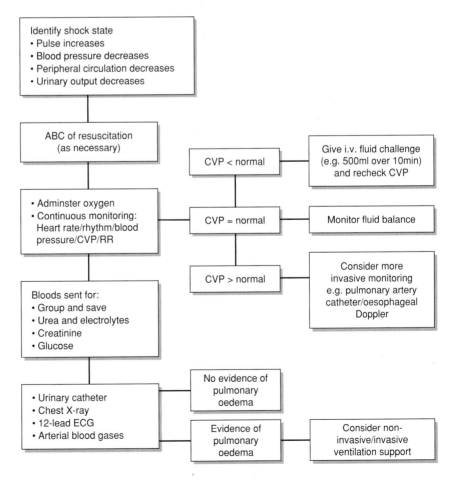

a urinary catheter and hourly measurements will give some indication of renal perfusion and, hence, cardiac output. An adequate cardiac output should support renal perfusion sufficiently to produce a urine output greater than 0.5 ml/kg of body weight per hour.

Other treatments and interventions that are likely to occur will depend on the cause of the low cardiac output (Figure 6.8).

Case example 6.2

Grace Wisdom, a 82-year-old lady, was admitted by her GP direct to the Medical Assessment Unit with a fever, abdominal discomfort and diarrhoea.

On admission her vital signs revealed a pyrexia but were otherwise unremarkable (temperature 38.8°C; blood pressure 110/80; pulse 82 bpm; respiratory rate 12/minute; SpO$_2$ 94%). However, her past medical history of hypertension and angina suggested that her cardiovascular status was slightly compromised.

Over the next 4 hours, her condition deteriorated, with her blood pressure progressively falling to 66/45 mmHg despite intravenous fluid replacement. She developed abdominal pain and distension was noted.

A surgical assessment was requested and a provisional diagnosis of abdominal sepsis was made necessitating an urgent laparotomy. However, in view of her deteriorating cardiac output, she was transferred to the intensive care unit for stabilization prior to theatre.

Cardiogenic shock

Cardiogenic shock or heart muscle pump failure is usually treated with positive inotropic drugs, such as dobutamine (see Box 6.3). These drugs need to be titrated to the individual's response and changing condition. ECG monitoring is essential. Patients need to be assessed (CVP, urine output) to ensure they are adequately 'filled' before inotropes are started. To prevent pulmonary oedema, diuretics may be needed. In order to minimize renal toxic effects, normal doses should be given and repeated according to response. If the cause is well established, then the medical team may decide that the placement of a pulmonary artery flotation catheter is not warranted.

Hypovolaemia

Replacement fluid will be the first-line therapy for hypovolaemia. Colloids are given rapidly in the form of either blood or plasma expander substances (e.g. Gelofusine, eloHAES). Generally, the packed cell volume or haematocrit is used as a guide to choice, although some units use haemoglobin (Hb) measurement. Blood should be given if the PCV is less than 30% or the Hb less than 10 g/dl. If large replacement volumes are needed, then blood products will also be required to prevent coagulation problems.

If possible, the amount of fluid that is lost should be measured to aid in the calculation of replacement fluid (e.g. fluid loss via post-operative drainage tubes or as a result of diarrhoea).

Dysrhythmias

A variety of causes may precipitate dysrhythmias that compromise cardiac output. The loss of an adequate circulating volume may be as a result of either an abnormally fast or slow heart rate. Excessively fast rates are seen, for example, with ventricular tachycardia, fast atrial fibrillation or flutter and with re-entrant tachycardias. These are usually treated initially with antiarrhythmic agents, such as amiodarone or adenosine, with the exception of pulseless ventricular tachycardia for which the definitive treatment is rapid defibrillation (Box 6.9).

Slow heart rates may be associated with parasympathetic (vagal) effects on the sinoatrial or atrioventricular nodes, or with varying degrees of atrioventricular block ('heart block'). This can be as a result of myocardial infarction, fibrosis of the conducting system associated with old age or cardiac surgery. Drugs with positive chronotropic (rate enhancing) effects may be used (e.g. atropine), which blocks parasympathetic activity. Temporary pacing may also need be initiated.

Temporary pacing

Artificial cardiac pacing is likely to be used for any condition resulting in failure of the heart to initiate or conduct an intrinsic electrical impulse at a rate adequate to maintain tissue perfusion throughout the body. Pacing is the repetitive delivery of very low electrical energies to the heart, thus initiating and maintaining the cardiac rhythm.

The different ways in which pacing may be undertaken as a temporary measure are described below.

Percussion pacing

Gentle blows to the patient's chest are applied over the precordium, lateral to the lower left sternal edge. This may be used to initiate contraction when there is a profound bradycardia (Resuscitation Council UK 2001). In this situation, a normal cardiac output can be maintained whilst preparations for temporary pacing are made.

Transcutaneous (external transthoracic)

First introduced by Zoll in the 1950s, this method is now used in emergency situations as a rapid, simple and safe method of maintaining cardiac output. It is non-invasive and relatively simple to commence following minimal training. With modern equipment, which uses a longer pulse duration (and thus lower amplitude), pacing is usually well tolerated, with little more than slight discomfort, such as tingling or tapping (Zoll

---

Box 6.9   Antiarrhythmics

Antiarrhythmic drugs can be classified clinically (British National Formulary 2004), according to which rhythms they act on:

1. Supraventricular arrhythmias, e.g. verapamil, digoxin, adenosine
2. Ventricular arrhythmias, e.g. amiodarone, disopyramide, flecainide
3. Both supraventricular and ventricular arrhythmias, e.g. lidocaine (lignocaine), bretylium

& Zoll 1985). However, if the patient does find the experience painful, analgesia (e.g. 2.5–5 mg diamorphine given intravenously) should be administered. Despite advances in technology, it remains a temporary measure until appropriate transvenous pacing can be undertaken.

Transvenous (endocardial)

A pacing lead is passed via a vein to the endocardial surface of the heart, most commonly the right ventricle. The wire is inserted in a similar way to a 'central line' via the subclavian vein, although the pacing wire is advanced into the ventricle. This is usually done under X-ray imaging guidance, with many coronary care units (CCUs) having an adjacent room set aside for pacing. Very occasionally and in emergency conditions, it may be inserted 'blindly'.

Epicardial

Following cardiac surgery, conduction disturbances may arise owing to oedema and manipulation of the conducting system. Temporary epicardial wires are frequently inserted during surgery; attached to the outer surface of the heart (epicardium), they are then brought out through the skin at the base of the sternotomy wound. They are usually removed 4 or 5 days after surgery.

Transoesophageal

This technique involves an electrode being inserted in a manner rather like a nasogastric tube. Although originally described in the late 1960s, it is used infrequently and is not very reliable (Jowett & Thompson 1995).

A summary of the nursing care required for a patient with a temporary pacing system and actions that may need to be taken if problems arise are given in Box 6.10. These aspects are discussed further in Thompson & Webster (1992: 194–198).

Case example 6.3

Ajay Shiva, a 40-year-old man, was brought to hospital with acute chest pain. He received analgesia, oxygen, sublingual glyceryl trinitrate and aspirin consistent with the emergency treatment of acute chest pain. His ECG showed an anterior myocardial infarction with marked S-T elevation and streptokinase was administered.

During the transfer from the casualty trolley to the coronary care unit bed, Mr Shiva lost consciousness, the ECG monitor showed ventricular tachycardia and no pulse could be felt. A single monophasic shock of 200 J was promptly administered to defibrillate the heart and sinus rhythm returned.

Four hours later, Mr Shiva complained that his chest pain had returned and an ECG confirmed that his myocardial infarction was extending. Complete heart block quickly developed with a heart rate of 10 beats/minute, loss of consciousness and unrecordable blood pressure. The defibrillator was modified, by the replacement of the defibrillator paddles with external pacing pads, to provide transcutaneous pacing. Mr Shiva had little chest hair, allowing easy adherence of the pacing electrodes. With the defibrillator in pacemaker function, the demand mode was selected. The pacing current was increased until transmission of an impulse was shown by the presence of a wide QRS following every pacing spike on the ECG. A pulse was now palpable. Mr Shiva was transferred to the cardiac pacing suite for an emergency transvenous pacemaker.

**Box 6.10   Nursing care for the patient with temporary pacing.
(Adapted from Nurse's Ready Reference 1992)**

Care of the patient will depend on the type of temporary pacing but will
include the following.

Assessing pacemaker function

- Settings should be recorded, battery life monitored and thresholds
  checked daily by an experienced nurse or doctor

Maintaining patient comfort and safety

- Ensure the wire is secured with an appropriate dressing
- Teach patients about their condition
- Respond to problems appropriately

Rhythm strips showing normal paced beat and two pacing problems

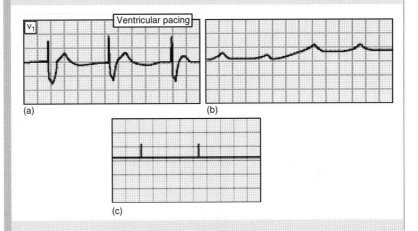

(a)   (b)   (c)

ECG	Action
(a) Ventricular paced beat Note 'pacing spike' followed by broad QRS complex	
(b) Failure to pace: P waves are not followed by a pacing stimulus or QRS complex **NB** May be caused by 'oversensing' of electrical impulses from pectoral muscles	Check connections Increase voltage
(c) Failure to capture: pacing spike seen but not causing depolarization of the ventricles (no QRS)	Move patient on to his or her left side Check connections Increase voltage

ADVANCED LIFE SUPPORT

In the event of a cardiac arrest, it is the nurse's first priority to call for help and commence basic life support (BLS) measures. Increasingly, nurses in both ward and high dependency areas are enhancing their skills to include advanced life support (ALS) techniques. Evidence suggests that the chances of a patient surviving are increased when defibrillation is implemented promptly (De Latorre et al 2001). It is now recommended that rapid defibrillation should take precedence over basic life support measures.

The majority of sudden deaths result from arrhythmias associated with acute myocardial infarction or chronic ischaemic heart disease. However, a significant number of 'arrests' also occur after medical interventions, such as line insertions or secondary to bleeding, as a result of trauma or surgery. The heart usually arrests in one of three rhythms:

- ventricular fibrillation (VF) or pulseless ventricular tachycardia (VT);
- asystole;
- pulseless electrical activity (PEA) – the presence of an electrical rhythm compatible with circulation but with no detectable cardiac output.

Successful resuscitation after cardiopulmonary arrest is most likely when the rhythm is VF or pulseless VT.

A cardiac arrest is usually unexpected and the ensuing events may easily become very chaotic. However, with high dependency patients in ward and specialist units, the level of monitoring may forewarn the nurse of changes in the patient's condition, enabling a potential arrest to be prevented or anticipated. The successful management of the situation requires an effective leader, and team members who are well rehearsed in basic and advanced life support skills. Nurses taking on expanded roles need first to be competent in BLS and have a good knowledge of arrhythmias associated with cardiac arrests (Inwood 1996). As studies have shown that the resuscitation skills of healthcare professionals are poor and that ability diminishes quickly over time (Cooper & Libby 1997, Young & King 2000), regular retraining and competence assessment are necessary.

> In the emergency of a cardiac arrest, nurses should not forget to be sensitive to the patient's family while being professional in a high-risk scenario.

During a cardiac arrest, nurses also need to be aware of their responsibility to the patient's family. Relatives may need to be telephoned and informed of the deterioration in the patient's condition. This should be done with sensitivity and a decision made about the exact extent of the information to be given based on the nurse's knowledge of the family. Relatives should be given realistic and honest information that enables them to decide how quickly and with whom to come to the hospital. If relatives are present when the patient arrests, they should not automatically be excluded from the ward or unit. There is increasing evidence, mainly from research carried out in accident and emergency departments, that many relatives find it beneficial to remain and witness the resuscitation (Royal College of Nursing 2002).

> Remember drugs that treat arrhythmias can also cause arrhythmias.

The UK and European Resuscitation Councils have produced standard guidelines for the management of a cardiac arrest (De Latorre et al 2001) including an algorithm to assist health professionals (Figure 6.9).

Figure 6.9 Advanced life support algorithm. (Reproduced with permission from De Latorre et al 2001, p. 213.)

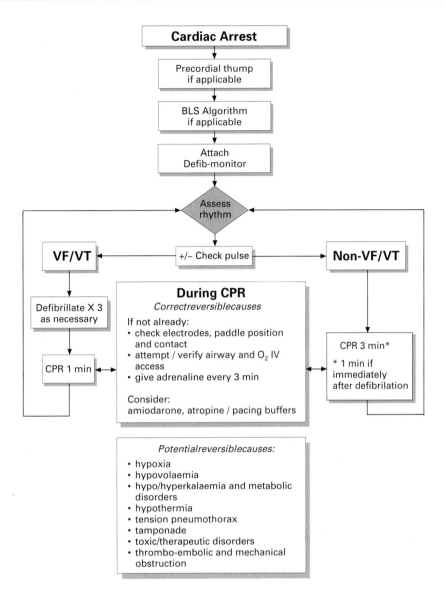

Although the initial drugs and dosages given during a cardiac arrest have been standardized, in a prolonged arrest, different inotropic and antiarrhythmic agents may be used (see Box 6.3 on page 130 and Box 6.9 on page 145).

CARING FOR THE PATIENT WITH CHEST PAIN

The prevalence rates for angina suggest that over 2 million people are living in the UK with a history of angina and an estimated 1.2 million people living in the UK have had a 'heart attack' at some time in their lives (Petersen et al 2004). Appropriate management of acute chest pain is essential to minimize the damage to the heart tissue and reduce the risk of death.

Chest pain is often referred to as being 'gripping' or 'tightening' in nature, and radiates to the arms, neck and jaw. Some patients (the elderly and those with diabetic neuropathy) may feel no pain and other symptoms have to be relied upon. This can lead to what is known as a 'silent infarction'. The chest pain usually comes on gradually (truly sudden-onset chest pain is more often associated with dissection of the aorta).

Breathlessness may occur as a result of exertion or at rest.

Light-headedness or syncope is a result of the reduction in cardiac output brought about by the inability of the heart to pump effectively without adequate oxygen supply. Some patients have reported these symptoms in the minutes leading up to a cardiac arrest.

Nausea is caused by congestion in the gastrointestinal tract following the diversion of blood to the vital structures.

Patients with chest pain require an immediate 12-lead ECG and cardiac enzyme tests in order to classify the acute coronary syndrome and to respond with appropriate early treatment. A 12-lead ECG recording is necessary as there is insufficient information from single monitoring leads. The ECG provides information about the area of ischaemia and myocardial damage present. The ECG will need to be performed promptly as part of the initial assessment of the patient's chest pain. It may need to be repeated every few minutes and will require repeating on subsequent episodes of chest pain. Therefore, it is important that nurses have the skills and ability to perform and accurately interpret the ECG (Quinn 1996). Generally speaking, ST segment depression suggests that there is ischaemia, whereas ST segment elevation is regarded as being an indication of an emerging myocardial infarction.

> Nurses should ensure accurate placement of chest and limb leads when recording a 12-lead ECG.

Pathophysiology

The build-up of fatty deposits in the coronary arteries (atherosclerosis) leads to the obstruction of blood flow and, therefore, a reduction of oxygen supply to the heart muscle. This imbalance between oxygen supply and demand causes pain.

Acute coronary syndromes are, most commonly, the result of a rupture of part of the atheromatous plaque that has built up in the coronary arteries. This causes a clot (thrombus) to be formed, at the site of lipid accumulation, which results in total (or near-total) blockage of the affected artery. The blood supply to this part of the heart is then reduced and tissue damage occurs. There are three levels of damage to the affected tissues:

- *ischaemia* – tissue damaged by lack of oxygen but potentially salvageable with an oxygen supply;
- *injury* – more jeopardized tissue but still potentially reversible;
- *infarction* – irreversible cell death.

STABLE ANGINA

Chest pain that occurs during exertion but is relieved by rest is termed 'stable angina'. The aim of care for these patients is to minimize the mismatch between the heart's oxygen demand and supply. In health, extra oxygen demands (e.g. as a result of exercise or anxiety) can be met by an increased supply of oxygen to the heart tissue. In angina, however, owing to the atherosclerotic changes causing narrowing of coronary blood vessels, the blood supply and, therefore, oxygen transport is reduced. Sufficient supply of oxygen to the heart tissue is thus not achieved. Attempts are made to address the imbalance by encouraging the patient to rest, giving oxygen and by the administration of a combination of medications. Typically, patients will have one or more of the following groups of drugs:

- vasodilators (Box 6.11; e.g. nitrates in intravenous, sublingual or sustained release tablet or patch form);
- beta-adrenergic blocking agents (e.g. atenolol);
- calcium-channel blockers (e.g. nifedipine);
- opiate analgesia (e.g. diamorphine).

ACUTE CORONARY SYNDROMES

There are three categories of acute coronary syndrome that represent the severity of coronary artery blockage, the causative mechanism of their chest pain:

1. unstable angina;
2. non-ST elevation myocardial infarction (NSTEMI); and
3. ST elevation myocardial infarction (STEMI).

Nurses caring for patients in acute care areas will be required to recognize the patient presenting with a myocardial event and, also, have an understanding of the diagnostic importance of ECG changes and diagnostic cardiac markers that may occur and the treatment required.

Unstable angina

This is characterized by chest pain, which usually manifests in one of the following ways:

- associated with exercise but increasing in frequency, and is initiated by less exercise over a few days;
- recurrent but short episodes of chest pain, not associated with exercise;
- a prolonged episode of chest pain without ECG or cardiac enzyme changes.

The ECG may be normal or show ST depression or T-wave inversion.

Box 6.11   Nitrates

Nitrates have been the mainstay in the treatment of angina for many years. Many different preparations have been developed to enable them to be used for treatment and prophylaxis, in oral, sublingual, transdermal and intravenous forms. They are also used intravenously in acute care settings to counteract hypertension and promote vasodilatation, e.g. after cardiac surgery.

Nitrates relax vascular smooth muscle, mainly in the venous system, and thus reduce pre-load to the heart.

Non–ST elevation myocardial infarction

In this case, a period of prolonged chest pain (greater than 20 minutes) is associated with raised cardiac markers and the ECG again shows ST depression or T-wave inversion. This is referred to as non-ST elevation myocardial infarction or non-Q wave myocardial infarction because these patients rarely develop Q waves on the ECG.

ST elevation myocardial infarction

Here the patient presents with prolonged chest pain, raised cardiac markers and ST elevation on the ECG. Over time, this ST elevation resolves and Q waves may appear (although less commonly with current treatment regimes). ST elevation myocardial infraction may also be referred to as *Q-wave myocardial infarction*. Figure 6.10 shows the typical sequence of changes in acute myocardial infarction. However, individual patients differ and any part or this entire spectrum may or may not be seen. Changes can occur over short periods of time, and highlight the dynamic and unstable nature of the patient. Box 6.12 indicates which leads of the ECG correspond to specific areas of the heart.

A rapid assessment of the patient that includes ECG monitoring, establishment of intravenous access, and the administration of diamorphine, oxygen, nitrates and aspirin form the initial treatment of all patients with chest pain (Box 6.13). The assessment should include consideration of the patient's condition and the environment. Patients must be nursed in a calm environment where they can be kept comfortable and avoid exertion. Further investigations will include blood tests for urea and electrolytes, glucose, cardiac markers and a full

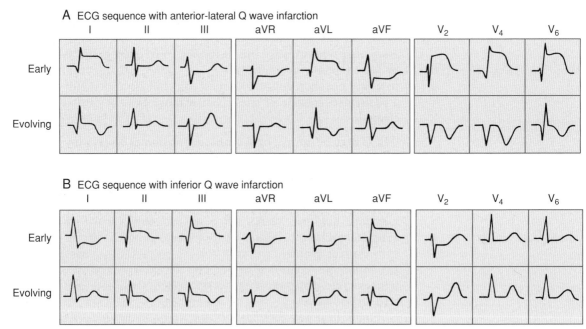

Figure 6.10 The sequence of ECG changes in myocardial infarction. (Reproduced from Braunwald et al 2001, Fig. 5-37, with permission from W B Saunders Co. After Goldberger 1999.)

Box 6.12   Identifying the area of infarction from the ECG

ECG changes indicating infarction will be seen in the leads lying over the area of damage.

Other leads may show mirror images or 'reciprocal changes' of these features, e.g. ST depression may be seen in the lead opposite to the area of infarction, where ST elevation is present.

Location of infarction	Leads showing changes
Anterior infarction	Some of the group V_{1-3}
Inferior infarction	II, III, aVF
Posterior infarction	V_1, V_2 but inverse of the usual changes. The images in V_1 and V_2 are reciprocal changes

---

Box 6.13   Immediate measures and nursing care in the treatment of a myocardial infarction

- Rapid assessment of the patient, e.g. shock, hypotension, signs of heart failure
- Establishment of intravenous access
- Continuous ECG monitoring
- Early thrombolysis, if not contraindicated, as soon as myocardial infarction is diagnosed

Morphine or diamorphine: repeated as necessary to control the pain, with an antiemetic, e.g. metoclopramide
Oxygen: in high concentration
Nitrates: glyceryl trinitrate (GTN) spray or sublingual tablet
Aspirin: 300 mg orally

- 12-lead ECG recording
- Portable chest X-ray
- Bloods for urgent urea and electrolytes, glucose, cardiac enzymes (e.g. troponin), full blood count and cholesterol levels
- Thrombolytic therapy (see Box 6.14)
- Calm and quiet environment, ensuring comfort and minimal exertion
- Explanations and reassurance to both patient and carers

---

blood count. A portable chest X-ray is also usually indicated to check on the size, shape and position of the heart. If ST elevation is present on the ECG (indicative of a ST elevation myocardial infarction), it is likely that thrombolytic therapy will be commenced (see Box 6.14). The patient may also have an echocardiogram to assess the left ventricular function.

CARDIAC MARKERS

Many substances are released from dead and dying cells. In cardiac muscle, four substances may be used to diagnose myocardial infarction:

- troponin;
- creatine phosphokinase (CPK or CK);
- lactate dehydrogenase (LDH);
- aspartate transaminase (AST), also known as serum glutamic oxaloacetic transaminase (SGOT).

Troponin is a sensitive marker for cardiac injury. It is a protein that is only released from cardiac cells and, unlike the other enzymes, is released by damaged as well as dead cells. The development of this marker has refined the management of patients who would have previously shown no raised cardiac enzymes. Troponin results are reported as positive or negative, and are used to provide both diagnostic and prognostic information that assist with risk stratification (Braunwald et al 2001).

Dead or damaged cardiac cells release the enzymes CK, AST and LDH; however, they are also released by skeletal cells where there is muscle damage and during vigorous exercise. Care needs to be taken when interpreting these enzyme results, as they may also be raised if the patient has had external chest compression (during cardiopulmonary resuscitation), intramuscular injections and/or surgery. Serial measurement of cardiac enzymes, such as CK, over 3 days following a cardiac event can give an indication of the amount of myocardial damage suffered. Under normal circumstances, these marker substances are only present in serum at low concentrations but this rises rapidly following cell death (Figure 6.11). Near-patient testing can be useful to speed up diagnosis and treatment. Nonetheless, it is important for nurses and doctors to ensure that blood/pathology test results are reviewed in a regular and timely manner.

THROMBOLYSIS

Thrombolytic therapy is the standard treatment for acute myocardial infarction [National Institute for Clinical Excellence (NICE) 2002]. The aim with this therapy is to unblock the coronary arteries and restore oxygen delivery to the heart muscle. For best effect, this must be done as soon as possible after the onset of symptoms. The criteria for administration of thrombolytic therapy relate to ST elevation, or the presence of new left bundle branch block on the ECG and absence of contraindications (Box 6.14).

MYOCARDIAL INFARCTION AFTERCARE

The aims of aftercare following an acute myocardial infarction (MI) are to minimize permanent damage to the heart, optimize cardiac function and promote the patient's return to normal activity. An integrated pathway of care, from presentation with chest pain to rehabilitation and secondary prevention, supports the seamless delivery of care to the patient with goals of risk stratification, intervention and flexibility to respond to individual needs.

Figure 6.11 Changes to enzyme levels after myocardial infarction. (Reproduced from Thompson 1997, p. 132, by kind permission of Churchill Livingstone.)

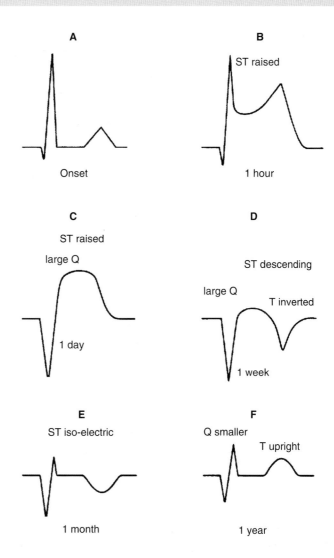

On the first day of admission, the priority of care is to establish an early diagnosis and initiate treatment (i.e. ECG, thrombolysis and analgesia, as appropriate). The patient will usually be kept on bedrest for about 24 hours to minimize cardiac workload. If pain-free after this time, early gentle mobilization will be encouraged to avoid the complications of bedrest (Jowett & Thompson 1995).

Medication post-MI usually includes aspirin, and beta-blockers should be initiated early in the post-MI phase and will usually be continued long term (NICE 2001). These drugs have been shown to reduce myocardial ischaemia and death in patients following myocardial infarction. ACE inhibitors (angiotensin-converting enzyme inhibitors) should also be initiated and titrated upwards, as tolerated, with close monitoring of renal function and blood pressure; these medicines have been shown to be beneficial for secondary prevention (Heart Outcome

---

Box 6.14   Thrombolytic therapy

Indications for thrombolysis

- ST segment elevation by two small squares (0.2 mV) in at least two adjacent chest leads
- ST segment elevation by one small square (0.1 mV) in at least two adjacent limb leads
- New left bundle branch block

Contraindications include

- Active bleeding
- Cerebrovascular accident (in the previous 6 months)
- Evidence or suspicion of aortic dissection

Thrombolytic agents are administered intravenously, some by bolus injection and others by infusion

- Streptokinase (infusion)
- Alteplase (complex infusion)
- Reteplase (bolus × 2)

Protection Study; HOPE Study Investigators 2000). The patient should also be prescribed a statin to assist with reducing serum cholesterol to less than 5 mmol/l (low-density lipoprotein to less than 3 mmol/l) or by 30%, whichever is the greatest (Hatchett & Thompson 2002).

By the second day, a risk-factor profile can be detailed and an action plan formulated to optimize patients' health promotion. Explanation about the rehabilitation following a myocardial infarction can begin in detail and be supported by patient information packs or leaflets. If patients have been pain free and haemodynamically stable for 24 hours, they will usually be allowed to sit in a chair. It is important that they understand that any episodes of pain or discomfort are to be reported to healthcare staff for investigation. Monitoring of vital signs will continue. Some patients may have an echocardiogram to assess left ventricular function.

Patients will gradually be reintroduced to exercise with walks to the toilet, building up to mobilization around the ward. Monitoring of the ECG will be discontinued subject to contraindications. Health promotion will be reinforced with lifestyle advice about smoking cessation, healthy eating, including a low-fat diet, alcohol intake and physical activity. Generally, patients will remain in hospital for 5–7 days following an uncomplicated myocardial infarction. Prior to discharge (this may be on day 5), patients may be given a 'modified Bruce exercise tolerance test' (ETT) to stratify risk and to look for signs of ongoing ischaemia. If positive, patients should be considered for angiography. They will continue on their prescribed medication and be given a supply of aspirin, a beta-blocker, ACE inhibitor and a statin to take home (where medications are not contraindicated).

In order to minimize the anxiety of patients and their family prior to discharge, it is important to ensure that patients understand specific short-term rehabilitation advice. Patients should expect to increase their participation in daily tasks progressively over a 4–6-week period, e.g. housework, avoiding heavy lifting for at least 6 weeks. Daily walking is to be encouraged, starting with trips to the bathroom (accompanied on stairs) and building up each day. Sexual activity should be avoided for 2–4 weeks and driving a car is prohibited for at least 4 weeks (patients should inform their insurer). Returning to work may be possible after 6 weeks if the job is light but may take 8–12 weeks for heavy manual work. A 6-week outpatient appointment and an invitation to the cardiac rehabilitation programme (exercise programme, lifestyle advice and support) will follow the patient's progress to normal living.

CONCLUSION

Cardiovascular disease remains a significant burden in the UK despite a reduction in deaths from heart disease over the last 5 years. Public health measures to encourage healthier lifestyles should continue this trend, and it is the role of all health professionals to promote optimum health and lifestyle options to patients, for example, diet, weight loss (where appropriate), exercise, smoking cessation, stress management, etc.

Nurses caring for patients with cardiovascular disease can continue to improve patient care by being equipped with the necessary skills to optimize patient outcomes. This will include the translation of government strategies, such as the National Service Framework for Coronary Heart Disease (Department of Health 2000), into care for patients.

References

Braunwald E, Zipes D, Libby P 2001 Heart disease, a textbook of cardiovascular medicine, 6th edn. WB Saunders, London

British National Formulary 2004 British Medical Association & Royal Pharmaceutical Society of Great Britain, London

British Vascular Foundation 2003 Conditions explained (http://www.bvf.org.uk/cond_explained.htm), accessed 10.3.03

Cooper S, Libby J 1997 A review of educational issues in resuscitation training. Journal of Clinical Nursing 6: 5–10

De Latorre F, Nolan J, Robertson C, Chamberlain D, Baskett P 2001 European Resuscitation Council guidelines for advanced life support. Resuscitation 48: 211–221

Department of Health 2000 National service framework for coronary heart disease. The Stationery Office, London

Department of Health 2004 National service framework for coronary heart disease. Winning the war on heart disease. Progress report. Department of Health Publications, London

Goldberger AL 1999 Clinical electrocardiography: a simplified approach, 6th edn. CV Mosby, St Louis

Guyton A C, Hall J E 1996 Textbook of medical physiology, 9th edn. W B Saunders, Philadelphia

Hartshorn J C, Sole M L, Lamborn M L 1997 Essential components for invasive monitoring using the brachial approach. Introduction to critical care nursing, 2nd edn. WB Saunders Co, London: 94

Hatchett R, Thompson D 2002 Cardiac nursing. a comprehensive guide. Churchill Livingstone, Edinburgh: 178

Hinchliff S M, Montague S E, Watson R 1996 Physiology for nursing practice, 2nd edn. Baillière Tindall, London

HOPE Study Investigators 2000 Effects of an angiotensin-converting enzyme inhibitor, Ramipril, on cardiovascular events in high-risk patients. New England Journal of Medicine 342: 145–153

Inwood H 1996 Knowledge of resuscitation. Intensive and Critical Care Nursing 12: 33–39

Jowett N I, Thompson D R 1995 Comprehensive coronary care, 2nd edn. Scutari Press, London

Lab Tests Online (www.labtestonline.org), accessed 21.3.03

National Institute for Clinical Excellence 2001 Prophylaxis for patients who have experienced a myocardial infarction. Inherited Clinical Guideline A. NICE, London.

National Institute for Clinical Excellence 2002 Guidance on the use of drugs for early thrombolysis in the treatment of acute myocardial infarction. Technology Appraisal Guidance no. 52. NICE, London

Nurse's Ready Reference 1992 Quick ECG interpretation. Springhouse Corporation, Pennsylvania

Park G R, Roe P G 2000 Fluid balance and volume resuscitation for beginners. Greenwich Medical Media Ltd, London

Petersen S, Peto V, Rayner M 2004 Coronary heart disease statistics. (http://www.heartstats.org), accessed 30.6.04. British Heart Foundation, London

Quinn T 1996 Myocardial infarction: the role of the nurse. Nursing Times 92(6 Suppl): 5–8

Resuscitation Council UK 2001 Advanced life support course provider manual, 4th edn. Resuscitation Council UK & ERC, London

Royal College of Nursing (RCN) 2002 Witnessing resuscitation. RCN, London

Singer M 1996 Better monitoring = better management: improved monitoring leads to more appropriate interventions. British Journal of Intensive Care 6(1): 24–32

Smith G 2000 ALERT™ course manual. University of Portsmouth, Portsmouth

Swan H J C, Ganz W, Forrester J S et al 1970 Catheterization of the heart in man with the use of a flow-directed balloon catheter. New England Journal of Medicine 283: 447–451

Thompson P L (ed.) 1997 Typical serum activity curves for biochemical markers after AMI. In: Coronary care manual. Churchill Livingstone, London: 132

Thompson D R, Webster R A 1992 Caring for the coronary patient. Butterworth-Heinemann, Oxford

Young R, King L 2000 An evaluation of knowledge and skill retention following an in-house advanced life support course. Nursing in Critical Care 5: 7–14.

Zoll P M, Zoll R H 1985 Non-invasive temporary cardiac stimulation. Critical Care Medicine 13: 925–926

Further reading

Houghton A R, Gray D 1999 Making sense of the ECG. Arnold, London

Iqbal Z, Chambers R, Woodmansy P 2001 Implementing the national service framework for coronary framework in heart disease in primary care. Radcliffe Medical Press, Abingdon

Shuldham C 1998 Cardiorespiratory nursing. Stanley Thornes, Cheltenham

Wagner G S 2001 Marriott's practical electrocardiography, 10th edn. Lippincott, Williams & Wilkins, London

Woods S L, Sivarajan Froelicher E S, Underhill Motzer S 2000 Cardiac nursing, 4th edn. Lippincott, Williams & Wilkins, Philadelphia

Useful internet sites

American Heart Association: www.americanheart.org
British Heart Foundation: www.bhf.org.uk/professionals/i
British Heart Foundation statistics site: www.heartstats.org

British Vascular Foundation: www.bvf.org.uk
Lab Test Online: www.labtestonline.org
Resuscitation Council UK: www.resus.org.uk

Chapter 7

Neurological care

Deborah Dawson and Sarah Shah

KEY LEARNING OBJECTIVES

- To provide a broad overview of the anatomy and physiology of the nervous system, and to relate that anatomy and physiology to pathophysiology
- To discuss the assessment of patients with neurological conditions
- To discuss the management of neurological conditions commonly requiring high dependency care
- To provide an overview of the common medications used in those conditions

INTRODUCTION

The human brain is by far the most complex structure in the known universe.
(Thompson 1993)

This quotation could be extended to include the whole nervous system, and it is that element of the unknown that ensures that the study and care of patients with neurological problems are both challenging and rewarding. The challenge includes the quick recognition of acute events and the unravelling of information to uncover the chronic condition. This chapter explores the care of patients with neurological pathology who might require high dependency care. It describes the assessment of these patients, and the care and medicines they may require. In order to care for them, it is important to have an understanding of the anatomy and physiology of the nervous system, so this is where we start.

ORGANIZATION OF THE NERVOUS SYSTEM

Prerequisite anatomy and physiology

- The neuron;
- the nerve impulse including saltatory conduction;
- electrical and chemical synapses;
- neurotransmitters;
- the skull and facial bones;
- the peripheral nervous system.

The nervous system is generally divided into two main functional units: the central nervous system (CNS) and the peripheral nervous system (PNS). The central nervous system consists of the brain and the spinal cord: these process new sensory information and combine that information with previous experience to provide appropriate motor responses. The peripheral nervous system consists of the cranial and spinal nerves, and their associated ganglia, which convey nerve impulses to and from the brain and the spinal cord.

THE BRAIN (ENCEPHALON)

The brain consists of three main areas: the cerebrum, the cerebellum and the brainstem. The major structures within these divisions are summarized in Box 7.1.

The cerebrum

The cerebrum consists of two cerebral hemispheres, which are partially separated by the longitudinal fissure and connected by the corpus callosum. The cerebrum is divided into dominant and non-dominant hemispheres. In approximately 90% of the population the dominant hemisphere is the left. The left side of the brain has been shown to control the right side of the body (spoken and written language, scientific reasoning and numerical skills), whereas the right side is more concerned with emotion and artistic and creative skills. However, at birth, the hemispheres are of equal ability, and very early injury to one side or another usually results in skills being acquired by the opposite side of the brain.

The surface area of the brain, the cerebral cortex (grey matter), is much increased by the presence of gyri (folds) and sulci (dips), resulting in

---

Box 7.1   The major structures of the brain

Cerebrum	Cerebellum	Brainstem
Cerebral hemispheres		Midbrain
Corpus callosum		Pons
Basal ganglia		Medulla
Diencephalon		
Hypophysis		

a 3:1 proportion of grey to white matter (Figure 7.1). 'White matter' refers to the areas that contain nerve processes, usually axons, which are frequently myelinated, that contain a high proportion of fat, hence the white colour, and 'grey matter' refers to areas that contain neuronal cell bodies. The cerebral hemispheres are divided into four lobes, the frontal, parietal, temporal and occipital, by the lateral sulcus (sylvian fissure) and the central sulcus (rolandic fissure). Box 7.2 summarizes the main functions of the lobes.

The diencephalon is located deep into the cerebrum, the major components being the thalamus and the hypothalamus. It connects the midbrain to the cerebral hemispheres. The thalamus is the relay and processing centre for all sensory information except smell. The hypothalamus is responsible for autonomic regulation, including temperature, appetite, blood pressure, sleep, thirst and emotional regulation; endocrine control, including glucostatic and hormonal regulation through the pituitary gland (hypophysis); and is the point where the two optic tracts cross (optic chiasma). Within the cerebral hemispheres are a number of masses of motor nuclei: the caudate nucleus, the putamen and the globus pallidus, collectively referred to as the basal ganglia or corpus striatum. The basal ganglia assist in the motor control of fine body movements by relaying information via the thalamus to the motor cortex in the cerebrum. Parkinson's disease, characterized by akinesia, rigidity and a resting tremor, and Huntington's disease, causing dyskinesia, are disorders of the basal ganglia. The cerebrum is divided from the cerebellum and brainstem by the tentorium cerebelli, which is an extension of the dura mater.

Figure 7.1 The surface area of the brain. (Reproduced from FitzGerald & Folan-Curran 2002 by kind permission of W B Saunders.)

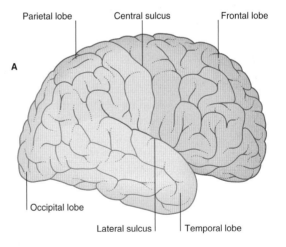

| Parietal lobe | Central sulcus | Frontal lobe |

A

Occipital lobe

Lateral sulcus | Temporal lobe

Box 7.2	The functions of the cerebral cortex by lobe		
Frontal	**Parietal**	**Temporal**	**Occipital**
Motor	Sensation	Auditory	Visual
Expression	Spatial	Equilibrium	
Moral		Interpretive	
		Intellectual	

The cerebellum

How might the symptoms of cerebellar dysfunction affect normal life?

The cerebellum is situated behind the pons and is attached to the midbrain, pons and medulla by three paired cerebellar peduncles. It consists of two lateral hemispheres, which are divided into three parts – the grey matter, the cortex and the white matter, which forms the connecting pathways for impulses joining the cerebellum with other parts of the central nervous system – and four pairs of deep cerebellar nuclei, which connect with the cerebellar cortex and with nuclei in the brainstem and thalamus. The cerebellum is the processing centre for coordination of muscular movements, balance, precision, timing and body positions. It does not initiate any movements and is not involved with the conscious perception of sensations. Disorders of the cerebellum, such as a tumour or cerebrovascular accident, may result in jerky movement, diminished reflexes, ataxia, slurring of speech, nystagmus and tremors. Symptoms of cerebellar dysfunction can be seen following overindulgence in alcohol! The symptoms occur on the same side as the lesion owing to impulses crossing in both the midbrain and lower medulla.

The brainstem

The brainstem is the connection between the cerebrum and the spinal cord, and is continuous with the diencephalon above and the spinal cord below. The brainstem has three main functions:

- it acts as a conduit for the ascending and descending pathways between the spinal cord and parts of the brain;
- all cranial nerves, except the olfactory and optic, emerge from the brainstem (Figure 7.2);
- it contains important reflex centres associated with respiration, the cardiovascular system and consciousness.

It is formed from three main structures: the midbrain, pons and medulla oblongata. The midbrain is the upper end of the brainstem, and connects the pons and cerebellum to the cerebrum. It arises from a small rigid opening of the tentorium cerebelli, which makes it vulnerable to trauma.

Figure 7.2 Brainstem, dorsal view. (Reproduced from Carola et al 1990, p 369.)

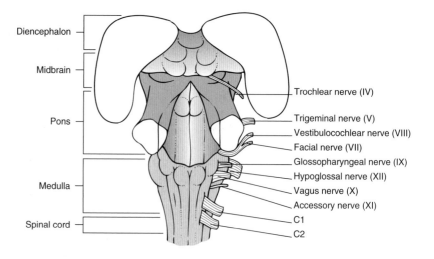

It is involved with visual reflexes: the oculomotor (III) and the trochlear (IV) cranial nerves arise from the midbrain. The oculomotor nerve controls the movement of the eyeball and eyelid, focusing and dilation of the pupils, and the trochlear nerve controls downward and outward eye movement. Damage to the parasympathetic nucleus of the oculomotor nerve produces a dilated pupil that does not react to light; this may indicate local damage or be a more sinister sign of global damage to the brainstem. Contained within the midbrain is a cavity called the cerebral aquaduct. This is a narrow channel connecting the third with the fourth ventricle. Compression of the cerebral aquaduct may cause hydrocephalus, an abnormal increase in the volume of cerebrospinal fluid within the brain.

The pons is located between the midbrain and the medulla oblongata, and serves as a relay station from the medulla to higher structures in the brain. The trigeminal (V), abducens (VI), facial (VII) and vestibulocochlear (VIII) cranial nerves arise from the pons. The trigeminal nerve controls mastication and facial sensation, the abducens enables abduction of the eye, the facial allows movement of the facial muscles, lacrimation, taste and salivation, and the vestibulocochlear is responsible for hearing and equilibrium. Damage by trauma, haemorrhage or a tumour will cause symptoms associated with the functions of these nerves.

The lowermost portion of the brainstem is the medulla oblongata. This connects the pons and the spinal cord; motor fibres cross from one side of the medulla to the other and this is known as the point of decussation of the pyramidal tract. In the deeper structures of the medulla are found the vital centres associated with autonomic reflex activity. These are the cardiac, respiratory and vasomotor centres, and the reflex centres of coughing, swallowing, vomiting and sneezing. The control of respiration is mainly found in the medulla and is regulated by the dorsal and ventral respiratory nuclei. The dorsal respiratory nucleus responds to carbon dioxide levels in the blood and enables the inspiratory part of the respiratory cycle, having an effect on the diaphragm, intercostal and accessory muscles. The ventral respiratory nucleus enables expiration. The glossopharyngeal (IX), vagus (X), accessory (XI) and hypoglossal (XII) nerves arise from the medulla oblongata. The glossopharyngeal nerve is responsible for taste and secretion of saliva. In conjunction with the vagus nerve, it is also involved with swallowing, respiration (they monitor oxygen and carbon dioxide levels in the blood) and blood pressure. The vagus nerve itself controls heart rate and innervates the smooth muscle of the lungs, pharynx, larynx and digestive system. The accessory nerve enables movement of the head and shoulders and voice production, and the hypoglossal controls movement of the tongue and swallowing.

The reticular formation is a complex of neurons that extend throughout the brainstem. It receives information from most of the sensory systems and it influences a wide range of activities including skeletal muscles, somatic and visceral sensation, the autonomic and endocrine systems, the biological clock and the reticular activating system. The reticular activating system (RAS) is responsible for arousal and level of consciousness. Sensory stimuli pass through the RAS, which in turn sends information to various parts of the cerebral cortex effecting conscious level.

The limbic system forms a border around the brainstem, which is important in the sensation and visceral response to emotions and for memory. Damage to the hippocampus, which is part of the limbic system, causes amnesia.

ASSOCIATED STRUCTURES

The meninges

The brain and the spinal cord are encased by three layers of membrane: the dura mater, the arachnoid mater and the pia mater, known collectively as the meninges (Figure 7.3).

The *dura mater* is a tough fibrous layer of tissue, which is generally fused with the periosteum, the lining of the skull, where it is not fused; these layers form the sinuses that drain venous blood from the brain. There are two folds of dura mater that extend into the cranial cavity to stabilize the brain; these are the falx cerebri and the tentorium cerebelli.

The *arachnoid mater*, in total contrast to the dura mater, is a fine serous membrane that loosely covers the brain. There is a potential space between this and the inner dura mater, known as the subdural space. Between the arachnoid mater and the pia mater is an actual space, known as the subarachnoid space; this contains the arachnoid villi, cerebrospinal fluid (CSF) and small arterial blood vessels.

The *pia mater* follows the convolutions formed by the gyri and sulci, and is attached to the surface of the brain. It consists of fine connective tissue, housing the majority of the blood supply to the brain.

The ventricles and cerebrospinal fluid

Within the brain there are four connected cavities called ventricles, which are lined with ependymal cells and contain cerebrospinal fluid. There are two lateral ventricles, the third ventricle and the fourth ventricle. The lateral ventricles lie one in each cerebral hemisphere, the third in the diencephalons and the fourth between the pons and cerebellum. The lateral ventricles are connected to the third ventricle by the interventricular foramen, sometimes known as the foramen of Munro, and

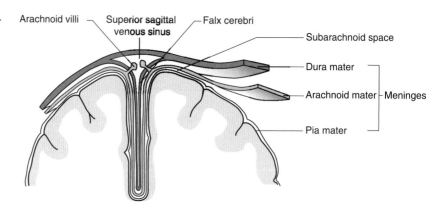

Figure 7.3 Cranial meninges. (Adapted from Hickey 1997, p. 46.)

> **Box 7.3   The blood–brain barrier**
>
> The blood–brain barrier protects the brain and maintains homeostasis. It is a diffusion barrier between the brain and vasculature, and the substance of the brain formed by tight junctions between capillary endothelial cells. The brain is further protected by an alliance between astrocytes and the capillary endothelial cells. This ensures that only certain substances can enter the brain.
>
> Water, carbon dioxide and oxygen pass readily through the blood–brain barrier, whereas glucose, which is the primary source of metabolic energy for nervous tissue, requires a lipid transporter. This can be a problem for clinicians attempting to deliver drugs to the brain.

the third ventricle is connected to the fourth by the cerebral aqueduct, sometimes known as the aqueduct of Sylvius (Figure 7.4). Ependymal cells assist in the circulation of CSF by the movement of their cilia, transport chemical substances from the CSF to the pituitary, and produce and secrete CSF from the choroid plexuses.

CSF is a clear colourless fluid composed of water, some protein, oxygen, carbon dioxide, sodium, potassium, chloride and glucose. CSF has several functions (Snell 2001):

- cushioning and protecting the CNS from trauma;
- providing mechanical buoyancy and support for the brain;
- serving as a reservoir and assisting in the regulation of the contents of the skull;
- nourishing the CNS;
- removing metabolites from the CNS;
- serving as a pathway for pineal secretions to reach the pituitary gland.

Figure 7.4 Ventricles of the brain, and circulatory path of cerebrospinal fluid through the cranial pathways. (Reproduced from Carola et al 1990, p 368.)

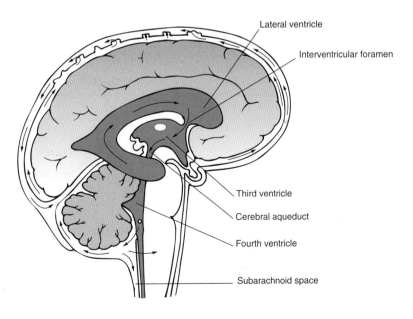

Lateral ventricle

Interventricular foramen

Third ventricle

Cerebral aqueduct

Fourth ventricle

Subarachnoid space

The major source of CSF is from the secretions of the choroid plexus, found in the ventricles. The choroid plexus produces approximately 500 ml of CSF daily, although the average adult brain only holds between 125 and 150 ml. CSF is renewed and replaced approximately three times daily, being reabsorbed through the arachnoid villi, which drain into the superior sagittal sinus, when the CSF pressure exceeds the venous pressure. Normal CSF pressure is 60–180 mm water in the lumbar puncture position (lateral recumbant) and 200–350 mm water in the sitting position.

Cerebral circulation

Cerebrovascular disease is the leading cause of neurological disability and the third leading cause of death in adults (FitzGerald Folan-Curran 2002); its diverse presentation requires an understanding of the cerebral circulation as well as cerebral anatomy. The brain is supplied with blood by four major arteries: two internal carotid, which supply most of the cerebrum and both eyes; and two vertebral, which supply the cerebellum, brainstem and the posterior part of the cerebrum (Figure 7.5). Before the blood enters the cerebrum, it passes through the circle of Willis, which is a circular shunt at the base of the brain consisting of the posterior cerebral, the posterior communicating, the internal carotid, the anterior cerebral and the anterior communicating arteries. These vessels are frequently anomalous; however, they allow for an adequate blood supply to all parts of the brain, even if one or more is ineffective (Figure 7.6).

The venous drainage from the brain does not follow a similar pathway. Cerebral veins empty into large venous sinuses located in the folds of the dura mater: bridging veins connect the brain and the dural sinuses and are often the cause of subdural haematomas. These sinuses

Figure 7.5 Major arteries of the head and neck: lateral view. (Reproduced From Carola et al 1990, p 368.)

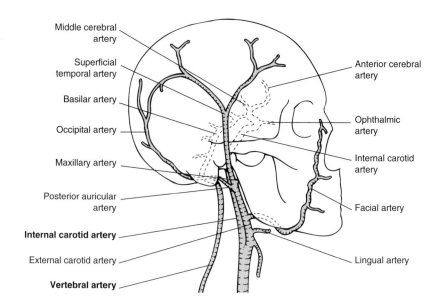

Figure 7.6 Major arteries of the head and neck: ventral view. (Reproduced from Carola et al 1990, p 587.)

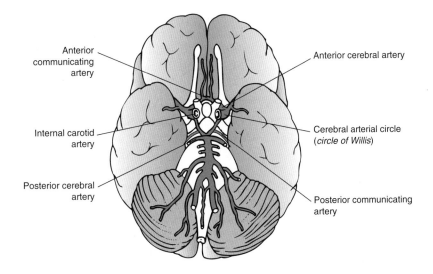

Anterior communicating artery

Anterior cerebral artery

Internal carotid artery

Cerebral arterial circle (*circle of Willis*)

Posterior cerebral artery

Posterior communicating artery

Figure 7.7 Major veins of the head and neck. (Reproduced from Carola et al 1990, p 591.)

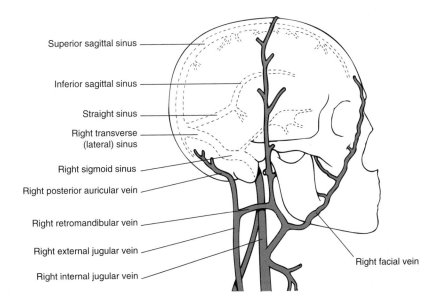

Superior sagittal sinus

Inferior sagittal sinus

Straight sinus

Right transverse (lateral) sinus

Right sigmoid sinus

Right posterior auricular vein

Right retromandibular vein

Right external jugular vein

Right internal jugular vein

Right facial vein

empty into the internal jugular veins, which sit on either side of the neck and return the blood to the heart via the brachiocephalic veins (Figure 7.7).

The brain – especially the grey matter – has an extensive capillary bed, requiring approximately 15–20% of the total resting cardiac output, about 750 ml/minute. Glucose, required for metabolism in the brain, requires about 20% of the total oxygen consumed in the body for its oxidation. Blood flow to specific areas of the brain correlates directly to the metabolism of the cerebral tissue. Blood flow in the cerebral vessels is controlled by autoregulation, by chemical or pressure response. Smooth muscle tone in the vessels is affected by levels of carbon dioxide in the blood. High levels of carbon dioxide result in vasodilation and reduced levels cause vasoconstriction. This response is supported by a myogenic response to intraluminal pressure, which maintains a steady perfusion of the brain in the range of 80–180 mmHg.

Spinal cord

The spinal cord is continuous with the medulla oblongata: it extends from the superior border of the first cervical vertebra (atlas) to the upper border of the second lumbar vertebra. The cone-shaped lower end of the spinal cord becomes the conus terminalis, located at the first lumbar vertebra (L1), which in turn becomes the filum terminale, consisting mainly of fibrous connective tissue. The cord is about 1 cm in diameter, except for two areas, the cervical and lumbosacral enlargements, from which the 31 pairs of spinal nerves emerge. The spinal nerves that emerge below the conus terminalis (L1) are known as the

Figure 7.8 The spinal cord and spinal nerves, and their relation to the vertebral column. (Reproduced from Carola et al 1990, p 337.)

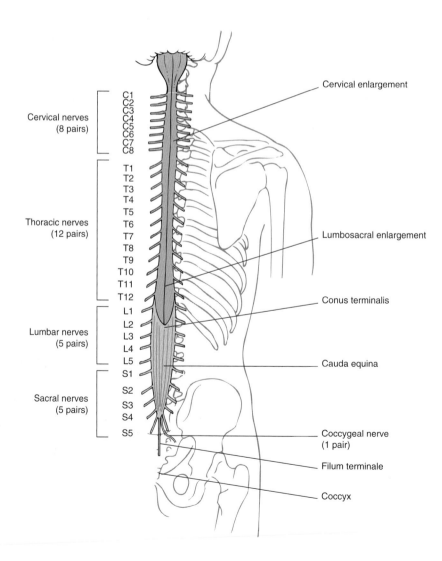

cauda equina. Figure 7.8 shows the spinal cord and nerves in relation to the vertebral column.

The cord is surrounded by the three layers of the meninges: pia, arachnoid and dura. Cerebrospinal fluid flows through the central canal – this is continuous with the fourth ventricle. The spinal cord has two functions. Firstly, it acts as a relay station between the peripheral nervous system and the brain, and secondly, as an activating centre in its own right, taking incoming sensory impulses and initiating outgoing motor signals, as in the reflex arc.

The spinal cord is composed of two layers: the outer white matter and the inner grey matter (this is the opposite to the brain where the grey matter is outermost). The white matter consists of mainly myelinated axons, and the cell body of these fibres can be in either the brain or the spinal cord. The grey matter consists of neurons and synapses. It is shaped like a letter 'H', which can be divided into three functional areas. The dorsal (posterior) horns carry sensory impulses, the ventral (anterior) horns carry motor impulses, and the middle zone undertakes association functions between the dorsal and ventral horns of the same and opposite sides (Figure 7.9).

> Think about the physiological effects of a whiplash injury, which normally affects the high cervical area.

NEUROLOGICAL ASSESSMENT

> What different challenges would be encountered when undertaking a neurological assessment of:
>
> - A sedated patient?
> - An uncooperative patient?
> - A patient who had suffered multiple trauma?

The spinal cord is protected by the spinal column. This is composed of 33 vertebrae, seven cervical, 12 thoracic, five lumbar, five sacral and the four fused bones of the coccyx.

Neurological assessment provides both the basic tool for diagnosis of neurological deficit and the means for measuring progress. It also provides a common language for clinicians to communicate symptoms and changes in condition. It is, therefore, essential that it is completed accurately, with any uncertainties communicated. This will ensure timely and appropriate patient care. Consciousness is defined by two functions:

Figure 7.9 A cross-section of the spinal cord.

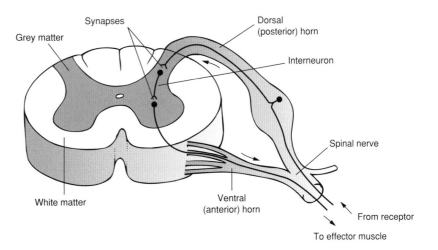

Table 7.1 Effects of the autonomic nervous system

Activity	Sympathetic	Parasympathetic
Heart rate	Increased	Decreased
Blood pressure	Increased	Decreased
Cardiac output	Increased	Decreased
Blood vessels in cardiac muscles	Dilated	Constricted
Blood vessels in abdomen and skin	Constricted	No effect
Blood vessels in skeletal muscles	Dilated	No effect
Respiratory rate	Increased	Decreased
Bronchioles	Dilated	Constricted
Blood sugar	Increased	No effect
Peristalsis (gastrointestinal)	Decreased	Increased
Bladder sphincters	Contracted	Relaxed
Sweat	Increased	No effect
Adrenals	Adrenaline and noradrenaline secretion	No effect
Pupils	Dilated	Constricted

Table 7.2 Functions of cranial nerves

Number	Name	Type	Function
I	Olfactory	Sensory	Smell
II	Optic	Sensory	Vision
III	Oculomotor	Motor	Movement of eyeball, elevation of upper eyelid, constriction of pupil, focusing of lens
IV	Trochlear	Motor	Downward and outward eye movements
V	Trigeminal	Mixed	Mastication, sensory regulation of ophthalmic, maxillary and mandibular areas
VI	Abducens	Motor	Abduction of eye
VII	Facial	Mixed	Taste, salivation, lacrimation, movement of facial muscles
VIII	Acoustic	Sensory	Hearing, equilibrium
IX	Glossopharyngeal	Mixed	Taste, secretion of saliva, swallowing
X	Vagus	Mixed	Swallowing, monitors blood levels of O_2 and CO_2, blood pressure regulation
XI	Accessory	Motor	Voice production, movement of head and shoulders
XII	Hypoglossal	Motor	Movement of tongue during speech, swallowing

- awareness or cognition (content of consciousness);
- arousal (level of consciousness).

These are determined by separate physiological processes. Coma is a disorder of arousal and depends on an intact ascending reticular activating system and diencephalon; whereas a persistent vegetative state is a disorder of awareness, which requires an intact cerebral cortex (Bateman 2001).

A complete neurological assessment should include:

- arousal;
- cranial nerves function;
- motor function;
- sensory function;
- pupillary reaction;
- vital signs;

but should not be independent of a history and a full general physical examination (Bateman 2001).

The neurological assessment should be completed on admission and thereafter at regular intervals to determine the patient's condition, although it may not be appropriate in an emergency situation. This type of full assessment would usually be performed by a clinician with neurological experience. Commonly, a reduced neurological assessment is performed, which includes:

- arousal;
- motor function;
- pupillary signs;
- vital signs.

In practice, this requires an assessment of the Glasgow Coma Scale (activity, awareness and arousal), a limb assessment (motor function), a pupil assessment and cardiorespiratory observations.

Glasgow Coma Scale

The Glasgow Coma Scale (GCS) was developed in 1974 by Teasdale & Jennett (Box 7.4). It forms a quick, objective and easily interpreted mode of neurological assessment, avoiding subjective terminology such as 'stupor', 'semi-coma' and 'deep coma'. The GCS records what you see, measuring arousal, awareness and activity by assessing eye opening (E), verbal response (V) and motor ability (M). Each activity is allocated a score, thus enabling objectivity, ease of recording and comparison between recordings. It also provides useful information for patient outcome prediction. The score is from 15 (fully conscious) to 3 (no response). The GCS arbitrarily defines consciousness as E2, V2, M4 (Bateman 2001).

As a stimulus is applied, it is good practice to commence with light pressure and increase to elicit a response. There is debate as to whether it is better to use a peripheral stimulus, for example, a pen pressed into the side of a finger near the nail (never press into the nailbed, as this can cause the nails to die) or whether to apply central pressure. A central stimulus can be applied in the following three ways (Shah 1999).

- *Trapezium squeeze*; this is least likely to cause any local injury and should be applied when ever possible. It is applied by using the thumb and two fingers, 2 inches of the trapezius muscle, where the head meets the shoulder are held and then twisted.

Box 7.4   Glasgow Coma Scale

Eye opening

4 **Spontaneously** This is when the patient's eyes open without stimulation of any sort.
3 **To speech** The patient's eyes open to verbal stimulation, which may need to be repeated, but no physical stimulation is required.
2 **To pain** The patient's eyes open either to vigorous shaking or following the application of a painful stimulus.
1 **None** The patient's eyes do not open, even with persistent verbal or adequate painful stimuli.

Verbal response

5 **Orientated** Patients are able to tell the assessor with complete accuracy the date, where they are and who they are.
4 **Sentences** The patient is not orientated, but formulates a full sentence or sentences. These may be inappropriate.
3 **Words** The response from the patient is restricted to words that are comprehensible, but may be inappropriate.
2 **Sounds** The patient makes sounds that are not recognizable as words.
1 **None** No sound is made by the patient in response to either verbal or painful stimuli.
    The patient may have difficulty in speaking (dysphasia). If so, the letter 'D' should be put in the 'none' column. If the patient is intubated, then the letter 'T' should be put in the 'none' column.

Motor response

6 **Obeys commands** The patient follows simple instructions, such as 'hold up your arms' or 'squeeze *and* release my hands'.
5 **Localizing** The patient raises his hands at least to chin level, in response to a stimulus applied above that level.
4 **Normal flexion** The patient's arms bend at the elbow in response to a painful stimulus, without rotation at the wrist.
3 **Abnormal flexion** The patient's arms bend at the elbow, the forearm rotates and the wrist is flexed, in response to a painful stimulus.
2 **Extension** The patient's arm straightens at the elbow and rotates towards the body, while the wrist flexes, in response to a painful stimulus.
1 **None** There is no response following the application of a deeply painful stimulus.
If the patient is receiving medicines to maintain muscle paralysis, record the letter 'P' in the 'none' column.

- *Supraorbital pressure*; this is applied by running a finger along the supraorbital margin – the bony ridge along the top of the eye – until a notch or groove can be felt. If pressure is applied here, it causes pain in the form of a headache. This is not recommended if the patient has facial fractures. Supraorbital pressure can make the patient grimace, leading to a closed eye rather than eye opening.
- *Sternal rub*; this is applied by grinding the centre of the sternum using the knuckles of a clenched fist. Assessment of motor function using sternal rub as painful stimuli is not ideal. The patient will not localize to the source of the pain correctly and the response could be confused with flexion to pain. Localizing to a painful stimuli requires the patient to move their arm to chin level.

However, it is the nurse who must decide the most appropriate stimulus for the situation. Applying central stimuli will always provide the most accurate response and should be used at all times when there is uncertainty, but mildly drowsy patients will not thank you for waking them up with a sternal rub!

Eye response

This shows that arousal mechanisms in the brainstem are intact. The best response is eye opening spontaneously; if the patient has their eyes closed, then their state of arousal can be assessed by the degree of stimulation required for them to open their eyes. Initially, this would be by using a verbal stimulus, saying their name and gradually repeating the stimulus and, finally, speaking in a louder voice (Shah 1999). If there is no response to a verbal stimulus, then a painful stimulus is applied as described above.

Verbal response

The verbal response measures awareness or cognition. For patients to be fully orientated, they must be able to report who they are, where they are and why they are there (Teasdale & Jennett 1974, Aucken & Crawford 1998). It is important to note that the verbal response may be affected by dysphasia. Dysphasia is a disorder of the comprehension and expression of speech (Bannister 1992). These are generally seen as distinct clinical symptoms; comprehension, which is sensory dysphasia, is often called receptive dysphasia and is due to damage in the Wernicke's speech centre. Here the patient is unable to comprehend what is being said to them. Expressive dysphasia is a motor disorder and is due to damage in the Broca's speech centre; in this case, patients are unable to respond appropriately to the spoken word (Shah 1999).

Motor response

Always record the best arm response. There is no need to record left and right differences – the GCS is not aiming to measure focal deficit, as this should be completed in the limb assessment. Within the GCS, there is no reason to measure leg response, as this may be measuring a spinal rather than a brain-initiated response.

When recording the GCS, it is important to record the individual scores as well as the total score (i.e. E2 V3 M4; GCS = 9), the motor response being the most reflective for determining prognosis. The GCS may be misleading in patients who have a high cervical injury or brainstem lesion, or who are hypoxic, haemodynamically shocked, fitting or post-ictal. These patients may be unable to move their limbs or show no responses at all. It is important to attempt to assess the spinal patient using facial movements, being aware of the possibility of a combined head and neck injury. Patients who show no response should be re-evaluated following correction of any shock or hypoxia.

Limb assessment

A limb assessment is useful to assess for focal damage; however, although it is usual for a hemiparesis or hemiplegia to occur on the opposite (contralateral) side to the lesion, it may occur on the same (ipsilateral) side. This is due to indentation of the contralateral cerebral peduncle and is known as a false localizing. Spontaneous movements are observed for equality: if there is little or no spontaneous movement, then painful stimuli must be applied to each limb in turn, comparing the result. It is most appropriate to complete this while assessing the motor component of the GCS. This may help in determining the site of the focal damage (Figure 7.10). Decerebrate rigidity is associated with bilateral extension of upper and lower limbs. This is usually due to a midbrain or pontine lesion. Decorticate posturing is associated with bilateral abnormal flexion of the upper limbs and extension of the lower limbs, and is usually due to an upper brainstem lesion. Unilateral lesions are associated with unilateral decorticate or decerebrate posturing (Bateman 2001).

Pupil assessment

Pupils are assessed for their reaction to light, size, shape and equality, cranial nerves II (optic) and III (oculomotor). Each pupil needs to be assessed and recorded individually. Assessment of the pupillary response is important in both localizing the site of coma and differentiating focal from toxic/metabolic causes, where the pupil response is usually intact (Bateman 2001). Pupils are measured in millimetres (normal range 2–6 mm in diameter) and are normally round in shape. Abnormalities are described as ovoid, keyhole or irregular (Hickey 1997). Initially, the nurse should look into the eye to assess the size of the resting pupil; size varies according to the time of the day and older patients usually have smaller pupils than younger patients. Then a bright light, preferably a bright pen torch, is shone into the side of each eye to assess the pupil's reaction to light; this should produce a constriction in both pupils, the consensual light reflex. Pupil response should be recorded as brisk, sluggish or no reaction, and recorded as

- brisk (+);
- sluggish (SL);
- no reaction (−).

Figure 7.10 Motor response to pain. (Adapted from Bateman 2001, Figure 3.)

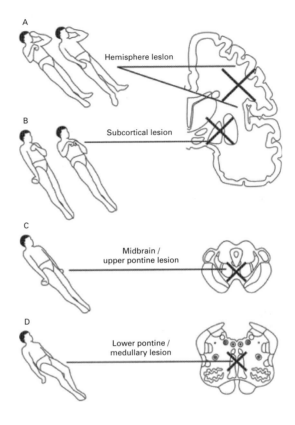

A

Hemisphere lesion

B

Subcortical lesion

C

Midbrain / upper pontine lesion

D

Lower pontine / medullary lesion

The reaction in the non-stimulated pupil may be less brisk than in the stimulated side. A common abnormality is a 'blown' pupil, where the pupil is large and usually unreactive to light. This follows herniation of part of the temporal lobe through the small space in the tentorium, which directly damages the oculomotor (third) nerve. Following damage to the pons, with the use of some eye drops (especially those for glaucoma), and during opiate administration, the pupils become pinpoint and unreactive. The magnification provided by an otoscope may be helpful to assess the response in small pupils. Drugs used for resuscitation, such as atropine, may have a prolonged effect on the pupil response (Bateman 2001). Cataracts and lens implants can prevent a pupil reacting to light (Aucken & Crawford 1998). Occasionally, a patient may have a pre-existing third nerve palsy, which may affect their pupillary response (Table 7.2). Alternatively an unresponsive patient may have a pupillary response; this may be due to a catatonic state, a pseudo-coma or locked-in syndrome.

Neurological assessments are usually recorded on a chart such that in Figure 7.11. It is important to record the GCS alongside vital signs, as this will graphically display events. For example, pressure on the brainstem

> Record vital signs alongside GCS to gain the fullest picture of events.

will cause not only neurological changes but changes in cardiac and respiratory patterns. The following are important points to remember.

- Hypotension is only of neurological origin in extremely dire circumstances; signs of hypovolaemia (or other causes of hypotension) should always be looked for in the hypotensive neurological patient.
- Hypertension, bradycardia and decreased respirations (Cushing's triad) are specific responses to a potentially lethal rise in intracranial pressure.

Figure 7.11 Observation chart.

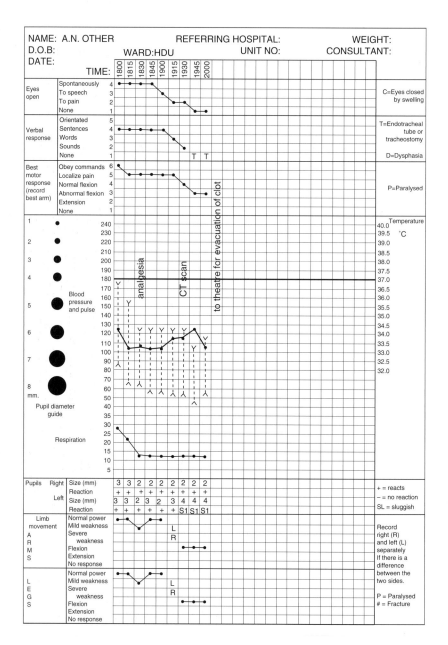

- Hypertension with or without hyperpyrexia may indicate autonomic dysfunction.

A computed tomography (CT) scan should be ordered for any of the reasons stated in the National Institute for Clinical Excellence (NICE) guidelines as shown in Box 7.5.

In patients with trauma, either as a precipitating event, for example, in head injury, or as a sequela possibly following a cerebrovascular accident, it is important to examine the patient physically, looking for signs of laceration or bruising. Deep lacerations could conceal evidence of depressed skull fracture; however, as it is easy to confuse the firm edges of a scalp haematoma with a fracture, a skull X-ray should be performed if there is doubt. Always ensure that the neck is fully examined and a collar applied, if there is any uncertainty regarding the integrity of the spine. Basal skull fractures are diagnosed clinically. Box 7.6 describes the clinical signs.

THE PHYSIOLOGY OF RAISED INTRACRANIAL PRESSURE

Intracranial pressure (ICP) is the pressure exerted by the cerebrospinal fluid within the ventricles of the brain (Hickey 1997). Normal ICP is 0–15 mmHg, with an average range of 0–10 mmHg, when measured from the foramen of Munro. Intracranial pressure varies with daily activities, such as coughing, sneezing and straining. To understand the physiology of

---

Box 7.5   Criteria for performing a CT scan on head–injured patients (NICE Guidelines 2003)

- GCS < 13 at any time since the injury
- GCS = 13 or 14 two hours after the injury
- Sign of basal skull fracture (battle signs, otorrhoea, haemotympanum, panda eyes)
- Vomiting more than once
- Person > 65 years with ↓GCS
- Therapy and decreased GCS
- Pedestrian hit by vehicle, fall from height > 1 metre
- Passenger in motor vehicle thrown from vehicle
- Suspected open or depressed skull fracture
- Post-traumatic seizure
- Focal neurologcial deficit
- Amnesia for > 30 minutes of events before the impact
- History of bleeding, anticoagulant

Box 7.6   Clinical signs of a basal skull fracture

- Rhinorrhoea
- Otorrhoea
- Bilateral periorbital haematoma (panda eyes)
- Subconjunctival haemorrhage
- Battle's sign (bruising over the mastoid)

raised intracranial pressure, it is useful to consider the modified Munro–Kellie hypothesis (Hickey 1997), which states:

The skull, a rigid compartment, is filled to capacity with essentially non-compressible contents; brain matter (80%), intravascular blood (10%) and CSF (10%). The volume of these three components remains nearly constant in a state of dynamic equilibrium. If any one component increases in overall volume, another component must decrease for the overall volume and dynamic equilibrium to remain constant; otherwise, ICP will rise.

There are limited ways for the brain to maintain normal ICP, by altering one or other component:

- increased CSF absorption;
- decreased CSF production;
- shunting of CSF to the spinal subarachnoid space;
- vasoconstriction – reduction in cerebral blood volume (CBV).

In the healthy brain, autoregulation and chemoregulation maintain a cerebral blood flow (CBF) sufficient to maintain the energy requirements of the brain tissue, while maintaining ICP (Figure 7.12). It is suggested by the Brain Trauma Foundation (2000) that intervention to reduce ICP should be initiated once the ICP has reached an upper threshold of 20–25 mmHg.

The cerebral perfusion pressure (CPP) is the pressure required to maintain CBF. Cerebral perfusion pressure needs to be above 70 mmHg (Goh & Gupta 2002) to maintain CBF; autoregulation fails below this point or above 160 mmHg (Lindsay et al 1997). Following head injury, autoregulation is impaired and it is vital to maintain cerebral perfusion pressure to ensure adequate oxygen to the brain tissue. To calculate cerebral perfusion pressure, the ICP needs to be subtracted from the mean arterial pressure (MAP):

$$CPP = MAP - ICP$$

According to the cause of the raised intracranial pressure, so symptoms may vary in acuity. A slow-growing tumour may grow to a larger size, as the three components of the brain have time to accommodate the additional tissue, before any symptoms of raised ICP are noted by the patient, whereas the sudden onset of a subarachnoid haemorrhage might cause many more symptoms, despite the overall volume being less. The common symptoms of raised ICP are as follows.

Figure 7.12 Vasodilatation and vasoconstriction. (Based on Lindsay et al 1997, p 74.)

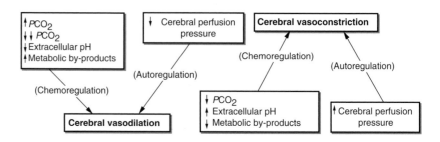

- Headache – this is due to traction on the pain-sensitive structures within the cranium. These can be aggravated by such activities as coughing or a change in position (Benarroch et al 1999).
- Nausea and vomiting – caused by increased pressure in the fourth ventricle, where the vagal motor centres are located (Benarroch et al 1999).
- Papilloedema – increased pressure on the optic nerve results in oedema of the nerve head. Papilloedema causes blurring of the optic disk margins when viewed with an opthalmoscope.
- Reduced level of consciousness – increased pressure results in hypoperfusion and pressure on the brainstem, resulting in a reduced level of consciousness.
- Cardiorespiratory signs – blood pressure may increase to enable CCP to be maintained as ICP rises. Bradycardia may occur owing to pressure on the vagus nerve. The respiratory pattern may change according to increased pressure in various areas of the brainstem (see Figure 7.22).

In head injury, ICP rises globally owing to cerebral oedema, with or without haematoma formation, and latterly a breakdown of autoregulation and chemoregulation. Figure 7.13 shows the cyclical nature of progressive brain swelling.

Once the compensatory mechanisms have been exhausted, a small additional change in volume results in a large pressure rise, as shown in Figure 7.14. It is, therefore, important to monitor for signs of rising ICP in the unresponsive patient.

Definitive management of an increased ICP requires monitoring of arterial, central venous and intracranial pressures, under neurosurgical direction.

THE MANAGEMENT OF NEUROLOGICAL CONDITIONS

The nursing management of neurological patients requires an understanding of the pathophysiology of both the disease process and complications that can arise as a result of the insult to the brain. The aim of management of patients with neurological conditions is:

Figure 7.13 Cycle for malignant progressive brain swelling. (Based on Hudak & Gallo 1994, p 677.)

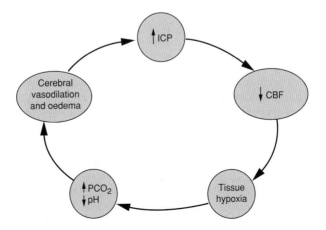

Figure 7.14 Volume pressure curve. (Based on Lindsay et al 1997, p 75.)

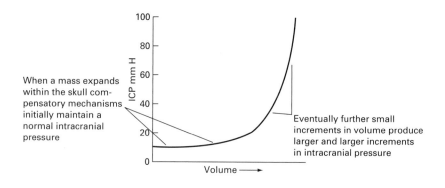

When a mass expands within the skull compensatory mechanisms initially maintain a normal intracranial pressure

Eventually further small increments in volume produce larger and larger increments in intracranial pressure

1. optimizing brain function;
2. preventing secondary damage occurring as a consequence of the disease process;
3. detecting and treating raised intracranial pressure;
4. monitoring neurological function;
5. optimizing patient recovery.

Table 7.3 describes the management of the unconscious patient with interventions aimed at reducing intracranial pressure. The principles of care can be applied to nursing patients with a variety of neurological conditions to optimize brain function and reduce secondary brain damage. It is intended to be read in conjunction with the subsequent sections describing the management of specific conditions.

> Think about the care of patients with problems in addition to neurological trauma.

HEAD INJURIES

Approximately 700 000 people per year attend accident and emergency (A&E) departments due to head injury (NICE Guidelines 2003). The majority (90%) of these are classified as minor (GCS 15) or mild (GCS 13 or 14), 5 % are moderate (GCS 9–12), and the remaining 5% are classified as severe with a GCS of 3–8 (Kay & Teasdale 2001). It is the moderate and particularly severe head-injured patients who require high dependency and critical care intervention.

Head injuries occur as a result of two forces: acceleration and deceleration, or sometimes a combination of both forces. Acceleration injuries occur when a moving object strikes a stationary head (e.g. a gunshot wound or a blow from a blunt object). Deceleration injuries occur when the head hits a solid object (e.g. a windscreen or the ground). These injuries can also occur at the same time: during an assault, for instance, a patient might be hit over the head and then fall to the ground. During the injury, the head may also be subjected to rotational forces, causing stretching and shearing of the white matter (nerve fibres in the brain) and brainstem (Box 7.8).

Head injuries can be further classified as open or closed.

- An *open head injury* (penetrating injury) may describe both a bullet lodged in the brain and a scalp laceration; thus it does not convey a degree of severity. It involves a rupture or break of the dura.
- A *closed head injury* (non-penetrating injury) results in damage to the brain without any breakage of the dura.

Table 7.3 The nursing management of the unconscious patient

Problem	Nursing intervention
Inadequate airway/poor gag reflex	Ensure clear airway through positioning patient on side with neck in neutral position or, if appropriate, use of nasal or oral airway Elevate head of bed to 30°. Care of tracheostomy/endotracheal tube
Ineffective clearance of secretions/	Assess patient's requirement for poor cough reflex suctioning, pre-oxygenate; if appropriate, limit active suctioning to 15 seconds Observe patient throughout suctioning for deteriorating cardiovascular signs, ensure recovery from suctioning
Poor respiratory pattern/deteriorating gas exchange	Observe rate, depth and regularity of respirations Listen to chest sounds, monitor tidal volumes and arterial blood gases Position patient appropriately, avoiding the use of prone positioning; regular change of position, if ICP allows, to dislodge pulmonary secretions Chest physiotherapy to reduce secretions and improve gas exchange Administer oxygen as required Monitor CO_2, via either arterial blood gases or end-tidal CO_2 (see Box 7.7)
Potential for alteration in normal cardiac status	Observe pulse rate, rhythm and regularity; blood pressure, where appropriate, CVP and skin colour of patient, including peripheries Maintain normal temperature Observe for signs of infection
Immobility	Reposition patient regularly, ensuring neck in neutral position, avoiding positions that may cause a rise in intracranial pressure (i.e. hip flexion); 6-hourly passive movements Assess Waterlow score, using the appropriate tools to prevent and treat pressure/skin damage. Use thigh-length pressure stockings/subcutaneous heparin (contraindicated in patients with cerebral bleeds) and monitor for signs of deep vein thrombosis
Neurological impairment	Regular Glasgow Coma Scale (GCS), pupil and limb assessments, increasing frequency, if any deterioration noted Avoid sensory deprivation/overload, planning workload to avoid clustering of activities, promote social interaction encouraging appropriate visitors to assist with care Consider patient's potential for pain, assessing any other injuries and managing appropriately
Maintenance of hydration and nutritional status	Monitor input and output of fluids – a catheter is usually passed in unconscious patients, especially if they are receiving diuretics. (A high ICP can cause inappropriate ADH production and urinary retention will increase ICP) Assess skin turgor, urine specific gravity, urine and serum osmolarity Administer fluids and nutrition enterally, where possible, to maintain gut integrity Fluid infusion should be isotonic and any electrolyte imbalance corrected (hypernatraemia promotes cerebral oedema)
Potential for seizure activity	Observe for origin, sequence of events and start/finish time. The patient should be placed in the left lateral position, when the seizure is over, and observation should continue. The GCS is affected by the post-ictal state, and should be completed regularly, until the pre-seizure status is regained. Anticonvulsants should be administered, in an attempt to stop the seizure, and subsequently administered regularly to inhibit seizure activity. Seizures will increase the ICP and, if continuous (i.e. status epilepticus), can cause severe cerebral oedema, occasionally causing brainstem death
Maintenance of hygiene requirements	Regular care of skin, ensuring particular care for mouth, eyes and areas around invasive catheters
Rehabilitation	Support and preparation of longer term carers; making discharge plans

ADH, antidiuretic hormone; CVP, central venous pressure; ICP, intracranial pressure.

> **Box 7.7   The role of carbon dioxide**
>
> Carbon dioxide (CO_2) in the blood causes dilatation of blood vessels. It is a potent cerebral vasodilator. In brain injury this can result in an increased cerebral blood flow (CBF) and, therefore, an increased cerebral blood volume (CBV) (hyperaemia), which in turn causes a rise in intracranial pressure (ICP). Severe hypocapnia results in cerebral vasoconstriction, a reduction in the blood flow to the brain and ischaemia. However, hyperventilation to reduce CO_2 levels to 30 mmHg or 4.0 kPa has been found to reduce cerebral blood flow, but not enough to cause ischaemia and further neurological injury (Diringer et al 2000). CO_2 rises owing to inadequate respiratory function are a major indication for mechanical ventilation. There has been much debate regarding the use of hyperventilation to reduce CO_2 levels to below normal. Most units will hyperventilate to control ICP (Matta & Menon 1996, Waldmann & Thyveetil 1998). Hyperventilation should aim to keep the PCO_2 between 4 and 4.5 kPa in order to prevent reducing CBF too far and so causing cerebral ischaemia. Mechanical ventilation remains an important method to control CO_2 and, in turn, reduce intracranial pressure (Oertel et al 2002).

> **Box 7.8   Stretching and shearing injuries**
>
> - A *stretching injury* involves pulling of the axons or nerve fibres in the brain, resulting in damage
> - A *shearing injury* involves damage through movement and rubbing of the nerve fibres over each other

These terms are commonly used, although there is no common agreement on their definition. 'Coup' (injury directly below the site of impact) and 'contracoup' (injury opposite the original site) are also common terms, but again describe location rather than severity of injury (Figure 7.15).

Gennarelli et al (1982) described the terms 'focal' and 'diffuse', in an attempt to relate outcome to location. These are very useful terms, especially if used in conjunction with the Glasgow Coma Scale. The GCS is commonly used in association with the terms 'mild', 'moderate' and 'severe', with 'mild' being a GCS score of 13–15, 'moderate' GCS 9–12 and 'severe' GCS 3–8.

Head injuries may be described as belonging to three anatomical sites: the scalp, the skull and the brain.

Scalp injuries

There are four types of injury to the scalp as shown in Box 7.9. Abrasions may not require any treatment but ice applied to the area may reduce any haematoma formation (Hickey 1997). Lacerations can bleed extensively, however, although bleeding from the scalp alone is unlikely to cause

Figure 7.15 Coup and
contracoup injury. (Based on
Hudak & Gallo 1994.)

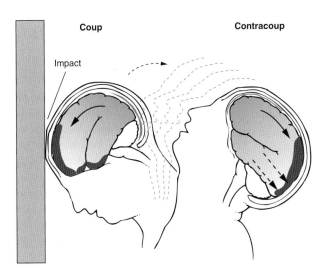

shock in an adult. In small children, a scalp laceration may be sufficient to
cause hypovolaemia. Scalp lesions should be explored under local anaesthetic for foreign bodies or skull fracture, with an X-ray examination if there
is any doubt in diagnosis, and any wound sutured or glued according to
depth and position prior to transfer out of the A&E department. There is
controversy surrounding the treatment of subgaleal haematomas because
of the risks of infection. Some doctors, therefore, argue that it is best to evacuate the haematoma, while others argue that it is best to let it reabsorb. If
the scalp injuries are only part of other injuries, it is important that they are
documented to allow further investigation at a more appropriate time.
They may need to be cleaned and dressed, or temporarily sutured.

Skull injuries

Only 2% of head injury casualty attenders will have a skull fracture;
however, the majority of the complications will occur within this 2%.
A skull X-ray should be performed with any of the following:

- loss of consciousness;
- post-traumatic amnesia;

Box 7.9   Types of scalp injury

- *Abrasions*: minor injuries that may cause a small amount of bleeding
- *Contusions*: here is no break in the skin, but bruising to the scalp may
  cause blood to leak into the subcutaneous layer
- *Laceration*: a cut or tear of the skin and subcutaneous fascia that
  tends to bleed profusely
- *Subgaleal haematoma*: a haematoma below the galea, which is
  a tough layer of tissue under the subcutaneous fascia and over the
  skull. The veins here empty into the venous sinus; thus any infection
  can spread easily to the brain, despite the skull remaining intact

- scalp damage;
- GCS < 15
- abnormal neurological signs;
- vomiting.

The development of an intracranial haematoma is 12 times more likely to occur with a skull fracture (NICE Guidelines 2003). Skull fractures are usually classified in four groups: linear, depressed, basal and comminuted. Linear are the most commonly occurring fractures. They are diagnosed following skull X-rays and will probably need no specific management unless they accompany other injuries (Hickey 1997).

Depressed skull fractures may be very evident clinically, but will require X-ray examination to discover the full extent of damage. They are managed according to their severity and whether there are any accompanying injuries. If there are no other injuries requiring surgical management, they may not be surgically elevated, owing to the risks of infection. However, if there is debris disturbing the brain tissue, then surgery will be required.

Basal skull fractures are often difficult to visualize on an X-ray and are usually diagnosed clinically (see Box 7.6). These are fractures of the skull that lies under the frontal lobes of the brain behind the eyes and under the temporal lobes. If there is any suspicion of a basal skull fracture and the patient requires stomach aspiration, then an orogastric tube must be passed, to avoid any risk of a nasogastric tube entering the cranium. When caring for head-injured patients, it wise to have a policy of only passing orogastric tubes routinely for these patients.

Brain injuries

Computed tomography scan is the primary radiological investigation that should be carried out in order to detect pathological brain injury (NICE Guidelines 2003).

Brain injuries may be focal or diffuse as shown in Figure 7.16.

Focal brain injuries

Contusion Cerebral contusions are bruises of the surface of the brain, most commonly the frontal and temporal lobes, diagnosed by CT scan. Bleeding may occur into contusions, and it is this that would cause an early decrease in the conscious level (Lindsay et al 1997). Unfortunately, the brain will swell around the sites of contusion and, if the contusions are large or widespread, the swelling may cause the ICP to rise, raising the mortality rate for this type of injury to 45% (Hudak & Gallo 1994).

Figure 7.16 Types of brain injury. (Adapted from Hickey 1997, p 386.)

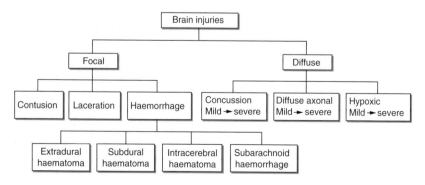

Cerebral oedema peaks 48 hours following injury (Toung el al 2002). Lacerations are tears of the cortical surface and occur in similar locations to contusions.

Haemorrhage There are four types of traumatic bleed: extradural (EDH), subdural (SDH), intracerebral (ICH) and subarachnoid (SAH). Subarachnoid bleeds are usually not traumatic in origin; however, they may be seen on CT scan following trauma. This is for one of two reasons. Either the patient has suffered an SAH prior to an incident (possibly the cause of the incident; Sakas et al 1995), or the vessels in the subarachnoid space have been damaged by shearing forces.

Extradural haematomas are situated between the periosteum and the dura mater (Figure 7.17). They are usually caused by a laceration to the middle meningeal artery or vein or, less commonly, the dural venous sinus, following a blow to the temporal–parietal region and skull fractures of the temporal bone. EDHs make up 16% of all haematomas (Lindsay et al 1997), and in 85% of patients the EDH will be accompanied by a skull fracture (Hudak & Gallo 1994; Hickey 1997).

Patients with EDHs present with a history of transient loss of consciousness. If the EDH is not diagnosed, they will then be lucid for a period of time – hours to days, depending on the rate of the bleed. They will then rapidly lose consciousness and deteriorate very quickly. A common presentation is patients who fall, get up after a short period of time, then go home to bed. The next morning their family or friends are unable to rouse them and they are taken to A&E.

Surgical treatment is to evacuate the haematoma and ligate the damaged blood vessel. Early signs of deterioration are irritation and headache, and later signs include seizures, ipsilateral pupil dilation and fixation, reduced level of consciousness and contralateral hemiplegia (Sherman 1990). Relatives or friends of these patients require a great deal of reassurance, as they often feel responsible for not bringing the patient

> How might a blockage by a tumour or a haemorrhage affect correct drainage?

Figure 7.17 Extradural haematoma. (From Hickey 1997, p 395.)

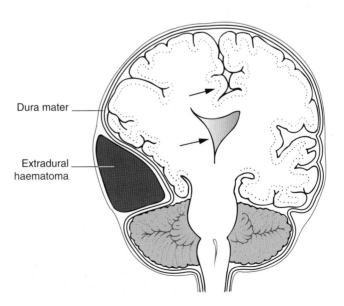

Dura mater

Extradural haematoma

to hospital earlier. An EDH on CT scan appears as a convex-shaped dense white area. The prognosis from an EDH is good and damage to the underlying brain from the blood clot is limited and, following removal of the EDH, the patient will make a good recovery. A delay in surgical treatment can have catastrophic results. The expanding haematoma, if left untreated, causes irreversible raised intracranial pressure, resulting in brain herniation and ultimate brain death.

Subdural haematomas are situated between the dura mater and arachnoid mater, and make up 22% of all haematomas (Lindsay et al 1997; Figure 7.18).

These haematomas are caused by the rupture of bridging veins from the cortical surfaces to the venous sinuses. SDHs can be seen in isolation, but are more commonly associated with cerebral contusions and intracerebral haematomas; this group totals 54% of all haematomas. SDHs are classified into acute, subacute and chronic. Acute refers to symptoms that manifest within 48 hours after injury, while chronic symptoms emerge after 2 weeks and subacute between 48 hours and 2 weeks. Subacute and chronic SDHs are often seen in the elderly and in alcoholics, as both groups can suffer regular falls and have a degree of cerebral atrophy, which puts strain on the bridging veins. Acute SDHs are associated with major cerebral trauma: the onset of symptoms, such as headache, drowsiness, slow cerebration and confusion, is slower than in EDH, but is often associated with other injuries and, therefore, the symptoms can become confused within a general head injury picture. Small SDHs may be treated conservatively, as they will reabsorb over time. Larger SDHs will require evacuation because of the secondary damage they will cause. A SDH on CT scan shows up as a concave, moon-shaped area of blood.

Intracerebral haematomas are found deep within the brain parenchyma. As mentioned before, they are related to contusions and

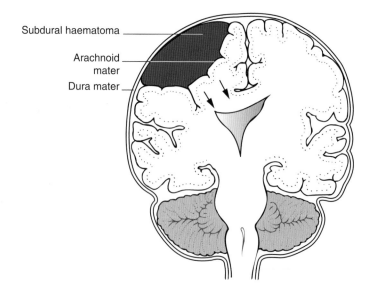

Figure 7.18 Subdural haematoma. (From Hickey 1997, p 395.)

Subdural haematoma

Arachnoid mater

Dura mater

are, therefore, usually found in the frontal and parietal lobes. Other causes include penetrating/missile injuries and a shearing of blood vessels deep within the brain following acceleration/deceleration injuries. They can also occur as a result of untreated longstanding hypertension. They are caused by bleeding within the substance of the brain (Figure 7.19). Symptoms include headache, contralateral hemiplegia, ipsilateral dilated/fixed pupil and a deteriorating level of consciousness, progressing to deep coma (GCS < 8).

Treatment tends to be conservative because of the associated injuries and the difficulty of evacuating a haematoma that is situated so deeply within the brain. Not surprisingly, mortality is high within this group of patients.

Diffuse brain injuries

Concussion   This is a mild form of diffuse injury, involving disorientation, headache, dizziness, inability to concentrate and irritability. This may occur with or without a loss of consciousness and/or memory for a short period of time. Recovery is usually within minutes to hours. Concussion is usually clinically diagnosed but, if performed, a negative CT scan would be produced. It is caused by shearing injuries from acceleration/deceleration forces.

Acute axonal injury   This occurs as a result of high-speed acceleration/deceleration injuries, typically road traffic accidents, causing a mechanical shearing of axons in the white matter.

Initially, there may be very little obvious injury on the CT scan. The patient is deeply unconscious, however, and with repeated scanning, small diffuse haemorrhagic lesions appear, commonly in the corpus callosum, midbrain and pons, accompanied by generalized cerebral oedema (Figure 7.20). Patients with this type of injury have high mortality or morbidity rates, the survivors requiring long-term care.

Hypoxic injury   This occurs when the brain is deprived of adequate

Figure 7.19 Intracerebral haematoma. (Based on Hickey 1997, p 395.)

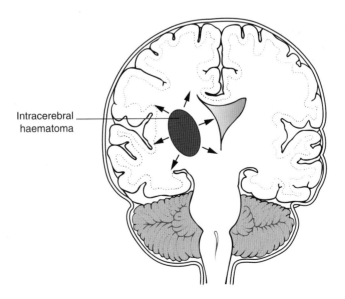

Intracerebral haematoma

Figure 7.20 Diffuse axonal injury. (From Hickey 1997, p 393.)

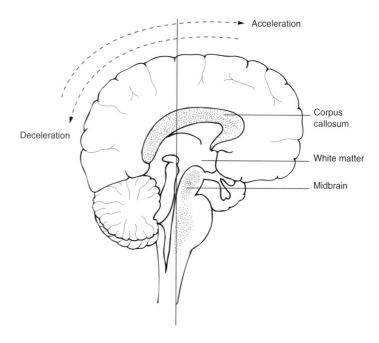

Acceleration

Deceleration

Corpus callosum

White matter

Midbrain

oxygen, for example, in cardiac or respiratory arrest, which may or may not be associated with head injury. Injury can be of varying degrees, according to the length of the hypoxic event, from mild cognitive deficits to death. The brain requires oxygen for metabolism. The hypoxic tissue leads to the development of cerebral ischaemia.

Secondary brain injury

Management of the head-injured patient is aimed at preventing or limiting secondary damage, as a result of oedema, haematoma, ischaemia and infection.

Cerebral oedema Cerebral oedema post-injury is the major cause of mortality and morbidity in patients following head injury (Toung et al 2002). It is not only seen in patients following head injury but can occur with a wide range of patients following an intracranial insult (e.g. subarachnoid haemorrhage, meningitis, encephalitis, encephalopathic liver failure). Oedema occurs as a direct result of the initial injury to the brain and damage to the blood–brain barrier. It also develops over time as a result of increasing demand for oxygen and nutrients by the damaged brain together with a reduction in the amount of blood flowing into the cerebral circulation. It can occur as a result of a variety of mechanisms. Vasogenic oedema occurs when there is damage to the blood–brain barrier (i.e. the capillary wall and protein-rich fluid moves from the blood to the extracellular space surrounding the cells in the brain). Cytotoxic oedema occurs when fluid moves into the actual brain cells (Lindsay et al 1997). Cerebral oedema peaks 48 hours post-ischaemia in both damaged and healthy brain tissue (Toung et al 2002). Ischaemia leads firstly to cytotoxic oedema and then vasogenic oedema, as the capillary becomes damaged.

Nursing management in the high-dependency unit includes regular assessment of neurological signs (as described in the section on assessment), vital signs, recognition of the signs of rising ICP, seizure control, management of fluid input and output, management of associated injuries and accurate documentation of events.

Nursing management

Nursing management specific to head-injured patients is shown in Table 7.4. For general principles of care, please refer to Table 7.3.

CEREBROVASCULAR ACCIDENTS

A cerebrovascular accident (CVA) or stroke occurs when there is either a blockage (ischaemic stroke) or bursting (haemorrhagic stroke) of a cerebral artery. It is characterized by either sudden or slow onset of a wide range of neurological deficits, which may vary in severity and permanence. It is the third largest killer in affluent countries, behind heart disease and cancer, and, in the UK, 150–200 per 100 000 population will suffer stroke annually, of which approximately one-third will be fatal (Lindsay et al 1997).

Ischaemic stroke

Ischaemic strokes make up about 85% of all strokes but carry a lesser mortality rate (about 25%) than haemorrhagic strokes (Lindsay et al 1997). They may be embolic or thrombotic in origin, with thrombosis carrying the higher mortality. The embolus or thrombus causes ischaemia, and latterly infarction and necrosis to the part of the brain supplied by that vessel. Thrombus formation in the cerebral arteries is the cause of transient ischaemic attacks (TIAs), and should be seen as a warning sign of a stroke. The signs and symptoms of a thrombotic stroke usually develop over a period of hours. Embolic strokes are usually secondary to atrial fibrillation, mitral stenosis or a mural thrombosis. These strokes are usually rapid in onset and may resolve quickly, if the embolus disperses.

Clinical presentation

The presentation will vary according to the area of brain involved and the severity of the stroke, but may include:

- reduced level of consciousness (the lower the GCS, the higher the mortality and morbidity);
- hemiparesis or hemiplegia;
- either left or right hemianopia (blindness of one side of both eyes);
- deviation of the head and eyes to one side (the same side as the stroke, the opposite side to the hemiparesis or hemiplegia);
- receptive and/or expressive aphasia (dominant hemisphere stroke);
- inattention to one side of the body (the opposite side to the stroke).

The patient's clinical history will commonly include TIAs, hypertension, cardiac disease, arteriosclerosis, diabetes mellitus or a family history of vascular disease.

Haemorrhagic stroke

These account for approximately 15% of all strokes; however, the mortality rate is high at 70% (Lindsay et al 1997). These haemorrhages can be:

Table 7.4   Nursing management specific to head-injured patients

Problem	Intervention	Rationale
Inability to maintain airway with decreasing GCS	Use of artificial airway (e.g. nasal/oral airway, intubation and mechanical ventilation Ensure airway is clear of debris (e.g. vomit, blood, sputum)	As GCS decreases, ability to maintain airway is decreased, cough reflex is suppressed; regurgitation of stomach contents
	Intubate and ventilate if: – GCS < 8 – PO_2 < 10 kPa – Spontaneous extensor posturing – PCO_2 > 6.0 – Flail chest – Marked oedema on CT scan – Spontaneous hyper-ventilation causing PCO_2 < 3.5 kPa (NICE Guidelines 2003)	Facial fractures – blood in oropharnyx
Poor respiratory pattern/ deteriorating gas exchange	Monitor respiratory rate and pattern Maintain oxygen saturations > 97% Regular blood gas analysis PCO_2 > 4.5 < 5.0 kPa (NICE guidelines 2003) Observation of type of secretions	Damage or pressure to the brain affects function of respiratory centres in the pons and medulla (Figure 7.21). This leads to abnormal breathing patterns
	Adequate sedation with drug such as propofol	Giving high levels of F_1O_2 post-injury ensures oxygen supply to brain and reduces lactate levels in brain tissue (Menzel et al 1999) Carbon dioxide is a potent cerebral vasodilator (see Box 7.7) Hyperventilation to control PCO_2 levels Patient may develop neurogenic pulmonary oedema, best described by Theodore and Robin (1975; see Box 7.10) Patient needs to be sedated to tolerate the endotracheal tube and may need a bolus of sedation to reduce the undesirable effects Drugs such as propofol have a short half-life and allow for quick reversal of the drug for neurological assessment (Kelly et al 1999)
Potential for alteration in cardiovascular function	Monitor heart rate, rhythm, blood pressure Maintain CPP > 70 mmHg	CPP < 60 mmHg causes ischaemia Inotropes can be used to increase MAP; in particular, use noradrenaline, which increases MAP without increasing ICP (Ract & Vigue 2001)
	ECG monitoring	Hypotension is rarely neurological in origin, but it is important to assess for any internal bleeding Cardiac arrhythmias may be due to brainstem irritation and raised ICP – inverted T waves, prolonged Q-T interval, S-T depression, S-T elevation (Syverud 1991)

Table 7.4 Nursing management specific to head-injured patients—cont'd

Problem	Intervention	Rationale
		Late signs of a very high ICP include a change in respiratory pattern, raised blood pressure and bradycardia, known as Cushing's triad
Raised intracranial pressure	Monitor ICP	
	Maintain head and neck in a neutral position	Promotes venous drainage from head
	30° head elevation	Optimum position that reduces ICP without reducing CPP (Moraine et al 2000)
	Hyperventilation	
	Diuresis usually with 20% mannitol ± (see p.209) furosemide	Mannitol is an osmotic diuretic, removing water from brain tissue and reducing cerebral oedema Furosemide decreases CSF production and increases its absorption
	Adequate sedation	Inadequate sedation leads to raised ICP (Matta & Menon 1996)
	Use of paralysing agents	Paralysing agents are used when other methods of reducing ICP are not working. Use of atracurium is effective in controlling raised ICP (McClelland et al 1995)
	Use of barbiturates	Drugs such as thiopentone can be used to reduce ICP and improve outcome (Eisenberg et al 1988)
	Treatment of pyrexia: – recording of temperature – use of antipyretics – patient-cooling measures – locate source of infection	Pyrexia increases cerebral metabolic rate and oxygen demand
Maintenance of hydration and nutritional status	Maintenance fluid – normovolaemia with isotonic saline	Fluid restriction has little effect on cerebral oedema
	Orogastric tube to reduce the chance of aspiration Enteral feeding	Early feeding within 72 hours linked with lower ICP (Wilson & Tyburski 1998)
Potential electrolyte deficiencies should be corrected	Monitor electrolytes imbalance	Trauma/damage to hypothalamus or pituitary can result in lack of ADH production – resultant hypernatraemia Hyponatraemia can occur owing to inappropriate ADH secretion
Pain control	Analgesics to reduce pain	Unresolved headache increases anxiety and blood pressure, which increase ICP
	Use of opiates, such as morphine/ dihydro-codeine in conjunction with paracetamol	Patients may be hypersensitive to touch, sound and light
	Reduce environmental stimuli	Familiar voice is shown not to increase ICP during short periods of time (Treloar et al 1991)

CPP, cerebral perfusion pressure; CSF, cerebrospinal fluid; CT, computed tomography; ECG, electrocardiogram; GCS, Glasgow Coma Scale; ICP, intracranial pressure; MAP, mean arterial pressure.

Figure 7.21 Respiratory patterns in neurological dysfunctions. (Based on Hudak & Gallo 1994.)

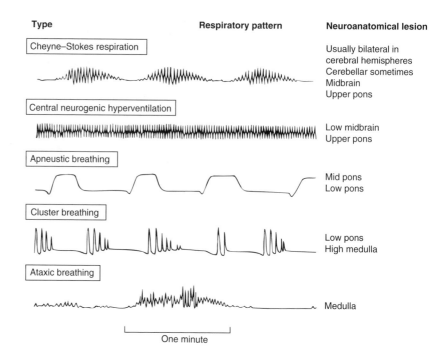

Type	Respiratory pattern	Neuroanatomical lesion
Cheyne–Stokes respiration		Usually bilateral in cerebral hemispheres Cerebellar sometimes Midbrain Upper pons
Central neurogenic hyperventilation		Low midbrain Upper pons
Apneustic breathing		Mid pons Low pons
Cluster breathing		Low pons High medulla
Ataxic breathing		Medulla

One minute

Box 7.10   Neurogenic pulmonary oedema

Neurogenic pulmonary oedema has the same symptoms as pulmonary oedema. However, the mechanism that causes it differs from that of pulmonary oedema. It is a condition that is associated with a variety of intracranial pathologies including head injuries, intracranial haemorrhage, uncontrolled generalized seizures, tumour and hydrocephalus. It can occur within minutes of the event or later after a few days (Pyeron 2001). The raised ICP causes a massive adrenergic (sympathetic) discharge; this leads to peripheral vasoconstriction and causes a rise in the systemic vascular resistance (SVR), resulting in a shift of blood from the systemic circulation to the pulmonary circulation with resultant damage to the pulmonary capillaries. The damage to the pulmonary capillaries results in movement of fluid out of the vascular bed into the lungs. Treatment is with ventilation with positive end-expiratory pressure (PEEP; although high levels of PEEP can increase intracranial pressure), osmotic diuretics (such as mannitol to normalize ICP) and positioning (sitting upright, if possible). Furosemide can also be used but its effects in relation to the patient's CPP would need to be monitored. Suctioning is not particularly helpful but may be unavoidable. It should, however, be kept to a minimum, as the distress caused by the trauma and change in gaseous exchange will cause the ICP to increase.

Box 7.11   Brainstem death

Unfortunately – and despite appropriate management – it is sometimes impossible to reduce the ICP sufficiently and maintain cerebral blood flow. The brainstem becomes starved of oxygen following herniation of the temporal lobe through the tentorium and consequent cerebellar tonsillar herniation through the foramen magnum.

The diagnosis of brainstem death is usually made in the intensive care unit, although, in some cases, this may occur in the high dependency unit. Certain initial pre-conditions must be fulfilled: that a known cause of irremediable structural brain damage exists, and that any reversible causes of apnoeic coma have been excluded. These are:

- Metabolic or endocrine disturbances
- Hypothermia
- Presence of CNS depressant drugs or neuromuscular blockade

Having satisfied the pre-conditions, the patient is tested to ensure the absence of brainstem reflexes and apnoea:

- The pupils are fixed and dilated, not responding to sharp changes in the intensity of light
- There is no corneal reflex when a piece of gauze or cotton wool is brushed across the cornea
- There are no vestibular–ocular reflexes. When 20 ml of ice-cold water is irrigated across the tympanic membrane, the eyes do not deviate (ensuring that the tympanic membrane is clear of debris and not ruptured).
- There is no gag or cough reflex
- There is no motor response
- There is no respiratory effort, despite allowing the PCO_2 to rise above the threshold for stimulus of respiration

Two senior doctors must perform these tests on two occasions. These may be documented on a pre-printed form, but must also be documented in the medical notes, the date and time of death being recorded when the second set of tests is completed. At this point, the patient may be disconnected from, or not reconnected to, mechanical ventilation. Also, at this time, the procedure for donating solid organs may be initiated, if wished.

The nurse is responsible for ensuring a clear communication of events to the patient's relatives during these procedures, and for providing appropriate reassurance and support.

intracerebral, as a result of the rupture of a small deep artery bleeding into the brain substance; *subarachnoid,* as a result of the rupture of an cerebral aneurysm causing bleeding into the subarachnoid space; or the result of a rupture of an *arteriovenous malformation,* causing either an intracerebral bleed or an intraventricular bleed (Box 7.12). Onset of symptoms is usually rapid, with further progression over the next few hours.

> **Box 7.12   Definition of type of haemorrhagic stroke**
>
> - *Subarachnoid haemorrhage* – rupture of a cerebral aneurysm causing bleeding into the subarachnoid space
> - *Arteriovenous malformation* – developmental anomaly of intracranial blood supply. Cerebral arteries feed directly into cerebral veins, bypassing the capillary network, which causes increased pressure in the venous circulation and subsequent rupture. They grow with time and are more common in younger patients. They rupture in 40–60% of patients, causing blood to be released into the ventricles or the brain tissue itself (Lindsay et al 1997)
> - *Intracerebral haemorrhage* – this comes from rupture of the arterial wall, which lies within the brain tissue. Hypertension accounts for 40–50% of these patients (Lindsay et al 1997). They can occur anywhere in the brain but most commonly around the area known as the basal ganglia/thalamus.

Clinical presentation

This is often similar to that of ischaemic stroke; however, typical presentation includes:

- sudden, severe headache – with a subarachnoid haemorrhage this is often likened to being hit over the head with a bat;
- a period of decreasing consciousness;
- nausea or vomiting;
- possibly seizures;
- hemiparesis or hemiplegia.

Diagnosis is based on clinical presentation and history. CT scanning may be useful to determine the area of stroke as might magnetic resonanace imaging (MRI), in suspected subarachnoid haemorrhage. Whenever raised intracranial pressure is suspected, a CT scan should be performed first; only in the absence of raised intracranial pressure is it safe to perform a lumbar puncture (Box 7.13, Figure 7.22). If a lumbar puncture is performed in the presence of raised intracranial pressure, herniation of brain tissue can occur, resulting in brain death. CT scan confirms the diagnosis of a subarachnoid haemorrhage in 95% cases when performed within 48 hours of the bleed (Lindsay et al 1997). Management is according to symptoms and aimed at reducing ischaemic damage and preventing further complications. The patient would be admitted to a high dependency unit to manage the airway and prevent aspiration, to manage hypertension/hypotension in order to maintain cerebral perfusion and for observation of neurological status. However, ultimately these patients would require neurosurgical intervention and the patient would need to be transferred to a regional neurocentre Table 7.5).

Nursing management

The management of patients will address the specific care for these conditions (Table 7.6). These patients can also suffer with the problems already

Box 7.13   Lumbar puncture

A sample of cerebrospinal fluid can be tested for many factors to assist in the diagnosis of many neurological diseases. The standard tests would be bacteriology (white blood cells < 5 mm^3) and biochemical, usually protein (normal value 0.15–0.45 g/l) and glucose (normal value 0.45–0.70 g/l). However, there are many other tests that can be performed: cytology, virology, fungal and parasitic tests, gamma globulin, human immunodeficiency virus (HIV), cryptococcus and Venereal Disease Research Lab (VDRL). A sample can be immediately observed for blood (normal CSF is crystal clear) – three consecutive samples are required to avoid contamination from the puncture site – and for pressure by connecting a manometer (normal pressure 100–150mm CSF).

To avoid injury, a lumbar puncture is performed below the second lumbar vertebrae, usually between L3 and L4. The spinal cord ends at about L1–L2. Patients lie on their side in the fetal position, with their knees drawn up to the chest and the neck flexed, as in Figure 7.22. This ensures the spine is flexed, separating the spinous processes.

If there is any suspicion of raised intracranial pressure or a space-occupying lesion, then a lumbar puncture should not be attempted. These circumstances could precipitate tentorial herniation and consequently death.

Figure 7.22 Position for lumbar puncture. (Based on Carola et al 1990, p 339.)

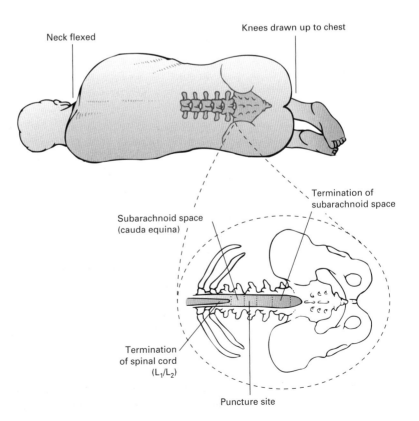

Neck flexed

Knees drawn up to chest

Termination of subarachnoid space

Subarachnoid space (cauda equina)

Termination of spinal cord (L$_1$/L$_2$)

Puncture site

Table 7.5 Treatment and complications associated with haemorrhagic stroke

Type	Complications	Treatment
Subarachnoid haemorrhage (SAH)	Rebleed Hydrocephalus Cerebral arterial vasospasm leading to brain ischaemia	Angiography to determine site of bleed Surgery to clip aneurysm Embolization of aneurysm by use of coils Insertion of drain/VP shunt to drain CSF /treat hydrocephalus
Arteriovenous malformation (AVM)	Raised intracranial pressure Hydrocephalus	Angiography to determine site of AVM Surgery to remove any haematoma Insertion of drain/VP shunt to drain CSF/treat hydrocephalus
Intracerebral haemorrhage	Haematoma Raised intracranial pressure	Angiography to rule out SAH or AVM Surgery to remove haematoma

CSF, cerebrospinal fluid; VP, ventriculo-peritoneal

Table 7.6 Nursing management of patients following haemorrhagic stroke

Problem	Intervention	Rationale
Potential rebleed with SAH (60% chance in first 24–48 hours; Hickey & Ryan 1997)	Strict blood pressure control (BP >130 mmHg < 180 mmHg) Treat hypotension Antihypertensives should be used with caution	Hypertension leads to further rupture of aneurysm Hypotension leads to cerebral ischaemia (Rees et al 2002). Antihypertensives can affect cerebral perfusion
Potential for neurological deterioration	Monitor GCS Hydration with SAH patients Maintain cerebral perfusion Use of calcium-channel blockers for patients with SAH Treat chest infections	Alerts to development of complications Calcium-channel blockers reduce cerebral vasospasm (Barker & Ogilvy 1996) Violent coughing increases risk of rebleed
Maintenance of hydration (particularly with SAH patients)	Adequate and accurate fluid intake/balance	3 litres of fluid/day for SAH patients prevents vasospasm Overhydration can increase intracranial pressure
Alteration in cardiovascular function	Monitor ECG	Cardiac arrhythmias can be due to raised ICP and are common with SAH patients
Headache	Analgesics to reduce pain Use of opiates such as morphine/dihydrocodeine in conjunction with paracetamol	Unresolved headache increases anxiety and blood pressure, which increases risk of further bleeds

BP, blood pressure; ECG, electrocardiogram; GCS, Glasgow Coma Scale; ICP, intracranial pressure; SAH, subarachnoid haemorrhage discussed in the section on nursing management of head injury. Please refer to this section (Table 7.4) and, for general principles of care, to Table 7.3.

BACTERIAL MENINGITIS

This acute inflammation of the meninges and subarachnoid space has three main causative organisms, as listed below.

- *Neisseria meningitides*, which usually occurs in children and young adults. Symptoms may include purpuric skin rash, a severity related to sudden onset, septicaemia, disseminated intravascular coagulation, and circulatory collapse. These symptoms indicate a poor prognosis.
- *Streptococcus pneumoniae*, which usually occurs in adults; associated with sickle-cell disease, pneumonia, alcoholism, splenectomy and ear infections. A poor prognosis is seen with sudden onset.
- *Haemophilus influenzae*, which is usually seen in small children; associated with upper respiratory tract and ear infections. There is generally a good prognosis.

Meningitis occurs when the causative organisms, which are commonly found in the nasopharynx, enter the bloodstream. It may also occur as a complication of sinus infection or head injury. Purulent exudate forms in the subarachnoid space causing inflammation of the meninges. The intact blood–brain barrier stops the body from defending itself against the bacteria and so allows for the bacteria to multiply in number (Lindsay et al 1997). The infection is quickly spread by the CSF around the brain and spinal cord. Intracranial pressure may rise as exudate inhibits the flow of CSF causing hydrocephalus, and irritates the vasculature causing a cerebral vasculitis or a thrombosis with resultant necrosis and haemorrhage.

Clinical presentation

- Headache: often frontal or occipital, and usually the first sign. This will be described as very severe.
- Fever.
- Meningeal irritation, including neck stiffness, photophobia and Kernig's sign (Figure 7.23).
- Reduced level of consciousness; initially loss of concentration, leading to disorientation and an inability to obey commands. Latterly, the patient is drowsy or unresponsive.
- Skin rash in meningococcal varieties.
- Seizure activity; may be general or focal, and indicates irritation of cerebral cortex.
- Increased ICP; often indicated by the onset of vomiting. If severe, may lead to tentorial herniation.
- Focal neurological signs: hemiparesis, dysphasia (speech problems).
- Cranial nerve dysfunction: II, III, IV and VI – difficulty moving the eye, ptosis (drooping upper eyelid), unequal pupils and diplopia; VII – facial paralysis; and VIII – tinnitus, vertigo and deafness (Hickey 1997).
- Endocrine disorders: inappropriate secretion of antidiuretic hormone; hyponatraemia.

Figure 7.23 Kernig's sign.
(From Hickey 1997, p 638.)

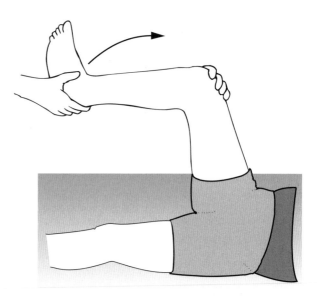

- Waterhouse–Friderichsen syndrome; adrenal insufficiency following infarction of the adrenal glands.

Kernig's sign is elicited by flexing the knee to 90°, bringing it up toward the body and then attempting to straighten the leg (Figure 7.23). This stretches the inflamed lumbar nerve roots, causing pain.

The disease is diagnosed from clinical signs and confirmed by lumbar puncture (Box 7.14). The source of the infection can be identified by taking X-rays of the patient's chest, sinuses and skull. The earlier appropriate antibiotics can be commenced, the better the outcome for the patient, reducing the risk of the more severe complications. After a diagnosis has been made, then treatment is aimed at antibiotic therapy, general supportive measures particular to the symptoms being displayed and care that the patient requires in order to recover from the disease, and recognition and management of complications (Hickey 1997).

Nursing management

Nursing management follows the principles of care of the unconscious patient (Table 7.3) and the principles of management of raised intracranial pressure that were discussed with reference to the care of head injuries (Table 7.4).

SEIZURES

Seizures describe intermittent abnormal neural activity in the brain, characterized by a number of stages, including predrome, aura, ictal (including tonic, clonic, unconscious) and post-ictal (Worthley 1994, Lindsay et al 1997). A seizure or fit is defined as a single event that results in an altered level of brain function. It can occur for a limited amount of time and, once the cause is treated, may not occur again. When seizures occur on several occasions (the time between the seizures can vary from minutes to years), they are described as being are chronic and are usually

Box 7.14   Cerebrospinal fluid analysis in meningitis

- Glucose level is low
- White cell count elevated: 100–10 000 cells/mm^3 (80–90% polymorphonuclear leucocytes)
- Gram stain positive cocci = pneumococcus infection
- Gram stain negative bacilli = *Haemophilus* infection
- Gram stain negative cocci = meningococcus

known as 'epilepsy'; however, this term still carries a stigma and should be used with caution (Hudak & Gallo 1994).

Seizures fall into three major categories: partial, generalized and unclassified.

Partial seizures

Partial seizures describe abnormal neuronal electrical discharge that is localized to one area of the cerebral cortex. This discharge may remain localized in one area of the brain or may progress to a generalized seizure. Partial seizures account for 80% of adult epileptic seizures (Lindsay et al 1997). A partial seizure may have its origin in the part of the brain that controls motor movement and so produce an abnormal jerking of a limb, or part of the face. Alternatively, it may come from the part of the brain that receives sensory information and so result in the patient feeling that their limb or face has altered sensation, whether it is felt as numbness or tingling in that area. Generally, the patient remains conscious during a focal or partial seizure, and can describe what is happening to them. This can be quite frightening to some patients. A patient suffering a partial seizure may have a warning (predrome and/or aura). A partial seizure indicates the presence of a lesion in the brain, such as a tumour, blood clot or abscess.

Another form of partial seizure is one where the focus of electrical discharge is in the temporal lobe of the brain. The result can vary from patients experiencing hallucinations in taste and smell to seeing flashbacks, feelings of déjà vu, hearing things or visual hallucinations to feelings of elation, depression and motor disturbances, such as fumbling, rubbing and semi-purposeful limb movements (Lindsay et al 1997). The patient during an attack is not fully conscious or aware of their surroundings.

General seizures

Generalized seizures can also be a primary event, and are commonly known as a 'grand mal seizure'. According to the area of the brain affected, different manifestations will occur; these can be motor, psychic, sensory or autonomic.

The most commonly recognized seizure is the convulsive generalized seizure. Here the patient will go through all the stages described above. Without warning, they will lose consciousness and fall to the ground – this is the tonic phase and the body becomes rigid. Following this, they exhibit clonic movements – rhythmic jerking of the body, which is bilateral – and then they will become flaccid, often being incontinent. A generalized seizure can last for several minutes. Patients then enter the post-ictal phase: their GCS may be below their normal and they may be confused, gradually returning to normal. Generalized seizures can also be non-convulsive. Occasionally, the seizure activity, either clinically or on EEG, will continue for 30 minutes or more. This is known as 'status epilepticus' and is a medical emergency (Hudak & Gallo 1994). If it is not treated, the patient can suffer hypoxic brain damage, as the brain is not allowed to recuperate. Seizures are associated with many causes, as shown in Box 7.15.

Nursing management

During the seizure   Maintain the airway but do not force an airway into the mouth of a patient who is having a generalized tonic–clonic seizure; observe respirations, observe type of seizure, duration and recovery, and ensure

---

Box 7.15   Causes of seizures (Reproduced from Worthley 1994, p 694, with kind permission of Churchill Livingstone)

- Idiopathic
- Multiple sclerosis
- Alzheimer's disease
- Febrile convulsion
- Electrocution, electroconvulsive therapy
- Eclampsia
- Pancreatitis
- Cerebrovascular diseases
  - hypertensive encephalopathy
  - embolism, infarction, atrioventricular malformation
  - subarachnoid haemorrhage
  - cerebral arterial or venous thrombosis, systemic lupus erythematosus, thrombotic thrombocytopenic purpura
- Structural cerebral defect
  - trauma, neoplasm, abscess, infarct
  - meningitis, encephalitis (particularly herpes simplex)
- Metabolic abnormality
  - hypocapnia, hypoglycaemia, hyponatraemia, hypocalcaemia, hypomagnesaemia, hypophosphataemia
  - uraemia, dialysis disequilibrium, hepatic failure, pyridoxine deficiency
- Drug withdrawal
  - antiepileptics, alcohol, barbiturates, benzodiazepines, opiates, corticosteroids
- Drug toxicity
  - aminophylline, lignocaine, phenothiazines, tricyclics, lithium
  - penicillin (CSF penicillin > 10 u/ml, 6 mg/ml), imipenem
  - isoniazid (due to pyridoxine deficiency)
  - insulin (due to hypoglycaemia)

patient safety. During status epilepticus, the first-line drug is diazepam, a benzodiazipine that suppresses brain activity. Phenytoin or muscle relaxants may be administered; these require documentation for effect.

Following the seizure   Reassure the patient, check for any injuries and record the event; if regular, record on a seizure chart to allow comparison and evaluation of any drug therapy.

Ongoing care   Ensure the patient is complying with the drug regimen, educate to any new regimen, and give information regarding the seizures and any investigations that may be required as in Table 7.7. Address the patient's pyschosocial concerns.

GUILLAIN–BARRÉ SYNDROME

This is an acute inflammatory polyneuropathy and is thought to be an autoimmune response to a viral infection with an incidence of 1–2 per 100 000 population (Lindsay et al 1997). It affects slightly more males than females, occurring in all age groups, although peaks have been noted in young adults and those in their 40s–70s (McMahon-Parkes & Cornock 1997). The disease usually proceeds rapidly, primarily affecting the motor component of the peripheral nerves.

Most patients survive and recover completely; those who deteriorate so as to require ventilatory support are more likely to have residual disabilities. Death may occur due to cardiac or respiratory arrest.

Guillain–Barré syndrome (GBS) is thought to be caused by an immune-mediated response to a viral illness. This causes destruction of the myelin sheath in both the spinal and cranial nerves, causing a loss of saltatory conduction and a resultant slowing of nerve impulses. The peripheral nerves become oedematous and inflamed, causing varying degrees of axonal damage. The greater the damage, the less the recovery.

Clinical presentation

There are four variants of Guillain–Barré syndrome: ascending, descending, Miller Fisher variant and pure motor GBS. The most common presentation is the ascending variety:

- ascending symmetrical weakness and numbness, commencing in the lower limbs and progressing upward to the arms, trunk and cranial nerves;

Table 7.7   Investigations

Investigation	Rationale
Serum biochemistry – glucose, sodium, calcium, magnesium, phosphate, acid–base balance, PCO_2	To ensure within normal limits
Drug levels	To establish cause
ECG, echocardiography	To assess for cardiac origin, such as cardiac syncopal, embolus
Electroencephalogram (EEG; see Box 7.16)	To establish a focus
CT scan/MRI scan	To identify structural brain disorders

> **Box 7.16 The electroencephalogram**
>
> The electroencephalogram (EEG) records the amplified electrical potential of the brain through approximately 20 electrodes placed across the patient's scalp. The first EEG was recorded by Berger in 1929, and the use of the EEG has greatly increased the understanding of seizure activity and its source (Lindsay et al 1997). It is recorded to show the location and type of cerebral disturbance and is used as a diagnostic tool in conjunction with patient history, clinical examination and biochemical results.
>
> The normal EEG shows alpha and beta waves. Alpha waves are recorded at rest from the parietal and occipital regions, and may be slowed by hypoglycaemia, hypercapnia and hypothermia. When an individual is concentrating, with the eyes open, there is more beta activity recorded from the anterior region of the brain. Alpha and beta waves are normally bilaterally symmetrical. The abnormal EEG displays delta and theta waves and spikes, with asymmetry (Worthley 1994, Hickey 1997). Figure 7.24 contrasts the normal EEG with an EEG during a convulsive seizure.
>
> The EEG is of reduced diagnostic value in the patient who is heavily sedated, which may be the case in the high dependency unit. It can, however, be of help in distinguishing between metabolic and hypoxic encephalopathies (Bion & Oh 1997).

- dysphagia;
- reduced vital capacity;
- hyperalgesia.

In 65% of patients, these symptoms occur 2–3 weeks following a viral illness or an immunization. Muscular weakness is at its maximum 3 weeks after the onset (Lindsay et al 1997).

Management is generally symptomatic, with emphasis placed on monitoring respiratory function. Respiratory support may be necessary and ventilation is necessary in 20% of all cases (Lindsay et al 1997). Patients can have autonomic disturbances, causing urinary retention, cardiac arrhythmias, hypotension and blurring of vision (Lindsay et al 1997). Plasmaphaeresis and immunoglobulins have been trialled with good effect, for use early after symptoms occur (Van der Mech & Schmitz 1992). Immunoglobulin therapy is presently preferred because of the risks of plasmaphaeresis, which seem to be heightened in GBS.

Nursing management

Respiratory function   Detailed observation of respiratory status is required in these patients, including vital capacity and tidal volume. Monitor cough and gag,

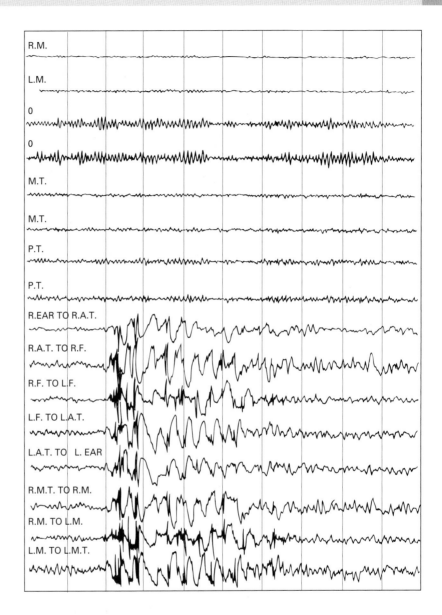

Figure 7.24 Comparison of a normal EEG (top) with that of an epileptic patient during a tonic–clonic seizure (bottom). (Based on Hickey 1997, p 96.)

encourage deep breathing and coughing. If doubt exists, measure arterial blood gases, administering oxygen as required and with caution. Ventilation and/or tracheostomy may be required, particularly if the vital capacity falls below 1 litre (Allen & Lueck 2002).

Neurological status   Motor and sensory assessments, including cranial nerves especially facial (VII), vagus (X), for autonomic dysfunction, and glossopharyngeal (IX).

Monitor autonomic dysfunction   Cardiac arrhythmias, hypotension/hypertension, urinary retention, inappropriate antidiuretic hormone secretion.

Pain control   Monitor characteristics of pain, positioning, analgesia, management of immobility. A pain chart is useful.

Immobility   Pulmonary embolism, ileus.

Psychosocial aspects   If the patient is unable to talk, establish a means of communication to ensure a level of independence, provide items to improve visual field, such as mirrors, and ensure a stimulating environment. Involve family and friends, where possible, and ensure that the patient's dignity and privacy are respected. This area of care is perhaps the most important, once respiratory, autonomic and pain management are agreed. The patient with GBS may be in hospital for a protracted period of time, in some cases a year or more. It is, therefore, important, especially in the high dependency area, to ensure that patients can take some degree of control in their care. This may require a great deal of planning and innovation on the part of the nurse and the multidisciplinary team.

PHARMACOLOGY

Many of the medicines used in the care of neurological patients are widely used for other conditions; these include sedatives and analgesics. In this section, only the most commonly used neurological medicines, such as anticonvulsants, osmotic diuretics and analgesia, will be described.

Phenytoin

Uses   Phenytoin is used in the prevention and treatment of generalized seizures. It is sometimes used in conjunction with other therapy for the treatment of localized seizures. When administered intravenously, it must be given slowly, thus limiting its use in status epilepticus, where diazepam is often the first-line treatment.

Dosage and administration   The initial intravenous dose is 10–15 mg/kg, delivered at no more than 50 mg/minute. This would be followed up by 300–400 mg daily in divided doses, either intravenously or orally. Patients receiving phenytoin intravenously should have cardiac monitoring throughout. Therefore, it is appropriate to move to the enteral route as soon as it is available. Phenytoin can be successfully given via the orogastric/nasogastric tube in its liquid form. There has been a lot of debate over whether giving enteral feeds should be stopped whilst giving phenytoin in order to allow absorption. However, recent studies have shown that even patients who have been having intravenous phenytoin have had low blood serum concentrations of the drug. Phenytoin concentration in the blood is not just influenced by its absorption from the gut but by a multitude of other factors (Randall & Tett 1994). Blood levels are monitored routinely and the dose adjusted accordingly to ensure therapeutic levels are maintained. Phenytoin is poorly and erratically absorbed from intramuscular sites; this route should, therefore, only be used with caution and as a last resort.

Contraindications   Phenytoin should be used with caution in patients who have respiratory depression, myocardial infarction or who are pregnant. Bradyarrhythmias may be exacerbated during intravenous administration.

Side effects These are frequent and wide ranging, particularly during intravenous administration. Rapid intravenous administration causes hypotension and can cause arrhythmias. Patients metabolize phenytoin at different rates, therefore, the dose is titrated against blood levels. Signs of toxicity include nystagmus, ataxia, diplopia, lethargy, drowsiness and, in severe cases, unconsciousness. Other side effects include nausea, vomiting, constipation, dysphagia, change in the patient's ability to taste, weight loss, blurred vision, dizziness, twitching, headache, shrinking of the gums, rashes, lymphadenopathy and haematological effects.

Carbamazepine

Uses Carbamazepine is used in the prophylactic management of localized and generalized seizures. It appears to be most effective in patients with complex localized seizures. It is also used for the control of neurogenic pain in a variety of conditions including trigeminal neuralgia, Guillain–Barré syndrome, multiple sclerosis, diabetic neuropathy and post-traumatic paraesthesia.

Dosage and administration Dosage is titrated according to individual requirements and response. The initial dosage is 400 mg daily in divided doses, increasing by 200 mg a day until an optimum response is achieved. Treatment with carbamazepine should be introduced or reduced slowly, usually at weekly intervals. Any previous treatment should be maintained or reduced as the carbamazepine is slowly increased.

Carbamazepine is available as a tablet or in suspension; the latter will provide higher peak concentrations and is prescribed in more frequent, smaller quantities. If administered via a nasogastric tube, it can be mixed with an equal volume of dilutant, water or 0.9% sodium chloride to prevent adherence to the PVC tubing.

Contraindications Carbamazepine should only be prescribed for patients with cardiac, hepatic, haematological or renal disease or in pregnancy after a risk–benefit analysis.

Side effects These are many and varied, but include decrease in platelet and leucocyte counts, adverse cardiovascular effects, including aggravation of hypertension, hypotension, congestive cardiac failure, syncope, aggravation of coronary heart disease, arrhythmias and atrioventricular block, abnormal liver function tests, urinary frequency/retention, impotence, drowsiness, fatigue, ataxia, confusion, blurred vision, visual hallucinations, hyperacusis, speech disturbances, nausea, vomiting, constipation and rashes.

Mannitol

Uses Mannitol is used to reduce raised intracranial pressure following trauma or during neurosurgery. Mannitol is an osmotic diuretic drawing water from both healthy and damaged brain tissue. Through its action as a diuretic, it decreases blood viscosity, making the blood thinner and able to travel through narrower vessels. It has also been shown to act as a neuroprotective agent as an oxygen free radical scavenger (Davis & Lucatorto 1994). There is evidence to show that there may be a rebound increase in intracranial pressure about 12 hours post-infusion and, if the blood–brain barrier is not intact, then mannitol could draw water back into the brain. For mannitol to work, renal blood flow and glomerular filtration must be appropriately high to enable the drug to reach the tubules. It should not be used if serum osmolarity is > 320 mosmol/l.

Dosage and administration

The dosage is 1.5–2 g/kg as a 20% solution, intravenously over 30–60 minutes.

Contraindications

Renal failure, pulmonary oedema, dehydration and congestive heart disease. Mannitol should only be used during pregnancy where clearly indicated.

Side effects

Electrolyte imbalance, dehydration, water intoxication (owing to fast administration or poor urine output) and pulmonary oedema are the most severe effects. Other effects include blurred vision, nausea, vomiting, hypotension, tachycardia and thrombophlebitis. Extravasation can cause localized oedema and possible necrosis of the surrounding tissues.

Nimodipine

This is a calcium-channel blocker similar to nifedipine. It has been unsuccessful in preventing vasospasm; however, it does seem to have a significant effect in reducing ischaemic complications (33% to 22%) by opening up the collateral circulation and blocking calcium influx (Lindsay et al 1997).

Uses

Nimodipine is used to reduce ischaemic neurological deficits following acute subarachnoid haemorrhage; it may also improve outcome following acute ischaemic strokes. In SAH, therapy should be commenced within 96 hours of the original bleed.

Dosage and administration

This is intravenously 1–2 mg/hour continuously, usually starting at a lower dose and increasing according the patient's ability to maintain blood pressure or orally 60 mg 4-hourly. Nimodipine is continued for 21 days to cover the period of vasospasm.

Contraindications

Nimodopine should only be used in pregnancy when the benefits outweigh the potential risks.

Side effects

These are hypotension, especially with intravenous use, flushing, headache and oedema.

Dihydrocodeine tartrate

Uses

Dihydrocodeine tartrate (DF118) is used in moderate to severe pain. It has a similar analgesic effect to that of codeine with minimal CNS depressant effects.

Dosage and administration   It is usually given intramuscularly 50 mg, or orally 30 mg 4-6-hourly. Listed under Schedule 2 of the Misuse of Drugs Act 1968, in intramuscular preparation.

Contraindications   Respiratory depression.

Side effects   Tolerance and physical dependence; CNS depression, especially in the older patient.

There is much debate regarding the use of opiates in neurological patients. It is commonly agreed that opiates should be given if the patient's pain requires them, including opiates such as morphine.

CONCLUSION

The nervous system is fascinating and, although complex, a basic understanding not only allows the nurse to provide well-planned and proactive care, but also provides insight into potential problems and, therefore, the ability to react appropriately to those situations. This understanding assists in the care of many patients who may not be admitted with a primary neurological diagnosis, but who have previous pathology of the nervous system or may be at risk of CVA or seizure. More detailed information can be found in the articles and books listed under References and Further reading for those who would like to discover more.

References

Allen C M C, Leuck C J 2002 Neurological disease. In: Haslett C, Chilvers E R, Boon N A, Colledge N R, Hunter J A A (eds) Davidson's principles and practice of medicine, 19th edn. Churchill Livingstone, Edinburgh

Aucken S, Crawford B 1998 Neurological assessment. In: Guerrero D (ed.) Neuro-oncology for nurses. Whurr, London

Bannister R 1992 Brain and Bannister's clinical neurology, 7th edn. Oxford Medical Publications, Oxford

Barker F, Ogilvy C 1996 Efficacy of prophylactic nimodipine for delayed ischaemia deficit after subarachnoid haemorrhage. Journal of Neurosurgery 84(3): 405–414

Bateman D E 2001 Neurological assessment of coma. Journal of Neurology, Neurosurgery and Psychiatry 71(Suppl 1): i13–i17

Benarroch E E, Westmoreland B F, Daube J R, Reagan T J, Sandok B A 1999 Medical neurosciences, 4th edn. Lippincott, Williams & Wilkins, Philadelphia

Bion J, Oh T E 1997 Sedation in intensive care. In: Oh T E (ed.) Intensive care manual, 4th edn. Butterworth Heinemann, London: 673

Brain Trauma Foundation 2000 The American Association of Neurological Surgeons. The joint section on Neurotrauma and Critical Care. Guidelines for the management of severe traumatic brain injury. Journal of Neurotrauma 17(6): 493–553

Carola R, Harley J P, Noback C R 1990 Human anatomy and physiology. McGraw Hill, New York

Davis M, Lucatorto M, 1994 Mannitol revisited. Journal of Neuroscience Nursing 26 (3): 170–174

Diringer M N, Yundt K, Videen T et al 2000 No reduction in cerebral metabolism as a result of early moderate hyperventilation following severe traumatic brain injury. Journal of Neurosurgery 92: 7–13

Eisenberg H M, Frankowski R F, Contant C F et al 1988 High dose barbiturate control of elevated intracranial pressure in patients with severe head injury. Journal of Neurosurgery 69: 15–23

FitzGerald M J T; Folan-Curran J 2002 Clinical neuroanatomy and related neuroscience, 4th edn. W B Saunders, Edinburgh

Gennarelli T A, Spielman G M, Langfitt T W 1982 Influence of the type of intracranial lesion on outcome from severe head injury. Journal of Neurosurgery 56: 26–36

Goh J, Gupta A K 2002 The management of head injury and intracranial pressure. Current Anaesthesia and Critical Care 13: 129–137

Hickey J V 1997 The clinical practice of neurological and neurosurgical nursing, 4th edn. J B Lippincott, Philadelphia

Hickey J, Ryan M 1997 Cerebral aneurysms. In: Hickey J (ed.) The clinical practice of neurological and neurosurgical nursing, 4th edn. J B Lippincott, Philadelphia

Hudak C M, Gallo B M 1994 Critical care nursing: a holistic approach. J B Lippincott, Philadelphia

Kay A, Teasdale G M 2001 Head injury in the United Kingdom. World Journal of Surgery 25. 1210–1220

Kelly D F, Goodale D B, Williams J et al 1999 Propofol in the treatment of moderate and severe head injury: a randomised, prospective double-blinded pilot trial. Journal of Neurosurgery 91: 1042–1052

Lindsay K W, Bone I, Callander R 1997 Neurology and neurosurgery illustrated, 3rd edn. Churchill Livingstone, Edinburgh

McClelland M, Woster P, Sweasey T, Hoff J T 1995 Continuous midazolam/atracurium infusions for the management of increased intracranial pressure. Journal of Neuroscience Nursing 27(2): 96–101

McMahon-Parkes K, Cornock M A 1997 Guillain–Barré syndrome: biological basis, treatment and care. Intensive and Critical Care Nursing 13: 42–48

Matta B, Menon D 1996 Severe head injury in the United Kingdom and Ireland: a survey of practice and implications for management. Critical Care Medicine 24(10): 1743–1748

Menzel M, Doppenberg E M R, Zauner A et al 1999 Increased inspired oxygen concentration as a factor in improved brain tissue oxygenation and tissue lactate levels after severe human head injury. Journal of Neurosurgery 91: 1–9

Moraine J J, Berre J, Melot C 2000 Is cerebral perfusion pressure a major determinant of cerebral blood flow during head elevation in comatose patients with severe intracranial lesions? Journal of Neurosurgery 92: 606–613

National Institute for Clinical Excellence (NICE) Guidelines 2003 Head injury – triage, assessment, investigation, and early management of head injury in infants, children and adults. NICE, London

Oertel M, Kelly D F, Lee J H, McArthur D L et al 2002 Efficacy of hyperventilation, blood pressure elevation and metabolic suppression therapy in controlling intracranial pressure after head injury. Journal of Neurosurgery 97(5): 1045–1053

Pyeron A M 2001 Respiratory failure in the neurological patient: the diagnosis of neurogenic pulmonary oedema. Journal of Neuroscience Nursing 33(4): 203–207

Ract C, Vigue B 2001 Comparison of the cerebral effects of dopamine and norepinephrine in severely head injured patients. Intensive Care Medicine 27: 101–106

Randall C T C, Tett S 1994 Phenytoin pharmcokinetics after intravenous administration to patients receiving enteral tube feeding. Pharmacy World & Science 16(5): 217–224

Rees G, Shah S, Hanley C, Brunker C 2002 Subarachnoid haemorrhage: a clinical overview. Nursing Standard 16(4): 47–56

Sakas D E, Dias L S, Beale D 1995 Subarachnoid haemorrhage presenting as a head injury. British Medical Journal 310: 1186–1187

Shah S 1999 Neurological assessment. Nursing Standard 13(22): 49–56

Sherman D W 1990 Managing an acute head injury. Nursing 20(4): 47–51

Snell R S 2001 Clinical neuroanatomy for medical students, 5th edn. Lippincott, Williams & Wilkins, Philadelphia

Syverud G. 1991 Electrocardiographic changes and intracranial pathology. Journal of American Association of Nurse Anesthetists 59: 230–232

Teasdale G, Jennett B 1974 Assessment of coma and impaired consciousness: a practical scale. Lancet ii: 81–84

Theodore J, Robin E 1975 Neurogenic pulmonary oedema. Lancet ii: 749–751

Thompson R F 1993 The brain: a neuroscience primer, 2nd edn. W H Freeman, New York

Toung T J K, Hurn P D, Traystman R J, Bhardwaj A 2002 Global brain water increases after experimental focal cerebral ischaemia: effect of hypertonic saline. Critical Care Medicine 30(3): 644–649

Treloar D M, Nalli B J, Guin P, Gary R 1991 The effect of familiar and unfamiliar voice treatments on intracranial pressure in head injured patients. Journal of Neuroscience Nursing 23(5): 295–299

Van der Mech F G A, Schmitz P I M 1992 The Dutch Guillain–Barré study group. A randomised trial comparing intravenous immunoglobulin and plasma exchange in Guillain–Barré syndrome. New England Journal of Medicine 326: 1123–1129

Waldmann C S, Thyveetil D 1998 Management of head injury in a district general hospital. Care of the Critically Ill 14(2): 65–70

Wilson R F, Tyburski J G 1998 Metabolic responses and nutritional therapy in patients with severe head injuries. Journal of Head Trauma and Rehabilitation 13: 11–27

Worthley L I G 1994 Synopsis of intensive care medicine. Churchill Livingstone, Edinburgh

Further reading

Crossman A R, Neary D 2000 Neuroanatomy: an illustrated colour text, 2nd edn. Churchill Livingstone, Edinburgh

Gentleman D, Dearden M, Midgley S, MacLean D 1993 Guidelines for resuscitation and transfer of patients with serious head injury. British Medical Journal 307: 547–552

Johnson B P 1995 One family's experience with head injury: a phenomenological study. Journal of Neuroscience Nursing 27(2): 113–118

Neuroscience nursing for the new millennium 1999 Nursing Clinics of North America 34: September

National Health Service Executive 1996 Admission to and discharge from intensive and high dependency care. Department of Health, London

National Institute for Clinical Excellence (NICE) Guidelines 2003 Head injury – triage, assessment, investigation, and early management of head injury in infants, children and adults. June. NICE, London.

Thomson R, Gray J, Madhok R, Mordue A, Mendelow A D 1994 Effect of guidelines on management of head injury on record keeping and decision making in accident and emergency departments. Quality in Health Care 3(2): 86–91

Chapter **8**

Post-anaesthetic and post-operative care

Guy Young and Rebecca Purdy

KEY LEARNING OBJECTIVES

The purpose of this chapter is to provide an insight into the needs of the patient following anaesthesia and surgery. The key objectives are that the reader will gain an understanding of:

- The importance of the pre-operative preparation of patients
- Anaesthetic techniques and their implications for post-operative care
- The use of supplemental oxygen in the post-operative period
- Airway management in the initial post-operative period
- The effective assessment and management of post-operative patients

Prerequisite knowledge

A general knowledge of anatomy, physiology and the disease process is assumed. The reader might find the chapter more rewarding if they have a more detailed understanding of the following.

The ABC of resuscitation (a basic life-support session would be particularly useful; see Chapter 9).
Respiratory physiology, including blood gas analysis (see Chapter 5).
Cardiovascular physiology, including ECG interpretation (see Chapter 6).

INTRODUCTION

Patients who are in the initial stages of recovery from anaesthesia and surgery are naturally highly dependent. Whether unable to maintain their own airway or in pain, they require a significant level of nursing intervention. Nurses working in this field need to have a high level of knowledge and skill in order to provide a high standard of care. While technical and analytical expertise is essential, humanistic skill and professionalism are vital. During this period, patients are extremely vulnerable and they rely very heavily on the nurse to act as their advocate.

The main focus of this chapter is the post-operative assessment and management of patients. Areas such as airway management, respiratory management, and nausea and vomiting will be examined in some detail. There is a strong emphasis on patient assessment, as this is seen to be key in providing appropriate and effective care. Assessment is approached from a systems perspective, as this has made presentation easier. Towards the end of the chapter, there are some brief pointers for the management of specific types of surgery. However, it is recognized that nurses working in these fields require a much deeper understanding of the specialty than will be covered in this chapter.

In order to make sense of much of the post-operative situation, it is necessary to provide some insight into the pre-operative phase and anaesthesia. This forms the basis of the first part of the chapter, which is then followed by more specific post-operative considerations.

For the purpose of this chapter, the term 'nurses' will be used to describe practitioners caring for the patient. However, the authors recognize that operating department practitioners may well carry out a comparable role.

PRE-OPERATIVE ASSESSMENT

The need for high dependency post-operative care can be largely predicted. By seeing patients pre-operatively, the nurse can help to ensure that the most appropriate post-operative care facilities are available.

Effective pre-operative assessment is vital in order to minimize the physiological changes and stresses that anaesthesia and surgery place on the patient (National Institute for Clinical Excellence, 2003). The anaesthetist or appropriately trained healthcare professional will take a detailed history looking at issues such as past medical history, chronic illness, reaction to previous anaesthetics and current state of health. The American Society of Anesthesiologists (ASA) classification (Box 8.1) is the most common grading system currently used, and gives an overall assessment of anaesthetic risk. Patients who are in categories 3 and above may be predicted to need high dependency care, throughout the peri-operative and/or post-operative episodes. Effective communication between medical and nursing staff is, therefore, important to ensure that this facility is available. Inevitably, there will be those cases where things do not go as planned and high dependency care is unexpectedly required. However, the need can often be predicted.

It is widely accepted that the giving of pre-operative information can enhance post-operative recovery (Hayward 1975, Droogan & Dickson 1996). For this reason, patients who are anticipated to require high dependency care should be given relevant information pre-operatively. Although the focus here is on post-operative care, it is suggested that the patient is prepared for the whole peri-operative episode and that information is not limited to what will happen when they wake up. Examples of the type of information that could be given are shown in Box 8.2.

> **Box 8.1   ASA physical status classification (Adapted from Dripps et al 1961)**
>
> ASA 1: Normal, healthy patient
> ASA 2: Patient with mild systemic condition, e.g. well-controlled diabetes, old age
> ASA 3: Patient with systemic disease that limits activity but is not incapacitating, e.g. angina, chronic airway disease
> ASA 4: Patient with an incapacitating disease that is a threat to life, e.g. advanced cardiac or pulmonary disease
> ASA 5: Moribund patient not expected to survive 24 hours, even with an operation

Particular emphasis should be placed on pain relief methods. It is crucial that patients understand that they need to inform staff if they are experiencing pain and that this is an appropriate thing for them to do. This will enable staff to ensure that they receive the best possible pain relief.

Much of this information can be given by ward staff. Ideally, they should themselves have some insight into the processes that take place within a high dependency area. This can be achieved by arranging short placements in high dependency areas for ward staff or by making it a part of any orientation programme.

Staff from the high dependency area could visit the patients pre-operatively. Although this can place considerable pressure on limited staff resources, every effort should be made to offer this facility. Patients themselves can visit the high dependency unit (HDU), although some may find the experience frightening (Watts & Brooks 1997). Therefore, the benefits of pre-operative visiting may vary according to the individual patient's needs and this should obviously be taken into account. Information can be given in other ways to those patients who would prefer not to visit the HDU. These include booklets and videos prepared by the post-operative area. The process of giving information to patients, including details of pain relief methods, should start as early as possible, preferably at the pre-admission stage. This is established practice in the field of day surgery and other elective surgery (e.g. diagnostic and treatment centres and some other in-patient areas), where nurses usually carry out the pre-operative assessment of patients.

ANAESTHESIA

Anaesthesia is the absence of normal sensation (Mosby's medical, nursing and allied health dictionary 2002). It can occur as a result of traumatic or pathophysiological damage to nerve tissue or be induced in order to allow pain-free surgery. Broadly speaking, there are two types of surgical anaesthesia: general and regional (local). General anaesthesia depresses the central nervous system, resulting in unconsciousness, loss of muscle tone and reflexes. Regional anaesthesia produces a loss of sensation in a specific area of the body without loss of consciousness.

> **Box 8.2   Pre-operative information**
>
> Discussing the following issues with patients may help to reduce pre-operative and post-operative anxiety
>
> **Pre-operative**
>
> - Fasting
> - Removal of prostheses and cosmetics
> - Pre-medication
> - Repeated checking of identity and proposed operation (including the specifics of the operation site, e.g. right or left side)
> - The anaesthetic room, including personnel and procedures carried out there, e.g. insertion of lines, pre-oxygenation, monitoring
>
> **Peri-operative**
>
> - The possible need for additional shaving, e.g. to accommodate a diathermy plate
> - Any particular position that they may be placed in or other intervention that would account for pain or discomfort post-operatively, e.g. a sore throat following intubation, or shoulder/back ache following laparoscopic surgery
> - The possible need for medication to be administered via the rectal route while under anaesthetic, e.g. analgesia. With this example, the patient's consent should be sought
>
> **Post-operative**
>
> - Attachments and monitoring, e.g. oxygen mask, endotracheal tube, intravenous lines, electrocardiogram (ECG) electrodes, urinary catheters and drains
> - Observations, particularly where they may be disruptive or unpleasant, e.g. neurological observations and pupillary reaction
> - Pain relief methods
> - What staff will be present and the degree of supervision the patient can expect
> - Whether family and friends can visit.
> - Patients should also be given the opportunity to ask their own questions.

General anaesthesia

Problems experienced by the patient during induction of anaesthesia can recur during emergence. Ask the anaesthetist about induction so that you can prepare for any likely or related problems during the post-operative phase.

General anaesthesia consists of four stages (Table 8.1). During induction of anaesthesia, the patients pass through stages 1–3. Stage 4 is considered to be overdose and should be avoided. As patients emerge from anaesthesia, they pass through the stages in reverse order. It is during stage 2 (excitement) that undesirable effects such as laryngospasm and vomiting may occur; this happens because voluntary control is temporarily lost. The patient becomes susceptible to uncontrolled and exaggerated response to almost any stimulus. Although modern anaesthetics have shortened stage 2, induction and emergence remain two of the most critical periods of anaesthesia.

It is important for the nurse caring for a patient during the immediate post-operative period to be aware of the patient's level of anaesthesia. By being able to assess that patients are still at a level of surgical anaesthesia because, for example, they require airway maintenance, the nurse can be prepared for any problems, such as vomiting, as they pass through stage 2. It is important that the anaesthetist relays any problems experienced during induction to the nurse caring for the patient post-operatively, as these may potentially recur on emergence.

General anaesthesia may be achieved using inhalational or intravenous agents (see Table 8.2 for examples). Inhalational agents can be gaseous or volatile (a vaporized liquid). These agents are easily absorbed and excreted through the lungs, resulting in rapid induction and emergence. Intravenous agents also produce rapid induction but, unlike inhalational agents, they need to be metabolized and excreted by the body, which can result in slower emergence. In practice, a combination of inhalational and intravenous anaesthetic is routinely used. Intravenous agents are used to produce rapid induction for the patient, which is more pleasant than breathing gas through a mask. Inhalational agents provide maintenance of anaesthesia and rapid emergence at the end of surgery. Alternatively, total intravenous anaesthesia (TIVA) is a technique where all anaesthetic drugs are given intravenously; propofol is commonly used for these techniques, with or without muscle relaxants. Respiration is controlled by administration of oxygen-enriched air. Target-controlled infusion (TCI) is another technique that

> Anaesthetic agents have a wide variety of physiological effects. Try waking the patient up before actively treating symptoms, such as hypertension and bradycardia.

Table 8.1 Four stages of anaesthesia. (Adapted from Boulton & Blogg 1989)

Stage	Effect	Patient response
1. Relaxation	Amnesia Analgesia	Drowsiness Dizziness Exaggerated hearing Decreased sensation of pain
2. Excitement	Delirium	Irregular breathing Increased muscle tone, motor activity Vomiting Breath holding and struggling Dilated pupils
3. Surgical anaesthesia	Sensory loss	Quiet regular breathing Jaw relaxed Loss of pain/auditory sensation Decreased muscle tone Eyelid reflex absent
4. Danger	Medullary paralysis	Paralysis of respiratory muscles Fixed dilated pupils Rapid thready pulse Respiratory arrest

uses a microprocessor-controlled infusion pump that has been programmed with a pharmacological model of the kinetics of propofol. If the patient's weight is entered into the pump, it will infuse propofol at varying rates to give a predicted blood level (Peck & Williams 2002). All anaesthetic agents can produce significant effects on cardiovascular, respiratory and neurological function. These will be covered later in this chapter. When emergency surgery is required, a technique known as rapid sequence or 'crash' induction is used (see Box 8.3 for more information).

Muscle relaxant drugs, such as suxamethonium and atracurium, are also used during anaesthesia and surgery. The main reasons for using these drugs are:

• to relax the vocal cords to allow endotracheal intubation;
• to relax the muscles involved in respiration to allow effective artificial ventilation;
• to relax striated muscle to facilitate surgery (e.g. laparotomy).

Insufficient reversal of muscle relaxants may lead to problems during the post-operative period. These are dealt with later in this chapter.

Regional anaesthesia

Regional anaesthesia aims to block nerve impulses temporarily from a particular area or region of the body. This can be very localized, such as

Table 8.2 Examples of anaesthetic agents

Name	Type	Advantages	Adverse side effects/considerations
Propofol	Intravenous	Smooth induction Rapid recovery, no hangover	Bradycardia Convulsions have been reported
Thiopentone sodium	Intravenous	Smooth, rapid induction	Irritant to tissues Effects may persist for 24 hours
Ketamine	Intravenous/ intramuscular	Analgesic properties Patient maintains a patent airway	Hallucinations Relatively slow recovery
Nitrous oxide	Inhalational Gaseous	Used for maintenance of anaesthesia Inexpensive	Cannot be used as sole agent, lack of potency
Sevoflurane	Inhalational Volatile	Very rapid induction Rapid recovery Pleasant to inhale	More expensive
Isoflurane	Inhalational Volatile	Rapid induction Fewer cardiovascular effects than halothane	Depressed respiration

Box 8.3   Rapid sequence induction

Rapid sequence (crash) induction is a technique used to anaesthetize patients who have a full stomach. Although seen primarily when dealing with emergency surgery, it is a technique that is likely to be used when it becomes necessary to intubate a patient in an HDU. The technique follows four stages: pre-oxygenation, intravenous induction, relaxation with suxamethonium and intubation. Rapid sequence induction is almost always accompanied by cricoid pressure, a technique used to occlude the oesophagus to prevent gastric regurgitation. Oesophageal occlusion is achieved by applying direct backward pressure on the cricoid cartilage towards the cervical vertebrae (see Fig. 8.1). Although it appears relatively simple, cricoid pressure is not a technique that a novice should attempt, particularly in an emergency. It is suggested that HDU nurses practise the technique in controlled situations, such as an anaesthetic room, under the supervision of an anaesthetist or skilled anaesthetic assistant before assuming competence.

infiltrating a wound prior to suturing, or widespread, such as a spinal anaesthetic. The injection of local anaesthetic (e.g. lidocaine, bupivacaine) around nerve fibres results in blockage of nerve transmissions from a specific area of the body. The resulting anaesthesia can last for hours and provides the opportunity for pain-free surgery without the risks of general anaesthesia. This makes regional anaesthesia a good choice for patients with pre-existing medical problems, such as chronic respiratory disease. It is not appropriate, however, for patients who are unable to cooperate or keep still, such as children, or those who are very anxious. Specific problems associated with regional anaesthesia are dealt with later in the relevant sections of this chapter.

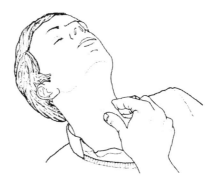

Figure 8.1 Cricoid pressure. (Reproduced by kind permission of BMJ Books from Colquhoun et al 1995.)

OXYGEN THERAPY

The administration of oxygen will be frequently referred to during this chapter. Therefore, before discussing the assessment and management of the post-operative patient, it is worth considering oxygen therapy in more detail. The use of oxygen in the immediate post-operative phase is necessary to enhance the patient's recovery and to prevent potentially serious complications. The nurse caring for the post-operative patient needs to be aware of the reasons for administering oxygen, the methods of administration (Box 8.4) and the potentially harmful effects. Traditionally, oxygen has been treated as a drug to be given only when prescribed by a doctor. With the development of high dependency areas, pulse oximetry and easy access to blood gas analy-

---

Box 8.4   Oxygen delivery methods

Face mask

The most common form of O_2 delivery. Many types are available to allow the administration of different concentrations. Some are dependent on adaptors (e.g. Ventimasks) to provide a fixed percentage, others use the flow rate of O_2 to adjust the concentration delivered to the patient. NB The flows suggested are only an approximation and the actual percentage the patient receives is influenced by factors such as the fit of the mask and the patient's inspiratory flow rate. Using a reservoir attachment can achieve more stable and consistently higher concentrations. Some patients become claustrophobic when wearing a mask and others find the smell of the plastic unpleasant.

Nasal cannulae

These devices deliver low flows of O_2 but this is often sufficient to prevent hypoxia. Although they are less claustrophobic, they can be uncomfortable and will dry out the mucous membranes of the nose. A more comfortable alternative is the nasal catheter, which is held in place by a small cylinder of sponge in a single nostril. The side of the nose used should be changed regularly, as this will reduce the drying effect. Both of these techniques can cause slight irritation to the nasal mucosa.

T-piece

This device is used to deliver O_2 to self-ventilating patients who have endotracheal tubes or laryngeal mask airways *in situ*. By attaching the T-piece, O_2 can be passed by the end of the tube/airway. Adding a short length of corrugated tubing creates a small reservoir of O_2 and helps to maintain a stable concentration. If use of the T-piece is required for any length of time, continuous positive airway pressure (CPAP) should be considered, as breathing against very little resistance can result in basal lung collapse.

sis, however, nurses should be able to make informed judgements about when additional oxygen is necessary, at what percentage it should be given, and when it can be reduced or discontinued. The administration of oxygen could also be covered via the development of a patient group direction.

By increasing the alveolar partial pressure of oxygen (PaO_2), the tension gradient of inhalational anaesthetic agents across the alveolar–capillary membrane is increased and, as a result, the elimination of anaesthetic is speeded up (Ashurst 1995). We will see later that hypoxia occurs for a variety of reasons following surgery and anaesthesia. The administration of supplemental oxygen in the immediate post-operative phase will help to reduce the risk of hypoxia occurring. The aim being to maintain SaO_2 at agreed levels (i.e. those prescribed by the anaesthetist). This may result in supplemental oxygen being requested for 24 hours or more following surgery. It is important to note that the aim is to maintain normal levels of arterial blood gases and peripheral oxygen saturations, not unnecessarily high levels. Running an abnormally high arterial partial pressure of oxygen (PaO_2) is of no benefit to the patient, as once the oxygen capacity has been reached, no further oxygen can be carried despite a rise in PaO_2.

The use of a heat and moisture exchange filter is recommended when patients are being given oxygen through a laryngeal mask or endotracheal tube. This filter warms, moistens and filters out any bacteria from the delivery system, effectively replacing the function of the nasal hairs.

Patients with chronic airways disease, such as emphysema, should have oxygen administered with care, as their stimulus to breathe is a low PaO_2. They should be closely observed for signs of a rising $PaCO_2$ (see respiratory assessment) and, where there is concern, arterial blood gas analysis should be performed. As long as this group of patients is monitored and oxygen is used carefully, there is no reason why they should not have it. They are equally at risk of becoming hypoxic following surgery, so the idea that they should not have oxygen at all because of their chronic health is outdated and not in their best interests. The only patients who do not routinely require additional O_2 are those who have had their operation under local or regional anesthesia. However, many of these patients have had some sort of sedation and, as a result, may have depressed respiration. If this is the case, then they may also benefit from added O_2 until fully alert.

POST-OPERATIVE ASSESSMENT

During the immediate post anaesthetic period, a key part of the nurse's role is to monitor and assess the patient. In carrying out continuous assessment, the nurse aims to establish when the patient has fully recovered from anaesthesia and is stable enough to leave the high dependency environment. Effective monitoring and observation will also pick up any problems promptly, such as hypoxia or haemorrhage. The Association of Anaesthetists of Great Britain and Ireland (2002) recommend that the following information should be recorded during this immediate post-anaesthetic period:

1. level of consciousness;
2. haemoglobin oxygen saturation and oxygen administration;
3. blood pressure;
4. respiratory frequency;
5. heart rate and rhythm;
6. pain intensity (e.g. a verbal rating scale);
7. intravenous infusions;
8. drugs administered
9. other parameters (depending on circumstances; e.g. temperature, urine output, central venous pressure, end-tidal CO_2, surgical drainage).

In practice, much of what is described in this section of the chapter will take place simultaneously and may involve more than a single practitioner. However, for the sake of clarity, the actions are described individually.

It should be made absolutely clear that this is a critical stage of the patient episode and patients are extremely vulnerable and highly dependent. Their condition can change rapidly and a seemingly manageable situation can very quickly become an emergency one. It is absolutely vital that the nurse calls for additional expert help if they are at all concerned about their patient's condition.

Patients should arrive in the post-anaesthetic care unit (PACU) accompanied by the anaesthetist and another member of the theatre team, preferably the anaesthetic assistant or scrub assistant. A handover to the PACU nurse should be given which should include:

- identification of the patient (and a name that they will respond to);
- relevant medical history (e.g. whether they suffer from respiratory disease or diabetes);
- allergies;
- details about the operation performed;
- type of anaesthesia used, and any problems at or before induction;
- baseline observations, goal setting;
- any peri-operative problems;
- analgesia and any other drug therapy already given, or to be given;
- the presence of drains, intravenous cannulae, catheters or wound packs;
- any specific post-operative instructions (e.g. that the patient may require additional oxygen for an extended period, or any specific messages to convey to ward staff).

This is also an opportunity for the PACU nurse to ensure that relevant documentation and prescription of analgesia, antiemesis, other drugs, oxygen and intravenous fluid therapy has been completed at sufficient levels to cover the short to medium term.

During handover the nurse can make a preliminary assessment of the patient's general condition. When doing this, it is useful to follow an ABC (Airway, Breathing, Circulation) model. The nurse should establish that the airway is patent and that the patient is breathing. Oxygen therapy and pulse oximetry monitoring should be commenced. The patient's respiratory rate and pattern should be noted. Baseline observations of heart rate and blood pressure should be made and recorded, and wounds and drains checked for excessive bleeding. The patient's level of consciousness and pain should be assessed. Following gynaecological and obstetric surgery, blood loss per vagina (PV) should be checked. If patients are unconscious and their condition allows, it is appropriate to position them laterally (the recovery position; Figure 8.2).

Once this initial assessment has taken place, and the nurse considers it safe, the anaesthetist may leave the patient. A more detailed and methodical assessment of the patient should then be made. It is suggested that the ABC model is still followed but it is recognized that individuals may use variations such as 'top to toe' assessment. The important thing is that the nurse follows a consistent assessment process that ensures nothing is missed. The method outlined here will be based on a systems model, although it is acknowledged that other models, adapted to the post-operative setting, may be equally effective.

> Using an ABC model of assessment will help the nurse to focus on the key priorities of care for a post-anaesthetic patient, irrespective of other issues (i.e. there is no point in checking the wound first if the patient does not have a patent airway!)

AIRWAY MANAGEMENT

Airway obstruction

Airway maintenance is of vital importance in the immediate post-operative phase. Unconsciousness, as a result of anaesthesia, means that the tongue can fall back and obstruct the airway. Even if anaesthesia has worn off, the peri-operative administration of opiates can have a similar effect.

Laryngospasm, as a result of upper airway irritation, causes airway obstruction even in a fully conscious patient. Regurgitation of stomach contents is possible during the immediate post-anaesthetic period and this is a real threat to airway maintenance. The patency of the airway is also at risk following any surgery in the region of the head and neck, as a result of oedema or haematoma formation. Haemorrhage or foreign bodies (e.g. gauze packs used during dental surgery) can also obstruct the airway.

Assessment

An initial overview of the patient's condition can give vital clues as to the patency of the airway. There may be cyanosis present. There may be no movement of the chest or paradoxical (see-saw) breathing, where

Figure 8.2 Recovery position. (Reproduced with permission form Resuscitation Council 2000)

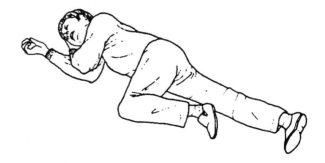

> Total airway obstruction is *silent*. A quiet patient is not necessarily a breathing patient: airway patency must be monitored continuously in an unconscious post-anaesthetic patient.

the abdomen 'sucks in' as the chest expands and vice versa. The trachea may appear to suck inwards during inspiration (tracheal tug). Any of these signs can indicate severe or total obstruction. The breathing may be noisy, as a result of soft palate obstruction indicated by snoring (stertor) or laryngospasm, which results in a loud crowing noise on inspiration (stridor). It is important to remember that total obstruction is silent and so the absence of noisy breathing does not mean that the airway is clear. Confirmation of a patent airway can only really be achieved by ensuring that air is moving in and out of the nose and mouth by listening with your ear close to the patient's face, feeling with your hand over the nose and mouth or by looking, for example, at whether condensation is forming on the inside of the oxygen mask during expiration.

Airway adjuncts

Patients may arrive from the operating room with an artificial airway *in situ* (Box 8.5). This should not be removed until patients show signs of being able to maintain their own airway. This would be indicated by, for example, an increase in conscious level, swallowing or gagging, or an attempt by the patient themselves to remove the airway. The removal of endotracheal tubes, laryngeal mask airways and Guedel airways must always be carried out under controlled and supervised conditions. If there is evidence that the airway is causing patients to gag, this is an indicator that they are likely to be able to manage without it, and it should be removed carefully. This is because the situation can result in the patient vomiting, which, in turn, could lead to serious airway and respiratory complications.

> A patient with an airway adjunct *in situ* must *never* be left unattended.

Intervention

When patients are experiencing problems with their airway, this should be dealt with immediately. In the unconscious patient, the airway should be manually supported until the patient is able to maintain it unaided. Airway obstruction can be life threatening and, for this reason, expert assistance must be sought without delay.

To open the airway, the nurse can move the tongue forward by using the head tilt/chin lift or jaw thrust methods (Box 8.6). If the patient does not already have one, a Guedel airway can be inserted. However, if the patient is not completely unconscious, this should be avoided because of the risk of stimulating a gag reflex and vomiting. The nurse should know that the successful insertion of a Guedel airway does not guarantee a patent airway, and that the patient, if still fully tolerant of a Guedel airway, will still require manual airway support. A nasopharyngeal airway may be used, but the risk of epistaxis and the fact that they can be difficult to insert do not make them ideal in a situation where an airway needs to be established quickly. It is important to note that, even if airway adjuncts are successful, patients who are unable to maintain their own airway should *never* be left unattended. Their condition can change rapidly and unpredictably and, also, synthetic airway adjuncts are not guaranteed to remain in place of their own volition.

Box 8.5   Artificial airways

Guedel (oropharyngeal) airway (Figure 8.3)

Curved plastic tubes with a flange at the oral end, they have a flattened shape so that they fit neatly between the tongue and hard palate. They come in a range of sizes and it is important to select the right one. Too large a size can cause vomiting and laryngospasm, too small will not maintain the airway. The patient's airway may still need to be manually opened even though a Guedel airway is inserted.

Nasopharyngeal airway (Figure 8.4)

These are made from malleable plastic with a bevel at one end and a flange at the other. They are inserted, where possible, into the right nostril (because of the angle of the bevel end), using plenty of lubricant. A safety pin should be inserted through the flange to prevent the airway disappearing. This is better tolerated than the Guedel airway but the risk of trauma is higher. Again, this may well require manual airway support as well.

Laryngeal mask airway (Figure 8.5)

This device is essentially a mini-face mask that sits over the laryngeal inlet. An inflatable cuff creates an airtight seal, allowing administration of anaesthetic gases and, if necessary, positive pressure ventilation. The major disadvantage is that, unlike a cuffed endotracheal tube, it does not protect the airway from aspiration of stomach contents. Left *in situ* following anaesthesia, however, it will prevent obstruction by the tongue. Although the manufacturers recommend that the cuff is deflated immediately prior to removal, this results in the displacement of secretions that have collected on the cuff, and the nurse should be prepared for the patient to cough and should have suction equipment ready. There is a developing trend, however, to leave the cuff inflated during removal, as this seems to remove pharyngeal secretions more effectively on the surface of the mask (Brimacombe et al 1996). This method should be used with care to avoid trauma to the teeth, mouth and the cuff itself. In practice the LMA is sometimes removed with the cuff partially deflated. This is less uncomfortable for the patient but retains most of the secretions. Again, this is a practised skill.

Figure 8.3 Oropharyngeal airway *in situ*. (Reproduced from Henry & Stapleton 1992, p. 102, with kind permission of W B Saunders.)

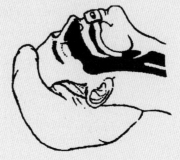

Figure 8.4 Nasopharyngeal airway *in situ*. (Reproduced from Henry & Stapleton 1992, p. 104, with kind permission of W B Saunders)

Figure 8.5 Laryngeal mask airway *in situ*. (Reproduced from Eaton 1992, p 43, with kind permission of the author.)

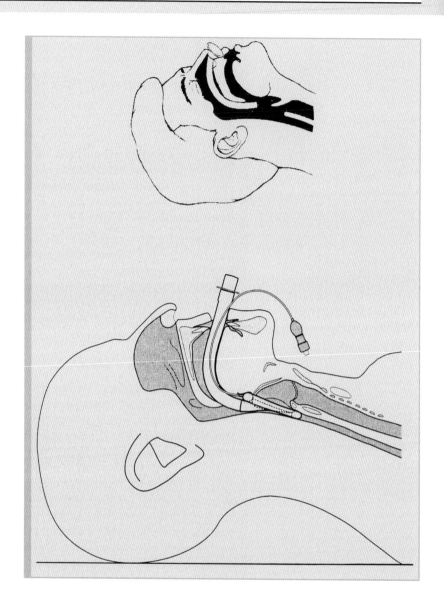

Laryngospasm

Laryngospasm is a protective reflex caused by irritation of the upper airway. It most commonly follows extubation or surgery in the area of the larynx or pharynx (e.g. tonsillectomy). It may also result from the presence of secretions or foreign bodies. It is characterized by a loud high-pitched and distinctive crowing noise on inspiration.

When laryngospasm is present, it is vital to get help and to ensure that emergency equipment necessary for intubation and resuscitation is at hand. The patient's condition can deteriorate very rapidly as hypoxia develops. Treatment is initially aimed at maximizing air entry and clearing the causative agent. If possible, and the patients' condition allows, they should be put in a sitting position to make inspiration more effective and, if not already doing so, encouraged to cough to try to clear any secretions or foreign bodies. Oropharyngeal suction with a large-bore (Yankauer) catheter should be performed if patients are unable to clear the irritant themselves. A high concentration of oxygen should be given via a face mask to reduce the risk of hypoxia. If it is certain that the air-

---

Box 8.6   Manual airway support (Resuscitation Council UK 1994)

Head tilt/chin lift (Figure 8.6)

1. Support the head on a small pillow
2. Extend the head on the neck by pushing the forehead backwards and the occiput forwards
3. Place two fingers under the tip of the mandible and lift the chin, displacing the tongue anteriorly

Jaw thrust (Figure 8.7)

1. Hold the patient's mouth slightly open by pushing the chin down with the thumbs
2. Place the fingers behind the angles of the mandible, and apply steady upward and forward pressure to lift the jaw forward

---

Figure 8.6 Head tilt/chin lift. (Reproduced from Henry & Stapleton 1992, p 51, with kind permission of W B Saunders.)

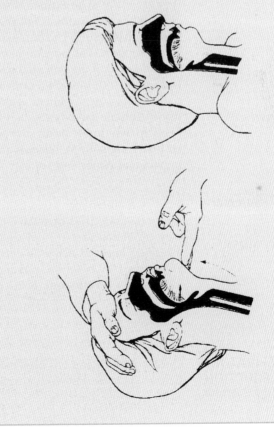

Figure 8.7 Jaw thrust. (Reproduced from Henry & Stapleton 1992, p 52, with kind permission of W B Saunders.)

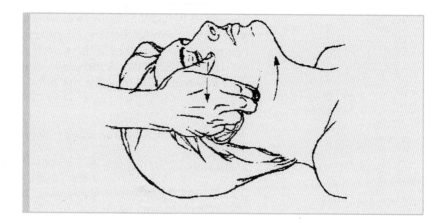

way is clear, then a bag and mask oxygen delivery system can be used to apply positive pressure in an attempt to relieve the laryngospasm (Murray-Calderon & Connolly 1997). In the semiconscious or unconscious patient, manual support of the airway should also be performed.

If these methods are unsuccessful, then the patient will require intubation and the condition allowed to settle before extubation is retried. It is important to remember that laryngospasm with moderate to severe airway obstruction can be present in conscious patients and, as a result, they are likely to be extremely frightened. Not only may patients experience difficulty breathing but they may also find the noise that they are making distressing. The nurse must be aware of this and provide appropriate support. The patient may be very sensitive to their surroundings and be aware of the potential severity of their condition, and it is important for the staff to remain calm and efficient, as this can help to make the patient feel safe. A patient with laryngospasm who starts to panic and hyperventilate can be extremely difficult to manage. This patient is more likely to deteriorate faster than one who is able to maintain a slow regular breathing pattern; hence the need for staff to remain calm in order to impart confidence and security to the patient.

Summary

Airway maintenance must be the prime objective for the nurse during the immediate post-operative period. If a patient is experiencing airway problems that are not easily dealt with, such as the presence of a foreign body or acute swelling of the neck, help should always be summoned. A potentially manageable situation can rapidly develop into a very serious one if an airway is not established quickly and effectively. This can be prevented by getting additional expert help at an early stage.

RESPIRATORY FUNCTION

Once a clear airway has been established, the patient's respiratory function needs to be assessed. Respiratory management is covered in detail in Chapter 5, and this section will focus on the immediate post-operative period and management specific to anaesthesia and surgery.

Anaesthesia depresses respiration and, as the deep stages of anaesthesia are reached, breathing will actually cease. Some surgery (e.g. abdominal) requires muscle paralysis, which, because of its effects on the respiratory muscles, causes respiratory arrest. Opiates given during surgery may depress respiration. The anaesthetist aims to have reversed these effects, with the exception of analgesia, by the time the patient leaves the operating room. Clearly, this is occasionally difficult to titrate accurately. However, there is potential for severe respiratory depression to be present in the immediate post-operative period if all of these things are not fully achieved.

Respiratory assessment

In order to make a comprehensive assessment of respiratory function, the nurse needs to view the patient holistically. The patient's general demeanour should be noted. Restlessness, confusion or a decreased level of consciousness can have many causes in the post-operative patient. However, hypoxia and hypercapnia (high plasma carbon dioxide levels) should be considered until proven otherwise. Pallor or cyanosis can indicate hypoxia. In patients with dark skin, the nailbeds and mucous membranes of the mouth should be looked at in order to make an accurate assessment. This is one of the reasons for removing nail varnish before surgery. As carbon dioxide causes vasodilatation, a patient with a flushed appearance and very warm peripheries may be hypercapnic.

The respiratory rate and pattern should be assessed. A slow rate may be caused by opiate overdose or deep anaesthesia, and this may be accompanied by shallow breathing with resultant diminished tidal volumes. Shallow respirations may also be associated with tachypnoea (a rapid respiratory rate) and this most commonly results from pain, particularly following abdominal or thoracic surgery. A shallow respiratory pattern may also be the result of the continuing effects of muscle relaxants. If the nurse suspects this, further information can be gained by asking patients, if conscious, to open their eyes wide, stick out their tongue or grasp the nurse's hand tightly. An inability to do these things or an obvious lack of power could indicate that there are some continuing effects from the paralysing agents. In an unconscious patient, assessment can be made using a nerve stimulator. This battery-powered device delivers small electric stimuli via two skin electrodes placed over a peripheral nerve. The resulting motor responses to stimuli give an idea as to the extent of neuromuscular blockade. This technique should only be used by people who have been trained to use the device safely.

Movement of the chest wall should be assessed. Both sides of the chest should move upwards and outwards during inspiration. Uneven movement indicates that one lung is inflating less effectively than the other. This can be due to lobar collapse as a result of sputum retention, pneumothorax or haemothorax. The position of the trachea should be noted, as a deviation from the midline can indicate a tension pneumothorax, which will develop into a potentially life-threatening situation if not treated promptly. Palpation of the chest wall can help to assess the symmetry of movement. One can also feel coarse crepitations, which indicate sputum in the larger airways. Surgical emphysema, a condition usually associated with pneumothorax (where air leaks from the pleural cavity into the subcutaneous tissues), may also be felt as a crackling sensation under the skin. Severe surgical emphysema around the neck can, in itself, cause airway obstruction.

Auscultation of the lung fields provides valuable information. In addition to confirming decreased air entry and the presence of loose secretions, fine crackles may indicate pulmonary oedema as a result of, for example, left ventricular failure or fluid overload. Wheezes or loud musical sounds indicate bronchospasm. This is most commonly associated with pre-existing respiratory disease, such as asthma and chronic obstructive airway disease, but may also result from anaphylaxis owing to drug or blood product administration.

Monitoring of oxygen saturation (SpO_2) is essential during the immediate post-operative phase and for those patients with ongoing oxygen therapy, invasive and non-invasive ventilatory support. An accurate measurement is, however, dependent on a good signal at the site of the probe. An unreliable reading may result from a patient with poor peripheral circulation (e.g. someone who is cold or shocked). Changing the monitoring site and using a dedicated probe on the nose or earlobe may produce a better signal. Ambient light sources can also interfere with the signal and a reduction in the amount of light interference, for example, by placing the hand under the bedclothes, can help to achieve a more accurate reading. It is essential to view the plethysmographic wave on the pulse oximeter produced by the patient's pulse in order to ensure that an accurate reading is being achieved. It is important not to accept the numerical display as being accurate, unless there is a clearly defined and supportive plethysmographic waveform. Although pulse oximetry gives useful information about oxygenation, it does not necessarily give any information about how well the lungs are being ventilated. There have been cases where patients with a normal SpO_2 have been found to have dangerously high blood levels of carbon dioxide as a result of hypoventilation (Davidson & Hosie 1993). Capnography should be available to enable monitoring of expired carbon dioxide levels, where indicated. Where hypoxia or hypercapnia is suspected, it is essential to confirm this by taking an arterial blood sample for blood gas analysis (see Chapter 5).

In order to complete the picture of the patient's respiratory status, a chest X-ray can be performed. This can confirm the cause of diminished respiratory function, in particular pneumothorax, lobar collapse owing to sputum retention and pulmonary oedema. It will also confirm the position of endotracheal tubes, pleural drains and central venous lines.

> Ensure that you have a clearly defined waveform on the pulse oximeter before you are confident that you have a correct numerical reading. Also remember that pulse oximetry measures O_2 saturation not CO_2 levels: a satisfactory SpO_2 does not necessarily mean that the patient is breathing effectively.

Respiratory management

While the majority of patients in the immediate post-operative period will not have respiratory problems, it is said that hypoxia is the most common and dangerous cause of damage to patients during this period (Hatfield & Tronson 1996). While nurses have a vital role to play in detecting respiratory insufficiency as outlined above, their main role must be to prevent it occurring in the first place. Where decreased respiratory function is present, it is important to establish the cause and treat it appropriately (Box 8.7). However, as every patient has the potential to develop breathing problems, nurses can reduce the risks substantially by intervening early.

Deep breathing can be encouraged to help prevent post-operative respiratory problems. Nurses can help the patient to deep breathe effectively by placing their hands on the chest wall and encouraging the patient to try to push the hands away by taking the deepest breath possible. When maximum inspiration is achieved, asking the patient to hold their breath, close their mouth and take a small 'sniff' will help to prevent areas of lung collapsing. In addition to this, the patient should be encouraged to cough, which will again help to prevent atelectasis (partial or full lung collapse) and reinflate collapsed areas of the lungs. When abdominal or thoracic surgery has been performed, patients should be instructed to hold their wound, having first covered it with a folded towel or small pillow, as this can make it less painful and helps to reduce patients' fear of 'bursting their stitches'. Both of these exercises are easier to perform with the patient in the sitting position unless this is contraindicated (e.g. following surgery on the spinal column). Unless otherwise specified or indicated, patients should be helped to sit up as soon as they are awake enough to do so. Sitting up will also improve expansion of the lung bases. It should be noted that, following certain types of surgery, such as ophthalmic or neurological, coughing should not be encouraged, as the resultant rise in local pressure can be detrimental to the patient's condition. This is important because the high intrathoracic pressures generated during coughing can be transmitted to, for example, the blood vessels in the brain. Following neurosurgery, where maintaining a low intracranial pressure is critical, this is clearly undesirable.

Deep breathing and coughing will be difficult, if not impossible, for patients to perform if they are in a lot of pain. This is particularly true following abdominal and thoracic surgery. The importance of adequate pain relief in preventing post-operative respiratory problems cannot be stressed strongly enough (Aitkenhead 1996).

> Encouraging early deep breathing and coughing helps to reduce post-operative respiratory complications.

CARDIOVASCULAR SYSTEM

Anaesthesia and surgery often affect the cardiovascular system. These effects can range from mild hypotension to serious levels of shock. Table 8.3 lists some of the more common cardiovascular effects.

Assessment

When first accepting a patient, the nurse should carry out a general assessment of the patient's cardiovascular status. Pallor, clammy skin,

> **Box 8.7   Causes of decreased respiratory function and initial interventions**
>
> **Anaesthesia**
>
> Maintain airway, give O_2, monitor SpO_2, provide stimulus to wake (shake patient gently and call name). Consider giving flumazenil, if benzodiazepines have been used in surgery or as pre-medication.
>
> **Opiate effects**
>
> Maintain airway, give O_2, monitor SpO_2, encourage patient to take deep breaths. Consider naloxone but expect patient to wake in pain; alternatively use doxapram to increase respiratory rate and depth.
>
> **Residual paralysis**
>
> Maintain airway, give O_2, monitor SpO_2, provide reassurance if patient awake. Give neostigmine to reverse paralysing agents.
>
> **Basal collapse**
>
> Give O_2, monitor SpO_2, encourage deep breathing and coughing exercises, sit patient up, change position regularly, consider CPAP, involve physiotherapist.
>
> **Pneumothorax**
>
> Give O_2, monitor SpO_2, prepare for chest drain insertion. If tension pneumothorax develops with acute deterioration in patient condition, consider needle thoracocentesis. Involve the physiotherapists.
>
> **Pain**
>
> Give O_2, monitor SpO_2, give adequate analgesia or consider alternative analgesia if present method not effective. Change patient's position, show patient how to support wound to aid deep breathing.
>
> **Heart failure**
>
> Give O_2, monitor SpO_2, sit patient up; consider diuretics, vasodilators and inotropic support.

weak peripheral pulses and cool extremities can all be signs of a poor cardiac output and/or hypovolaemia. Wounds should be checked for any obvious bleeding or haematoma formation, and volumes of blood in any drainage systems should be noted. The patient's temperature should be taken, preferably using a tympanic thermometer, to ensure that the patient is not hypothermic. There is a vast range of techniques available for monitoring cardiovascular parameters, such as ECG monitoring and automated non-invasive blood pressure measurement, and choice depends upon patient need and the availability of equipment. It is

Table 8.3 Cardiovascular effects

Effect	Possible cause
Dysrhythmias	Anaesthetic agents and drugs
	Hypoxia
	Hypokalaemia
Hypotension	Anaesthetic agents and drugs
	Hypovolaemia/haemorrhage
	Epidural/spinal anaesthesia
Hypertension	Fluid overload
	Peripheral vasoconstriction
	Pain/anxiety
	Pre-existing hypertension
Haemorrhage	Incomplete surgical haemostasis
	Ruptured suture line/slipped tie
Heart failure	Fluid overload

important, however, that nurses do not become overdependent upon technology and forget, for example, how to use the manual palpation of pulses, manual auscultation of blood pressures and water central venous pressure manometers as measurement tools. It will, after all, be these techniques that will have to be employed in the event of equipment failure or non-availability. Nevertheless, the bare minimum is regular monitoring of heart rate and blood pressure, as these give fundamental information about cardiovascular status. Changes in these parameters can be a good indicator of impending problems. The frequency of these measurements is really dependent on the condition of the patient, but the important thing is to measure and record them regularly so that any trends can be seen. 'One-off' measurements can be highly subjective and give little useful information.

Advanced cardiovascular monitoring is covered in more detail in Chapter 6.

Dysrhythmias

The majority of dysrhythmias seen immediately post-operatively tend to be sinus tachycardia or bradycardia. These are normally related to drug therapy, hypovolaemia, pain and anxiety. The main aim of management should be to treat the causative factor, not the rhythm. It is also worth looking at the pre-operative ECG, if available, as this can save a lot of anxiety for the staff, as the patient may have a pre-existing abnormal ECG. Many patients with hypertension are treated with beta-blockers and bradycardia is normal for them. Again, the important thing is whether or not the patient's condition is compromised. Patients with a heart rate of 120 who are otherwise stable should be observed and the tachycardia not treated unless there is deterioration in their condition. Patients with a heart rate of 50 who are hypotensive and complain of feeling light-headed may need to have the rate speeded up with drugs such as atropine or glycopyrrolate. However, in such an instance, the opinion of a medical colleague should be sought.

Atrial fibrillation is frequently seen and its treatment depends on the patient's pre-operative state, and whether or not it is causing problems. The serum potassium should be checked and digoxin given, if necessary. Ventricular extrasystolic beats (ectopics) are usually due to hypokalaemia and this should be corrected with prescribed potassium therapy. Antiarrhythmic drug therapy is only usually used if the extrasystoles are frequent and may potentially compromise the patient's condition. Very often, the more common dysrhythmias are benign and do not need treatment (Aitkenhead 1996).

Less common arrhythmias associated with pre-existing heart disease or peri-operative myocardial infarction are covered in Chapter 6 and so will not be dealt with here.

Hypotension and hypertension

Hypotension is often directly related to anaesthesia and, as such, usually ceases to be a problem as the anaesthesia wears off. It can, however, also be due to haemorrhage, or the effects of spinal or epidural anaesthesia or pain relief. The overall condition of the patient needs to be assessed before treatment of hypotension is initiated. A sleeping patient who is stable, except for a systolic blood pressure of 80 mmHg or below, should be allowed to wake before a decision to treat the blood pressure is made.

Patients having spinal or epidural anaesthesia are often hypotensive, as the blocking of the sympathetic nerves owing to this technique can cause peripheral vasodilatation. The reason that these patients should not sit up until they regain feeling in their legs is that they lose the ability to vasoconstrict and would, therefore, be at risk of postural hypotension. As chronic respiratory or heart disease is often the reason for using spinal anaesthesia, it is not wise to treat the hypotension with large volumes of fluid. More commonly, ephedrine, a vasoconstrictor, is used to raise the blood pressure. However, it must be remembered that this is achieved synthetically (i.e. via medication) rather than occurring naturally.

Patients who are cold following surgery can become hypotensive as they warm and peripherally vasodilate. This is managed by giving colloid solutions, preferably while monitoring central venous pressure. Where hypotension is a result of cardiac insufficiency, it may be necessary to use inotropic agents (see Chapter 6). A rare but serious cause of hypotension is malignant hyperpyrexia (Box 8.8). Although most commonly seen during anaesthesia, it is important for the post-operative care nurse to be aware of it and its treatment.

The two most common causes of *hyper*tension in the immediate post-operative period are pre-existing peripheral vascular disease and pain. Antihypertensive medications should not be omitted prior to surgery because the patient is fasting. Evidence suggests that taking a small volume of fluid (i.e. a sip to swallow) with their tablets prior to surgery does not increase the risk of vomiting (Greenfield et al 1997).

Following certain types of surgery (e.g. cardiac and vascular), it is important to keep the blood pressure below a certain level to protect the integrity of vascular suture lines. However, if doubt prevails, this must

> Patients who have had spinal anaesthesia should be sat up gradually to avoid dizziness and syncope. They should not stand up until full sensation has returned to their legs.

> Unless specifically requested, regular medications should not be omitted on the grounds that the patient is 'nil by mouth'.

Box 8.8   Malignant hyperpyrexia

Malignant hyperpyrexia is a hereditary disorder of calcium metabolism. Following administration of a triggering agent, usually inhalational anaesthetic agents or depolarizing muscle relaxants, there is an excess release of calcium ions in the muscle tissues. This results in massive and continuous skeletal muscle contraction with associated build-up of heat. The temperature can rise rapidly by as much as 6–8°C/hour. Left untreated, the patient is likely to die. The only effective treatment is sodium dantrolene, which inhibits calcium ion release. The nurse working in the post-operative care unit must be aware of where the stock of this drug is kept, as, when it is required, it is required immediately. Other measures include stopping the administration of the triggering agent and active cooling of the patient. This is immediately life threatening and expert medical help should be summoned without delay.

---

be discussed with the anaesthetist/surgeon beforehand, and the decision clearly documented.

Haemorrhage

Nearly all surgery involves some degree of blood loss and the degree of post-operative bleeding is dependent on the type of surgery. For example, one would expect more blood loss following hip replacement than following thyroidectomy.

When assessing post-operative bleeding, the overall cardiovascular status should be taken into account rather than simply looking at the volume of ooze or drainage. For example, take a patient who is cardiovascularly stable and peripherally warm following hip/knee joint surgery, but continues to drain 200 ml/hour into vacuum drains. This patient would cause no real concern as long as he or she is given blood to replace the losses. However, there should be great concern about a patient following laparotomy who is persistently tachycardic, hypotensive, cold and oliguric despite continued colloid filling.

The management of haemorrhage should aim at preventing complications by maintaining an adequate circulating volume and haemoglobin content. Observed losses (e.g. into drains) should be replaced with colloid, preferably blood. Where bleeding is less obvious, filling should be guided by vital signs and, where possible, central venous pressure measurements. Haemoglobin levels should be measured, particularly when large volumes of plasma (or plasma substitutes) have been infused. If felt appropriate, a clotting screen should be performed and, where indicated, clotting agents such as fresh-frozen plasma given.

Obvious oozing from a wound should be treated by applying a pressure dressing, which should then be monitored closely. When bleeding from a wound is heavy or sudden, direct manual pressure should be applied and maintained while a surgeon is summoned. If this does not stem the flow, it is likely that exploration of the wound in theatre will be required. A return to theatre may be necessary where bleeding is suspected but not visible (e.g. intra-abdominally). In certain cases, wounds may need to be opened quickly as haematoma formation may put the patient at risk (e.g. following thyroidectomy), where a patent airway could be threatened. For this reason, wounds for this type of surgery are often closed with clips or staples, which are easier to remove than sutures, especially in an emergency. The nurse caring for these patients should have clip/staple removers easily to hand. Occasionally, sudden catastrophic haemorrhage may occur (e.g. following vascular surgery). As well as the measures outlined above, rapid fluid administration will be necessary, including non-cross-matched blood (O negative), if indicated and prescribed. It may also be necessary to initiate cardiopulmonary resuscitation if the patient either becomes pulseless or ceases to have an effective cardiac output. It is important to remember that bleeding will not always be obvious (e.g. if it is intra-abdominal). The importance of regular and thorough monitoring and recording vital signs must not be underestimated.

If large volumes of stored blood need to be given because of a major haemorrhage, patients can become hypothermic and it is best to give the blood through a warming system where possible. Clotting problems may also develop, as stored blood is depleted of clotting factors. In view of this, it is common to give fresh-frozen plasma after every few units of blood to try to reduce this problem.

Clearly, as in all situations involving body fluids, the nurse caring for a bleeding patient should observe universal precautions.

Hypothermia

Hypothermia is said to exist when the body temperature drops to 35.8°C or less (Surkitt-Parr 1992). There are many reasons why hypothermia develops in the surgical patient, including the effects of anaesthesia, insufficient covering, the ambient temperature of operating theatres (21–24.8°C), the length of surgery and pre-operative fasting (McNeil 1998). Although measures are often taken in theatre to reduce the risk of hypothermia, such as the use of warming mattresses and blankets, it is common for patients to be hypothermic post-operatively. It is important to monitor the patient's temperature frequently during the initial period. Mild hypothermia (35.8°C) can be managed by using woollen blankets and ensuring that the patient is not unnecessarily exposed (e.g. ensure that arms and shoulders are covered with bedclothes). At temperatures below 35.8°C, active warming should be performed. This can be done using forced warm-air technology. This involves the use of a warm air blower and a disposable inflatable quilt. The quilt is placed next to the patient and warm air escapes from the underside. This has been shown to be the most effective way of warming post-operative patients (Giuffre et al 1991) and is becoming increasingly popular. However, because the technique is so effective, care should be taken not to overheat the patient and so avoid the problems of sudden rewarming, as mentioned earlier. Where possible, warming should be achieved by more conventional (non-technological) approaches.

NEUROLOGICAL STATUS

Assessment

During anaesthesia, there is obviously a marked change in neurological status. At the lower stages of anaesthesia, the patient is deeply unconscious and loses many of the normal reflexes. When anaesthesia is stopped, the patient emerges from unconsciousness, passing through the stages of anaesthesia in reverse. This is important, as it gives the nurse dealing with a waking patient an idea of what stage of recovery has been reached. It also gives some insight into the reasons for the patient's behaviour. Generally, the lines of distinction between the stages are blurred and the patient simply wakes up without difficulty. Reactions are sometimes very marked, however, and it is important to remember that a restless, confused or aggressive patient may simply be passing through the delirium stage.

In the event of the surgical procedure taking less time than anticipated, the patient may be paralysed and, therefore, have to be maintained in an unconscious state until the muscle relaxant drugs that have been administered wear off.

Formal assessment of a patient's neurological function is only really necessary if he or she does not wake as expected or remains confused or distressed. Neurological assessment is dealt with in detail in Chapter 7 and so will not be discussed here. From the point of view of immediate post-anaesthetic assessment, the patient's name should be called and, if necessary, he or she can be gently shaken by the shoulders. If this fails to elicit a response, then the patient should be left to sleep and another attempt made to rouse him or her a few minutes later. Painful stimuli (e.g. rubbing the sternum, twisting ear lobes or even slapping the face) should *never* be used to wake the patient up! Indeed, nurses should, in general, avoid these altogether. They are extremely painful and potentially harmful and, if not done for a justifiable reason, are tantamount to assault. Also, the application of controlled painful stimuli, such as applying pressure to nailbeds or testing palmar reflexes, should be used only as part of a full neurological assessment when there is genuine concern about the patient's level of consciousness. In addition, these techniques should only be carried out by staff who are proficient and skilled in this area. The point at which one should become concerned about the patient not waking up is dependent on many factors. These include the type and length of anaesthetic, whether or not pre-medication was given, what analgesia was given in theatre and the patient's age, general health and pre-operative neurological state.

It is important to make the distinction between the sleeping and the unconscious patient. Where reflexes are present, the airway is being self-maintained and there is some response to stimuli, it is likely that the patient is in a deep sleep, possibly due to opiate analgesia. It could also be due to pre-medication still having an effect or merely because the patient is physically exhausted. It tends to be forgotten that patients may have very little rest in the days leading up to surgery, often as a result of anxiety, sleeping in an unfamiliar environment and constant interruptions. If they have undergone emergency surgery, they may well have endured days of discomfort or pain. It should not be surprising then, that when it is all over and their pain is well controlled, they can sleep deeply

Painful stimuli should be used only as part of a formal neurological assessment: never use them simply to wake a patient up.

for a considerable time. Sleeping patients may stir from time to time and respond to stimuli, although they may not be able to keep their eyes open or talk coherently. However, the unconscious patient will not respond and may well require assistance to maintain a patent airway. For example, an unconscious patient will tolerate a Guedel airway while a sleeping patient will tend not to. It is the patient who remains unconscious for a long time who should give cause for concern and must be closely and constantly attended to until the situation corrects itself.

Serious neurological problems following anaesthesia are rare (Hines et al 2002), but some people do have oversensitive reactions and can remain unconscious for hours; this is sometimes referred to as delayed emergence (Hatfield & Tronson 1996). Treatment of this condition is mainly supportive, including artificial ventilation, if necessary. More commonly, the combination of pre-medication, anaesthetic and opiate analgesia can be the cause of prolonged unconsciousness. If it is felt necessary, the administration of naloxone will usually reverse the effects of the opiate either partially or fully. Naloxone acts by blocking the effects of opiates, which means that, unless used very carefully, the patient can wake rapidly in considerable pain. Its judicious use can, however, establish that there is no serious neurological problem. It is important to appreciate that naloxone has a very short half-life and repeated doses may be required to maintain satisfactory levels of neurological and respiratory function. Naloxone can also be administered as a controlled infusion. The use of benzodiazepines (e.g. diazepam) as pre-medication can also delay a return to consciousness, particularly if they are given very near the time of surgery. If this is suspected, flumazenil (Anexate) may be used as an antagonist to reverse the effects of the drug.

As in every situation, the level of consciousness should not be viewed in isolation and the patient's general condition should be assessed carefully before treatment is initiated. For example, in a patient who is profoundly hypotensive, restoring normal blood pressure is more likely to improve the conscious level than administering naloxone. This also avoids the undesirable reversal of analgesia.

Neurological assessment during the immediate post-operative period is not confined to the central nervous system. A large range of regional and local blocks may be used instead of general anaesthesia or as post-operative pain relief. These should be assessed not only to make sure that they are working but also to protect the patient from injury. Following spinal anaesthesia, for example, patients should not be allowed to stand until full sensation has returned to their legs and they are able to weight bear fully, otherwise they are at serious risk of injury/falling. Because of reduced sensation and mobility, these patients are also at risk of pressure-related injuries, in the same way as a paraplegic might be. It is essential for the nurse to ensure that areas at risk, for example, heels and the sacral area, are assessed diligently using a validated assessment process, e.g. Waterlow. Where necessary, pressure-relieving devices, such as low airloss beds, should be considered.

However, as the effects of the block are transient, regular monitoring and changes of position should be effective. Where local blocks have been used, the affected area should be protected until sensation returns in order to avoid injury. The nurse should be particularly aware of this, as it is all too easy to trap an anaesthetized hand between a bed and trolley without any reaction from the patient. This is all part of the advocacy role of nurses on behalf of their patient.

FLUID MANAGEMENT

The management of fluid balance will be covered in detail in Chapter 10. There are certain things that should be borne in mind when looking after the post-surgical patient. It is important to establish the amount and type of fluid that has been given and lost in theatre, as this can have a bearing on the patient's overall condition. Colloid will only normally be given if there has been significant blood loss in theatre. Generally, crystalloid, such as Hartmann's solution (compound sodium lactate), is given as necessary to maintain the patient's blood pressure, replace insensible losses and to rehydrate them following a period of fasting.

Post-operative fluid regimens are dependent on factors such as weight, age, measured blood loss and the anticipated time before oral fluids will be taken. It is now fairly standard practice following major surgery to give fluid based on measurement of central venous pressure and urine output, where appropriate, rather than simply giving a certain volume over a period of time. This approach is often safer, more effective and better geared to the individual.

Following major surgery, it is common for the patient to have an indwelling urinary catheter. This allows better assessment of fluid requirements and cardiovascular status. The urine output may be low following surgery. This is often due to the fact that no fluids have been taken by the patient for up to 16 hours, as it is still common practice, although largely unnecessary, to allow nothing by mouth from midnight on the day before the operation. If the urine is very concentrated or volume is small, it is usually no real cause for concern as long as the patient is not cardiovascularly compromised. It is likely that it will improve as the patient starts to take oral fluids or is intravenously rehydrated. It may be necessary to increase the rate of intravenous fluids or give a fluid challenge, if the urine output is very low. As a rule of thumb, the aim is to achieve a urine output of 0.5–1.0 ml/kg per hour.

When there is no urine output at all, it is best to check for mechanical problems before administering large volumes of fluid to the patient. The position of the catheter should be checked to make sure it is correctly sited. A bladder washout with saline can be performed in case a blood clot or debris is blocking the catheter lumen. If fluid can be injected but not aspirated, it indicates that there is some form of obstruction. This may be caused by the retaining balloon and removing a few millilitres of water from it may improve the situation. If the problem persists, then the catheter may well need changing.

If the urine output remains poor despite the patient being adequately filled, with a reasonable blood pressure and a patent catheter, a dopamine infusion at a rate that will improve renal perfusion (2–5 μg/kg per minute) may be commenced. Diuretics, such as urosemide, should only be used if there is evidence of fluid overload or retention or signs of heart failure. Using diuretics simply to improve the figures on the chart without resolving the cause results in a dehydrated patient who will stop passing urine later on and is not good clinical care.

PAIN CONTROL

Good pain control is vital following surgery. Uncontrolled pain not only is distressing for the patient, but delays recovery and increases the risk of post-operative complications (Hauer et al 1995). Pain assessment and management will be dealt with in detail in Chapter 11. This section will focus on the relief of immediate post-operative pain.

Analgesic drugs are usually given during surgery to keep the patient pain free during the procedure and, in an ideal situation, this should continue into the immediate and later post-operative periods. In practice, analgesia given in theatre, apart from epidural and spinal, will have lost some of its effectiveness by the time the patient wakes up. The anaesthetist has to balance the positive side of good post-operative analgesia against the negative aspects of the patient not waking up or breathing effectively. It is, therefore, common for nurses to have to deal with patients waking up in some degree of pain, varying from mild to very severe. Dealing with pain often becomes the priority, as the distress it causes makes any accurate assessment of the patient's condition impossible. Assessment and management of pain is an essential element of nursing care. To assess pain and evaluate the effects of pain control administered, scoring tools are used. These vary from hospital to hospital; however; the prerequisites of all tools are that they are easy to understand and that they are accompanied by a protocol for appropriate intervention.

Fortunately, there are a number of types of pain control available that are very effective in the immediate post-operative period:

- non-steroidal anti-inflammatory drugs (NSAIDs);
- opiates;
- regional and local blocks.

NSAIDs

This group of drugs, which includes paracetamol, coproxamol and diclofenac, is useful for mild to moderate pain. Although they are not the first choice in treating acute severe pain, they are extremely effective in treating deep aching pain, as seen following orthopaedic or gynaecological surgery, for example. Given either during surgery or at the same time as opiates, they can provide an excellent long-lasting combination of analgesia. There are many preparations available and they can be given by a variety of routes. One of the most commonly used is diclofenac (Voltarol). Voltarol may be given rectally as well as orally, which is useful if the patient is nauseated or vomiting.

Opiates

Opiates are by far the most common type of analgesia used for acute post-operative pain. Although there are many preparations, the two most commonly used are morphine and diamorphine. The usual routes of administration are intramuscular, intravenous and epidural. Intramuscular (i.m.) injection remains popular. It gives good pain relief for moderate to severe pain within 15–30 minutes of administration. The duration of analgesia is dependent on the preparation but i.m. morphine, for example, can last for up to 3–4 hours. The drawback to the intramuscular route is that there are peaks and troughs of effectiveness. Ideally, the drug should be given regularly whether the patient has pain or not. What tends to happen, however, is that the doses are given when the patient requests them, meaning that the patient has to experience pain in order to obtain analgesia, which is far from ideal.

More even or constantly titrated analgesia can be achieved by running a continuous infusion. The infusion can be run subcutaneously but the intravenous route is felt to be slightly more effective for acute post-operative pain. The problem with using opiates by continuous intravenous infusion is that the effect is cumulative and the risk of overdose is high unless the patient's conscious level is carefully monitored. As this would effectively mean waking the patient every 30–60 minutes, it rather defeats the object of providing good analgesia. A technique rapidly growing in popularity in the area of post-operative analgesia is patient-controlled analgesia (PCA). This involves intravenous opiate being delivered via a device that allows patients to administer regular analgesia, as they require it. There are many different devices on the market but effectively they all do the same thing, which is to allow the patient to deliver a fixed dose of analgesia at set intervals. These parameters either are fixed, as in some of the disposable systems, or may be determined by nursing and medical staff. The great advantage of PCA over continuous infusion is that it puts the patient in control. It also makes overdose virtually impossible, as the patient has to be conscious in order to deliver a dose. It is important to note that, in order for this method to be fully effective, the patient will require full, and quite possibly repeated, explanation of how it works. It is also essential that nurses undertake regular assessment of patients' pain, nausea and sedation levels, and the effectiveness of the analgesia. The fact that analgesia is patient controlled does not mean that the nurse is not or must not be involved in its management; quite the reverse is true.

Giving statutory intravenous doses of opiate has a place in the immediate post-operative period in order to control pain rapidly. The doses should be small and given regularly until the pain is relieved. It is important to achieve good analgesia by this method before commencing continuous infusion or PCA, otherwise they will simply not be effective. In the case of continuous infusion, this will allow the rate to be set at a reasonable level. The temptation otherwise will be for the nurse to increase the rate to the maximum prescribed dose and, as a result, patients receive far more of the drug than they actually need. If patients in pain are simply connected to a PCA system, they will end up demanding doses more frequently than they are able to receive them. Not only will the pain not be controlled, but they will grow increasingly more frustrated and disillusioned with the system. Most modern PCA systems will allow nurses and doctors to assess how many times a patient is requesting a dose of analgesia versus the number of viable doses that have been delivered. This helps to assess the efficacy and adequacy of the prescription.

Epidural administration of opiates, usually by continuous infusion, is particularly effective for surgery of the lower limbs, pelvis and abdomen. Pain from thoracic surgery can also be well controlled by an epidural sited at cervical level. Less commonly, epidural analgesia is managed with a PCA system, although this tends to be most often used with obstetric patients.

Opiates depress the central nervous system. Of particular importance is depression of the respiratory centre. Patients receiving opiates, particularly by continuous infusion, should have their conscious level and respiratory function closely and regularly monitored at a very minimum. Where possible, the peripheral oxygen saturation should be continuously monitored. It is standard practice for a patient having an opiate infusion to be prescribed naloxone. This is often instructed to be given if the respiratory rate falls below a certain level; however, this is often an arbitrary figure, and it is wise to perform a thorough assessment of patients and to try to rouse them before giving naloxone. Obviously, if patients are unrousable with a slow respiratory rate that is potentially compromising them, then the opiate effects should be reversed. Whenever the nurse is attending to post-operative patients, particularly those having opiate analgesia, it is good practice to encourage them to take a few deep breaths and to cough. This will greatly reduce the risk of atelectasis (collapse of alveoli) and chest infection.

Regional and local blocks

Epidural administration of opiates has already been mentioned; however, local anaesthetic can also be given by this route. This blocks pain impulses in the peripheral nervous system and so has the advantage of not creating drowsiness or respiratory depression. It does, however, produce paraesthesia and so decreases patient mobility and, as mentioned earlier, can cause hypotension. In practice, epidural infusions tend to be made up of local anaesthetic and opiate mixed together. This allows smaller doses of each to be used, reaping the benefits of both, but minimizing the unwanted side effects.

Local or regional blocks are achieved by infiltrating the area around a nerve with local anaesthetic. These can be very localized, such as a ring block, or can cover a wider area, such as spinal anaesthetic. These blocks are very effective and aim to numb the area completely. This means that the actual surgery can be performed using them, so avoiding the risks of general anaesthesia. Even if the patient does have an anaesthetic, they provide good analgesia post-operatively. The effects last anything up to 4–6 hours, but it is wise to commence some other form of analgesia once sensation starts to return, so that the pain does not get out of control. In certain situations, a catheter can be left *in situ* through which local anaesthetic may be given by continuous infusion. This is particularly effective following thoracic surgery, where the tip of the catheter is situated near the nerves supplying a specific area of the chest wall (paravertebral block). A growing practice is for surgeons to instil the tissues with local anaesthetic before the wound is closed. This can mean that the patient is completely pain free for a couple of hours post-operatively, which is a great benefit, particularly to aid the necessary deep breathing and coughing in the initial recovery phase.

Pain control is one of the most important aspects of post-operative care and the nurse has a primary role in ensuring that it is achieved. Patients in pain can be difficult to manage and this can make other aspects of their condition harder to assess. By effectively controlling pain, recovery can be quicker and complications reduced.

WOUND CARE

Wound management is a huge subject and detailed examination is beyond the scope of this book. There is a massive range of proposed strategies (Moore 1997, Courtenay 1998, Lait & Smith 1998) and of products available on the market. Every hospital is likely to have an infection control team who are instrumental in developing local wound-care protocols. In addition to this, surgeons will have their own preferences as to how wounds should be managed. With this in mind, this chapter will not go into specifics, but will concentrate on the basic principles of management of fresh surgical wounds and the more common post-operative complications.

Wounds should be checked regularly as part of the overall post-operative assessment. More often than not, this is a cursory glance at the dressing to make sure that there is no obvious bleeding, swelling or reddening of the skin. Immediately following surgery, there are unlikely to be any signs of infection, but reddening may occur because of an allergic reaction to the dressing itself and/or the skin preparation.

> Make sure not to confuse skin reddening owing to the type of skin preparation used with an allergic reaction. However, check with a senior nurse or doctor if unsure.

Although most dressings are now hypoallergenic, Elastoplast is still used where it is necessary to apply pressure to the wound, and many people are allergic to this. If an allergic reaction is suspected, the dressing should be removed and an alternative used. Care should be taken when removing the dressing, as skin can be pulled away at the same time, particularly in the elderly or where blistering has occurred.

The main complication associated with fresh wounds is haemorrhage. This may be obvious or may result in haematoma formation. Where there is overt bleeding from the wound, direct pressure should be applied and a surgical opinion sought. Initially, the pressure should be applied over the existing dressing, but this may have to be removed for either better assessment or renewal. The aim should be to keep any contact with the wound aseptic. If the bleeding is heavy, however, the priority is to stop it and so a clean technique is acceptable. At the very least, universal precautions (such as wearing gloves) should be followed to protect both the patient and staff in the best way possible under such urgent circumstances. Often a period of direct pressure application, followed by some form of pressure dressing, is sufficient to stop the bleeding. If this is not the case, then re-exploration of the wound in theatre may be necessary. It should be remembered that a little blood goes a long way and that what may appear to be a significant bleed may only amount to a few millilitres. Surgical dressings are designed to absorb blood, thereby taking it away from the wound; a bloodstained dressing pad is best left alone, as it is doing what it is supposed to do. Only if blood is seeping through should one consider changing it. Even then, it may be better to apply a pad over the top of the existing dressing, rather than remove the original. Each time a fresh wound is exposed, it increases the risk of infection to the patient.

Haematoma formation can be very obvious and, again, direct pressure should be used to prevent the haematoma becoming larger, and a surgical opinion sought. Where drainage devices are present, their patency should be confirmed, and vacuum systems should be checked to ensure that a vacuum is present. Removing a proportion of the wound closure system can sometimes allow the haematoma to drain but, more often than not, the wound will require surgical re-exploration. Early detection and treatment of haematoma formation is particularly important following surgery around the head and neck (e.g. carotid endartarectomy or thyroidectomy), as the patient's airway can be compromised. If this occurs, the nurse may often have no option but to remove some or all of the wound closure in order to prevent a life-threatening situation. However, this is an extreme situation with significant consequences, and should only be carried out by a skilled operator.

POST-OPERATIVE NAUSEA AND VOMITING

Nausea and vomiting are two of the most common complications following anaesthesia and surgery (Naylor & Inall 1994). The physiology of post-operative nausea and vomiting (PONV) is multifaceted and complex, and beyond the brief of this chapter. A number of factors are thought to affect its incidence, such as age, gender, obesity, anxiety and previous history of PONV (Tate & Cook 1996a). The type of surgery also has an effect (e.g. laparoscopic procedures have been found to have a high incidence of PONV; Fortier et al 1998). Drugs used during anaesthesia and opiate analgesia are thought to be major contributory factors in PONV (Palazzo & Evans 1993).

Although often seen as a relatively minor complication, PONV is distressing for patients and potentially dangerous, as it increases, for example, intracranial and intraocular pressure. This is particularly so, if the surgery has been performed in these areas. Prevention of PONV is desirable and anaesthetists will often give prophylaxis before or during surgery.

Treatment of PONV with antiemetic drugs is common (Box 8.9) and often very effective. There are, however, measures that the nurse can take to reduce PONV. These include keeping movement to a minimum, ensuring adequate pain relief and reducing anxiety. Maintaining oxygenation, hydration and blood pressure will also help prevent PONV. Less orthodox treatments, such as acupressure, herbal remedies and aromatherapy, have been shown to be effective (Tate & Cook 1996b), but do not appear to be widely practised in the acute hospital and immediate post-operative setting.

Post-operative nausea and vomiting is unpleasant and distressing for the patient. It is not a 'minor' complication or something that can be left to get better on its own. Make treating it a priority.

Box 8.9   Antiemetic agents

Phenothiazines

Most common is prochlorperazine. It can cause Parkinsonian-type symptoms at high doses. It is also known to cause sedation and hypotension, particularly if given intravenously.

Dopamine antagonists

An example is metoclopramide. Metoclopramide can also cause extrapyramidal effects but can be given intravenously without hypotension, and so is useful for rapid treatment.

Butyrophenones

Examples are droperidol and haloperidol. These have an antiemetic effect but are major tranquillizers and so will produce drowsiness. They tend to be used for prophylaxis rather than treatment.

Antihistamines

Cyclizine is sometimes used for PONV but its duration is short, and it can cause sedation.

5-HT$_3$ antagonists

These drugs have already been widely used in the prevention of chemotherapy-induced nausea and vomiting. Their use in the treatment of PONV is becoming more common, although they are not always the first choice because of their high cost. The most commonly used are ondansetron and granisetron.

Patients experiencing PONV should have their airways closely monitored, as they are at risk of obstruction and aspiration. Patients who have vomited should be given the opportunity to rinse out their mouth or brush their teeth. Efforts should be made to make them comfortable and any vomit should be removed. The smell of vomit does nothing to help a nauseated patient. If patients are diaphoretic (sweaty), they should be washed and the bedclothes changed, although very often patients will prefer to be left alone and not moved around too much. Clearly, this will vary according to the specific desires or needs of the patient at the time.

FACTORS SPECIFIC TO TYPE OF SURGERY

Whatever type of surgery has been performed, the basic principles of management as outlined in this chapter will apply. However, there will be certain areas that will require special consideration depending on the type of surgery. The following information is provided for guidance only and is not meant to be exhaustive.

Abdominal surgery

Abdominal wounds are common following general and gynaecological surgery, making good pain relief vital in order to prevent respiratory problems secondary to hypoventilation. Epidural analgesia is particularly effective. Significant fluid imbalance can occur following major gut surgery, and central venous pressure and urine output should be closely monitored during the immediate post-operative period. If surgery is likely to prevent eating and drinking for some time, then parenteral feeding should be considered sooner rather than later. If paralytic ileus is anticipated, a nasogastric tube must be inserted (Field & Bjarnason 2002).

Thoracic surgery

Good pain relief is again particularly important in order to facilitate chest expansion. Sitting patients up and encouraging deep breathing as soon as they are conscious is also useful in maximizing ventilation. An early visit from the physiotherapist can be very beneficial. The patients will have underwater seal drains (see Chapter 5) and may well require early chest X-ray to check for lung re-expansion.

Vascular surgery

Haemorrhage, sometimes major, is the most important complication associated with vascular surgery. Wounds and drains should be closely monitored and the blood pressure maintained within any prescribed limits. Formation of thrombus at the site of operation can cause ischaemia. Circulation to the limbs should, therefore, be closely monitored following surgery on the vessels in the lower part of the body, and pulses distal to the site of the surgery, for example, pedal, should be checked regularly. The use of a Doppler machine may be necessary if pulses are weak. Regular neurological observation should be carried out following carotid endartarectomy. The urine output should be closely monitored following abdominal aortic aneurysm repair, especially where the aorta has been clamped above the renal arteries during surgery.

Orthopaedic surgery

Blood loss tends to be great during and after orthopaedic surgery, particularly joint replacement. Wound and drains should both be closely monitored. Checking the haemoglobin level post-operatively will indicate whether or not blood transfusion is required. Correct positioning of these patients is vital, particularly following spinal and hip surgery. Expert advice should be sought, if there is any doubt. It is worth noting that many emergency orthopaedic operations are on the elderly and so particular care will need to be taken when moving them. Following orthopaedic surgery, many patients will also have plaster casts and it is important to check regularly for good circulation to the distal limb. As this type of surgery often imposes a degree of immobility, close attention to pressure areas and the use of pressure-relieving devices is, therefore, vital.

Gynaecological surgery

It is important to check for any bleeding from the vagina as well as from wounds and drains. It is best to avoid tipping these patients head down, as this can result in blood pooling in the vagina and hence going unrecognized. Emergency gynaecological surgery is often as a result of miscarriage or ectopic pregnancy and, therefore, signifies the loss of a baby. Patients and partners will be very distressed and require tactful and sensitive support.

Genitourinary surgery

Careful management of fluid balance is obviously required following renal surgery. Surgery on the prostate gland may result in major bleeding and this needs careful monitoring. Continuous bladder irrigation is required to prevent clots forming in the bladder and urinary retention. Cold irrigant can significantly lower body temperature and this should be measured regularly. Irrigant can also be absorbed, resulting in fluid overload and hyponatraemia (TURP syndrome). This is potentially life threatening and requires rapid treatment.

Plastic surgery

There are many types of procedures undertaken within the field of plastic surgery; however, the key post-operative issue is wound management. Where flaps have been grafted, it is important to monitor their temperature and circulation. Keeping the patient warm, well hydrated and well oxygenated will give the flap the best chance of success. When surgery is on the head or neck, the airway should be closely monitored.

Ear, nose and throat surgery

The major consideration following ear, nose and throat (ENT) surgery is maintenance of the airway. Nursing patients on their side and with the head slightly down, until the patient is conscious, helps prevent inhalation of blood. Bleeding can also be masked if it is going into the patient's stomach; excessive swallowing is a sign of bleeding and should be investigated further. This tends to be seen most often following tonsillectomy or septorhinoplasty. Following surgery of the inner ear, nausea and vomiting are common and distressing problems. Antiemetics should be given as appropriate.

Cardiac and neurological surgery are not discussed here, as their management is very specific and detailed. The principles involved are covered in Chapters 6 and 7.

CONCLUSION

This chapter has aimed at providing an insight into the needs of the patient during the initial post-operative period. It can be seen that patients are highly dependent throughout the whole peri-operative process. Nurses caring for patients during this time need to possess a broad range of human, clinical and technical skills in order to provide the highest quality care. The ability to act as the patient's advocate is essential, as this is a time when the patient is particularly vulnerable. The nurse must be aware of and be proactive in ensuring the patient's safety, comfort and welfare.

> Technology usually enhances the delivery of nursing care – it does not replace it. However, it is not good practice for nurses to become over-reliant upon it (e.g. automated blood pressure machines), as this often leads to the loss of ability to undertake manual assessments. Remember, machines get it wrong too!

The modern operative process involves a considerable use of high technology. It is essential that the post-operative nurse be technically knowledgeable and skilled. However, it should be remembered that technology is there to enhance the delivery of nursing care, not replace it. The skilled high dependency nurse will selectively utilize technology to make the fullest assessment possible and provide the most appropriate patient interventions. However, only by using the fundamental assessment and practice skills, such as looking and listening, manual observation (blood pressure, pulse, respiration, etc.) checks, as well as nurse's own experience and intuition, will he or she be able to provide the highest standard of care.

References

Aitkenhead A R 1996 Postoperative care. In: Aitkenhead A R, Smith G (eds) Textbook of anaesthesia, 3rd edn. Churchill Livingstone, London

Ashurst S 1995 Oxygen therapy. British Journal of Nursing 4: 508–515

Association of Anaesthetists of Great Britain and Ireland (2002) Immediate postanaesethetic recovery. The Association of Anaesthetists of Great Britain and Ireland, London

Boulton T B, Blogg C E 1989 Ostlere and Bryce-Smith's anaesthetics for medical students. Churchill Livingstone, Edinburgh

Brimacombe J K, Brain A I J, Berry A M 1996 Instruction manual on the use of the laryngeal mask airway in anaesthesia, 3rd edn. Intravent Research Limited, Maidenhead, Ch 16

Colquhoun M C, Handley A J, Evans P R 1995 ABC of resuscitation, 3rd edn. BMJ Publishing Group, London

Courtenay M 1998 Choosing wound dressings. Nursing Times 94(9): 46–48

Davidson J A, Hosie H E 1993 Limitations of pulse oximetry: respiratory insufficiency – a failure of detection. British Medical Journal 307: 372–373

Droogan J, Dickson R 1996 Pre-operative patient instruction: is it effective? Nursing Standard 10(35): 32–33

Field J B, Bjarnason K 2002 Feeding patients after abdominal surgery. Nursing Standard 16(48): 41–44

Fortier J, Chung F, Su J 1998 Unanticipated admission after ambulatory surgery – a prospective study. Canadian Journal of Anaesthesia 45: 612–619

Giuffre M, Finnie J, Lynam D, Smith D 1991 Rewarming postoperative patients: lights, blankets, or forced warm air. Journal of Post Anaesthesia Nursing 6(6): 387–393

Greenfield S M, Webster G J M, Vicary F R 1997 Drinking before sedation. Preoperative fasting should be the exception rather than the rule. British Medical Journal 314: 162

Hatfield A, Tronson M 1996 The complete recovery room book, 2nd edn. Oxford University Press, Oxford

Hauer M, Cram E, Titler M et al 1995 Intravenous patient controlled analgesia in critically ill postoperative/trauma patients: research based practice recommendations. Dimensions of Critical Care Nursing 14: 144–153

Hayward J 1975 Information – a prescription against pain. Royal College of Nursing, London

Hines R, Barash P G, Watrous G, O'Connor T 2002 Complications occurring in the postanesthesia care unit – a survey. Anesthesia and Analgesia 74: 503–509

Lait M E, Smith L N 1998 Wound management: a literature review. Journal of Clinical Nursing 7(1): 11–17

McNeil B A 1998 Addressing the problems of inadvertent hypothermia in surgical patients. Part 2: Self learning package. British Journal of Theatre Nursing 8(5): 25–31

Moore Z 1997 Continuing education: wound care. World of Irish Nursing Series of articles Feb 1997–Oct 1997

Mosby's medical, nursing and allied health dictionary, 5th edn. 2002 Mosby, St Louis

Murray-Calderon P, Connolly M A 1997 Laryngospasm and noncardiogenic pulmonary edema. Journal of Peri-Anesthesia Nursing 12: 89–94

National Institute of Clinical Excellence (NICE) 2003 The use of routine preoperative tests for elective surgery. NICE. London

Naylor R J, Inall F C 1994 The physiology and pharmacology of postoperative nausea and vomiting. Anaesthesia 49(Suppl): 2–5

Palazzo M, Evans R 1993 Logistic regression analysis of fixed patient factors for postoperative sickness: a model for risk assessment. British Journal of Anaesthesia 70: 135–140

Peck T E, Williams M 2002 Pharmacology for anaesthesia and intensive care. Greenwich Medical Media, London

Resuscitation Council 2000 Resuscitation for the citizen, 6th edn. Resuscitation Council UK, London

Surkitt-Parr M 1992 Hypothermia in surgical patients. British Journal of Nursing 1(11): 539–545

Tate S, Cook H 1996a Postoperative nausea and vomiting. 1: Physiology and aetiology. British Journal of Nursing 5: 963–973

Tate S, Cook H 1996b Postoperative nausea and vomiting. 2: Management and treatment. British Journal of Nursing 5: 1032–1039

Watts S, Brooks A 1997 Patients' perceptions of the preoperative information they need about events they may experience in the intensive care unit. Journal of Advanced Nursing 26: 85–92

Further reading

Aitkenhead A R, Smith G (eds) 1996 Textbook of anaesthesia, 3rd edn. Churchill Livingstone, London

Ellis H, Feldman S 2004 Anatomy for anaesthetists, 8th edn. Blackwell Scientific Publications, London

Hutton P et al 2002 Fundamental principles and practice of anaesthesia. Dunitz, London

Chapter 9

Clinical emergencies

Helen O'Keefe

CHAPTER CONTENTS

KEY LEARNING OBJECTIVES

- To enable the early recognition of acute illness
- To develop an understanding of thorough patient assessment
- To enable patient centredness in the delivery of care
- To facilitate the use of evidence-based interventions
- To develop an understanding of common clinical emergencies and their management in acute clinical care

INTRODUCTION

As the role of nurses in general wards in acute settings becomes more technically complex, with the shift towards increased acuity of patients and the reality of higher levels of care required by the in-patient population, it has become increasingly necessary for nurses to expand their knowledge. Responsibility for caring for acutely ill patients receiving Level 2 care on a ward is a reality for many nurses and, daunting though this may seem to many, the importance of focused patient care remains paramount. The role boundaries of nurses and the concept of critical care have become blurred with the growing recognition during the 1990s that patients may deteriorate at any stage during their hospital admission. From the time of arrival in the accident and emergency (A&E) department to discharge, the patient is reliant on the clinical expertise and judgement of an array of healthcare professionals and, with nurses spending the highest proportion of their time with patients, it has never been more important to hone skills of clinical assessment and recognition of deterioration to improve the delivery of appropriate care, regardless of the patient's location in the hospital, and positively affect patient outcomes.

RAPID ASSESSMENT

A systematic approach to patient assessment should be used in order to provide an accurate picture of the presenting clinical emergency. This should be both simple and logical in order to enable rapid patient assessment and guide subsequent action.

Norman & Cook (2000) suggest a three-stage rapid assessment framework based on 'know, see and find' (Table 9.1). This 'snapshot' assessment simply requires basic nursing assessment skills and is within the capability of every nurse working in an acute clinical area.

Following the initial 'know, see and find' assessment, the next step is to gather more information to inform judgement and enable prioritization of care and appropriate referral. Smith (2000) recommends a structured more thorough system of assessment using the 'look, listen and feel' approach, which, if used following the 'know, see and find' approach, will enable a fuller understanding of the patient's status to be gained.

The combination of the 'know, see and find', and the 'look, listen and feel' approaches to patient assessment enables the nurse to gather the 'whole' picture of the patient's status, which is essential in order to make sense of and interpret the findings. This allows nurses to prioritize their response and take the appropriate action. Subsequent alert of appropriate

Table 9.1 Rapid assessment. (Adapted from Norman & Cook 2000)

Element	Definition	Data
Know	What the nurse is told	Present and past medical history Social history Previous medical interventions, e.g. surgery Patient's usual respiratory rate, heart rate and blood pressure
See	Quick visual assessment	Airway patency Pallor Sweating Mental state Posture Facial expression General condition
Find	Quick vital signs assessment	Respiratory rate Adequacy of oxygenation Pulse Blood pressure Urine output Conscious level Monitor for changes or trends in any of the above

Table 9.2 The 'look, listen and feel' approach. (Adapted from Smith 2000)

Assessment step	Look for	Listen for	Feel for
A – Airway	Patent airway	Obstruction/stridor Ability to speak	Breath/movement of air
B – Breathing	Respiratory rate depth and pattern Chest movement Adequacy of oxygenation	Audible wheezes and crackles Breath sounds using stethoscope	Tracheal position Vibrations on chest wall, indicating sputum retention
C – Circulation	Pallor Haemorrhage Manifestations of reduced renal, cerebral or cardiac perfusion, i.e. oliguria, drowsiness, angina	Does patient feel faint or dizzy?	Reduced peripheral perfusion Capillary refill Heart rate regularity and volume Blood pressure
D – Disability	Altered conscious level		
E – Expose to examine	Previously unseen haemorrhage or wound/drain leakage Peripheral oedema	Does patient report pain?	

personnel could be further facilitated by using an early-warning scoring tool, with nurses able to articulate their concerns more thoroughly to orientate the medical team to the clinical urgency.

Local early-warning scoring systems provide specific criteria for calling a doctor or critical care outreach personnel and, whether these are used across a whole Trust or in designated areas, they undoubtedly enable nurses to alert appropriate help. However, they may not be applied in practice, and require further debate and validation (McArthur-Rouse 2001). Patients who become acutely ill present with a complex picture, which the nurse at the bedside is in a prime position to assess, make an interpretation of findings and articulate the problem to the appropriate medical team. The investment in critical care skills education nationwide would suggest that there is now an expectation that nurses are encouraged to use and develop their skills in clinical assessment to improve patient care.

The clinical emergencies included in this chapter are those commonly arising, whether the patient presents in the A&E department, has been admitted to a ward, or has been transferred from Level 3 care. It is important to acknowledge that, with timely appropriate intervention, a patient who is deteriorating and requiring Level 2 care may not proceed to escalation to Level 3 care, but show improvement and return to Level 1 care requirements. The aim of this chapter is to present clinical emergencies as they occur in practice, with the reader presented with patient information in scenario format and subsequent interventions explained.

ASTHMA

Case example 9.1 The patient with asthma

A 48-year-old man, Mr D, is admitted to a medical ward with an acute exacerbation of his asthma. He presented in the A&E department 2 days ago following an acute asthma attack, was given salbutamol nebulizers and required 35% oxygen, intravenous (i.v.) hydrocortisone 200 mg, and commenced oral prednisolone 30 mg a day. He took self-discharge from the A&E department saying he did not want to be admitted to hospital. His peak expiratory flow (PEF) recording at best is 400 litres/minute. He is under the care of a chest physician but missed his last clinic appointment 2 months ago.

The initial impression on seeing Mr D is that:

- he is extremely frightened and asks you not to leave him;
- he has removed his oxygen mask and is profoundly cyanosed;
- he is unable to say more than a few words at a time before gasping for breath;
- he is breathing through pursed lips;
- he is using accessory muscles;
- he has a notably prolonged expiration time with an audible expiratory wheeze.

Clinical assessment reveals:

- he is alert and orientated;
- he has a respiratory rate of 34/minute;
- his SpO_2 is 88% on room air;
- unable to perform peak expiratory flow recording as he is too breathless;
- a loud expiratory wheeze on chest auscultation;
- his heart rate is 118/minute;
- his pulse is thready but regular;
- he has warm peripheries with a capillary refill of < 3 seconds;
- his blood pressure is 150/90 mmHg.

Can you interpret the above data and identify priorities of care?

Interpretation of data and recognition of clinical emergency

This patient has several features of acute severe asthma (e.g. he is unable to complete sentences in one breath, his respiratory rate is > 25/minute and his pulse is >110/minute). In addition, he has several features of life-threatening asthma (e.g. SpO_2 < 92%, cyanosis and exhaustion).

Many definitions of asthma exist, and the clinical diagnosis of asthma is not always simple:

A chronic inflammatory disorder of the airways...in susceptible individuals, inflammatory symptoms are usually associated with widespread but variable airflow obstruction and an increase in airway response to a variety of stimuli. Obstruction is often reversible, either spontaneously or with treatment

(British Thoracic Society 2003a)

The disease process creates an airflow obstruction that affects both inspiratory and expiratory air movement. Expiratory airflow obstruction causes alveolar hyperinflation as a result of gas-trapping (increased auto-PEEP).

Most patients who die of asthma have chronically severe asthma and death occurs before admission to hospital. Many deaths are associated with inadequate treatment with inhaled steroid or steroid tablets, inadequate monitoring of response to treatment, and increasing use of β_2-agonist therapy. Behavioural and adverse psychological factors are also commonly found:

Patients at risk of developing near-fatal or fatal asthma

- Patients with severe asthma, recognized by one or more of the following:
  - previous ventilation or respiratory acidosis;
  - previous hospital admission/A&E department attendance for asthma in the last year;
  - heavy use of a β_2-agonist inhaler;
  - brittle asthma.
- Adverse behavioural or psychological features are indicated by a history of:
  - non-compliance with treatment or monitoring;
  - self-discharge from hospital;
  - psychiatric illness;
  - obesity;
  - alcohol or drug abuse.

Increasing levels of severity of acute asthma exacerbations are shown in Box 9.1.

Immediate treatment and priorities of care

- Give high-flow oxygen, usually 40–60%, to achieve oxygen saturations of at least 92%. CO_2 retention is not usually aggravated by oxygen therapy in asthma.
- Give nebulized salbutamol 5 mg (or terbutaline 10 mg) plus ipratropium bromide 0.5 mg via an oxygen-driven nebulizer. Salbutamol can be given more frequently (i.e. 5 mg up to every 15–30 minutes). Consider a continuous salbutamol nebulizer if no improvement is seen.
- Position the patient to aid chest expansion. An electric frame bed will aid patient positioning, although many patients will prefer to sit in a chair during a period of acute breathlessness.
- Test arterial blood gas (ABG), if $SpO_2 < 92\%$, to ascertain the acid–base status, degree of hypoxaemia and adequacy of ventilation. ABG in severe airflow obstruction will show increased $PaCO_2$.
- Administer oral prednisolone 40–50 mg or i.v. hydrocortisone 100 mg, or both if the patient is very ill.
- No sedatives of any kind should be given.
- An i.v. infusion of magnesium sulphate 1.2–2 g should be given over 20 minutes.
- Intravenous β_2 agonist or i.v. aminophylline may be used if the patient is not improving.

> **Box 9.1   Increasing levels of severity of acute asthma exacerbations (British Thoracic Society 2003a)**
>
> **Moderate asthma exacerbation**
>
> - Increasing symptoms
> - PEF > 50–75% best or predicted
>
> **Features of acute severe asthma**
>
> - PEF 33–50% best or predicted
> - Respiratory rate ≥ to 25 minute
> - Pulse ≥ 110 beats/minute
> - Can't complete sentences in one breath
>
> **Life-threatening features**
>
> - PEF < 33% best or predicted
> - SpO_2 < 92%
> - Silent chest, cyanosis or feeble respiratory effort
> - Bradycardia, dysrhythmia or hypotension
> - Exhaustion, confusion or coma
>
> **Near-fatal asthma**
>
> - Raised $PaCO_2$ requiring mechanical ventilation with raised inflation pressures

- An early-warning scoring system should be used for referral to critical care outreach for support or advice, or a request made to the intensive care unit (ICU) team for review.
- Transfer to ICU in preparation for intubation should be considered, if PEF deteriorates further, hypoxia worsens, or if exhaustion, feeble respirations, confusion or drowsiness develops.
- The patient should be accompanied at all times and not left alone.

Subsequent management and interventions

- Repeat PEF measurement 15–30 minutes after starting treatment to determine the severity of airflow obstruction and to assess the effectiveness of treatment.
- Maintain SpO_2 > 92%. Avoid oxygen desaturation when administering nebulized β_2 agonist bronchodilators by administering nebulizers through oxygen rather than air
- Repeat blood gas measurement within 2 hours of starting treatment, if initial PaO_2 < 8 kPa, unless SpO_2 is subsequently > 92%, $PaCO_2$ is normal or raised above 4.6 kPa, or if the patient deteriorates.
- Respiratory assessment including recording of SpO_2 should be carried out regularly.

- Rehydration with intravenous fluids and correction of electrolyte imbalance, especially K^+ disturbances, should be performed, as acidosis causes hyperkalaemia and salbutamol can cause hypokalaemia.
- Peak expiratory flow rate recordings before and after nebulizer use should be made at least four times per day. PEF should be compared with the patient's baseline. Less than 60% of the baseline for PEF is an indication of severe airflow obstruction.
- A chest X-ray may be performed if pneumothorax or consolidation is suspected or if patient requires intubation and ventilation.
- Patients should be woken to receive salbutamol nebulizers. They should not be omitted if the patient is sleeping

The main goals of treatment are to improve oxygenation and reverse airflow obstruction. This is achieved through prompt administration of high-flow oxygen, reduction of airway inflammation and relief of bronchospasm through the use of bronchodilators and steroids.

Asthma management

- Unlike patients with chronic obstructive pulmonary disease (COPD), there is little danger of causing carbon dioxide retention (hypercapnia) with high-flow oxygen. Hypercapnia indicates the development of near-fatal asthma and the need for emergency intubation and mechanical ventilation.
- There is no evidence for any difference in effectiveness between salbutamol and terbutaline, although patients may express a preference (British Thoracic Society 2003a).
- Inhaled β_2 agonists are at least as effective as i.v. β_2 agonists, and the use of i.v. salbutamol, terbutaline and aminophylline is generally only required for patients in whom nebulizers cannot be tolerated or used reliably.
- Steroid tablets are as effective as i.v. steroids as long as the patient can reliably swallow the tablets. If oral steroids are used, they should be continued for at least 5 days or until recovery. Steroid tablets can be stopped and do not require tapering off as long as the patient is receiving inhaled steroids
- Combining nebulized ipatropium bromide with a nebulized β_2 agonist provides improved bronchodilation leading to a shorter recovery time.
- Intravenous magnesium sulphate, thought to relieve bronchospasm, as a single dose should be considered for patients with acute severe asthma who have not responded well to inhaled bronchodilator therapy, or those with life-threatening features.
- Routine prescription of antibiotics is not indicated for acute asthma.
- Non-invasive ventilation (NIV) using expiratory positive airway pressure (EPAP) and inspiratory positive airway pressure (IPAP) in the presence of outflow obstruction may exacerbate alveolar hyperinflation, even if the inspiratory:expiratory ratio is manipulated to allow extended expiratory time to enable alveoli to empty. NIV is, therefore, not normally recommended in acute severe or life-threatening asthma, even in the presence of hypercapnia. If used, low EPAP pressures are necessary to reduce the risk of further alveolar hyperinflation.

Hypercapnic respiratory failure (Type II respiratory failure) in asthma is an indication for urgent admission to ICU for intubation and mechanical ventilation.

Intravenous bronchodilators

Salbutamol

- 5 mg salbutamol in 500 ml 0.9% sodium chloride or dextrose 5% to give a 10 µg/ml solution.
- Dose range is 3–20 µg/minute (180–1200 µg/hour).
- Rate of infusion is 18–120 ml/hour.

Terbutaline

- 2.5 mg terbutaline in 500 ml 0.9% sodium chloride or dextrose 5% to give a 5 µg/ml solution.
- Dose range is 1.55 µg minute (90–300 µg/hour).
- Rate of infusion is 18–60 ml/hour.

Aminophylline

- Loading dose is usually only given if the patient is not on oral theophylline or aminophylline. Loading dose is 5 mg/kg in 250 ml 0.9% sodium chloride or dextrose 5% over 20 minutes.
- For maintenance infusion, add 500 mg aminophylline to 500 ml 0.9% sodium chloride or dextrose 5% to give 1 mg/ml and set rate at 0.5 mg/kg per hour (half patient's weight in kilograms = number of millilitres/hour of infusion).

ACUTE PANCREATITIS

Case example 9.2 The patient with pancreatitis

Mrs W is a 55-year-old woman admitted yesterday with a 1-day history of severe epigastric pain radiating to her back. She was diagnosed with gallstones 6 months ago and is awaiting an appointment for an oesophagogastroduodenoscopy (OGD) to investigate recent intermittent epigastric pain occurring mainly after eating. She is normally fit and healthy and takes no regular medications.

On admission, she was commenced on i.v. fluids, kept 'nil by mouth' (NBM), a nasogastric tube was inserted and placed on free drainage and a urinary catheter was inserted. Overnight, she has received very little i.v. fluid because her peripheral cannula 'tissued', and she has developed profuse diarrhoea. This morning the, Health Care Assistant informs you that Mrs W does not look well. The initial impression on seeing Mrs W is that:

- she is tachypnoeic;
- she has severe epigastric pain, which is radiating to her back;
- she is nauseated and has just vomited;
- she looks pale, slightly jaundiced and unwell.

Clinical assessment reveals:

- she is very drowsy;
- her respiratory rate is 38/minute;

Case example continues

- she has an SpO$_2$ of 89% on air;
- she has reduced breath sounds on chest auscultation;
- her heart rate is 130/minutes;
- her pulse is thready but regular;
- she has cool skin with ice-cold hands and feet;
- she has a delayed capillary refill of > 5 seconds;
- her blood pressure is 85/60 mmHg;
- she has a rigid distended abdomen with absent bowel sounds;
- her urine output for the last 3 hours is 20/20/10 ml;
- she has a pyrexia of 38.9°C (tympanic).

Can you interpret the above data and identify priorities of care?

Blood results show:

White blood cells (WBC)	22 IU/l × 10^9/l
Amylase	2583 IU × 10^9/l
Glucose	15 mmol/l
Calcium	Low
Magnesium	Low
Liver function tests	Normal
Coagulation	Raised fibrin
ABG	pH 7.47, PCO_2 1.7 kPa, PO_2 8.4kPa, HCO$_3$ 19mmol/le, O$_2$ saturation 88%, base excess −12

Interpretation of data and recognition of clinical emergency

This lady is hypoxic and in shock, caused by hypovolaemia and myocardial depression. Compensatory mechanisms are fully active, and she has responded with tachypnoea, in an attempt to improve oxygenation, and tachycardia, in an attempt to improve organ oxygen delivery. Peripheral vasoconstriction, oliguria and tachypnoea in the presence of such extreme hypotension and hypoxia indicates probable hypoperfusion at organ level with metabolic acidosis, and associated compensatory hyperventilation developing in an attempt to raise arterial pH.

Mrs W is extremely ill. She has all five features of critical illness (i.e. drowsiness, tachypnoea, tachycardia, hypotension and oligura). It is essential to inform a senior member of her surgical team quickly and contact the critical care outreach team or ICU for further advice and support.

- Theophylline levels should be monitored 18–24 hours after starting the infusion.
- Potassium levels should be checked as aminophylline causes hypokalaemia.

Pancreatitis is an inflammatory disease of the pancreas caused by an autodigestive process of pancreatic tissue by its own enzymes. Pancreatic enzymes are stored in their inactive form in acinar cells, which, when damaged by obstruction of the pancreatic duct, trauma or ischaemia, are released and activated by trypsin. Autodigestion occurs as these enzymes come into contact with pancreatic tissue, and further spillage causes chemical peritonitis and third spacing of vast amounts of fluid within the peritoneum.

Acute pancreatitis creates a catabolic state promoting a systemic inflammatory response with vascular damage at microcirculatory level, causing release of vasoactive mediator substances from the endothelial cell wall, which contribute to capillary leakage and depressed myocardial function. Increased capillary permeability causes large losses of intravascular water and non-protein molecules into the interstitial space, leading to hypovolaemia, interstitial oedema and poor oxygen delivery at the microcirculation/organ cell interface, which leads to organ dysfunction and ultimately failure. The frequency of acute pancreatitis requiring hospitalization has increased over the last decade (Fiorianti et al 2003), with mortality from pancreatitis as high as 70% when necrosis and haemorrhage of pancreatic tissue occurs.

Causes

- Alcohol abuse is present in over 60% of cases. Alcohol triggers excess hydrochloric acid production in the stomach, which can cause spasm and inflammation at the sphincter of Oddi and obstruct the flow of both pancreatic enzymes and bile.
- Obstructed pancreatic ductal flow, owing to biliary tract dysfunction. Gallstones are present in over half of patients with acute pancreatitis.
- Viral or bacterial infection (e.g. hepatitis, mumps).
- Hyperlipidaemia.
- Trauma to pancreas (e.g. abdominal injury, complication of endoscopic retrograde cholangiopancreatography).
- Ischaemia, owing to prolonged severe shock or vasculitis.

Complications

Respiratory failure is a common complication, owing to acute lung injury as a result of the inflammatory response. Mechanisms are unclear but the inflamed pancreas is known to release phospholipase, which destroys surfactant. During the inflammatory process, immature neutrophils are released from bone marrow and cause endothelial injury in the lung microcirculation, resulting in pancreatitis-induced acute lung injury. Other life-threatening complications include disseminated intravascular coagulation, renal failure, circulatory collapse and sepsis. The most common sign of acute pancreatitis is sudden onset of sharp abdominal pain, which may radiate to the back. Other signs include nausea, vomiting, fever, tachycardia, dyspnoea, hypotension, restlessness and confusion.

Immediate treatment

The patient is hyperventilating secondary to an extreme metabolic acidosis caused by inadequate tissue oxygen delivery.

- Give O_2, preferably humidified and commencing at 40%, via a face mask.
- Monitor SpO_2 continuously, titrating FiO_2, aiming to achieve SpO_2 of at least 95%.
- Institute aggressive fluid replacement – i.v. crystalloid and colloids to improve circulating volume and restore blood pressure.
- Monitor for cardiac and haemodynamic instability by assessing pulse rate, volume and regularity, blood pressure, capillary refill, peripheral warmth.
- Monitor urine output hourly – aim for 0.5 ml/kg per hour. If the patient is not fully fluid-resuscitated, hypovolaemia may lead to renal hypoperfusion and acute renal failure.

- Perform arterial blood gas analysis to ascertain the acid–base status, arterial oxygen tension and degree of microcirculatory hypoperfusion, which provides a guide for fluid replacement therapy.
- Move the patient to bay 1 or an area where she can be more easily monitored closely. The bed space should have a wall oxygen supply.
- An early-warning scoring system should be used for referral to critical care outreach for support and advice or, if the patient does not show immediate improvement, a request should be made to the ICU team to review.

Investigations

- Haematology and biochemistry:
  - the raised WBC is indicative of the presence of an inflammatory process;
  - amylase is raised but may be low as a result of pancreatic necrosis;
  - hyperglycaemia results from damage to pancreatic β cells – this damage impairs carbohydrate metabolism and may lead to diabetes mellitus;
  - hypocalcaemia is frequently found as a result of hypoalbuminaemia and altered fat metabolism because calcium binds to proteins and free fatty acids;
  - normal LFTs indicate that the pancreatitis is not caused by alcoholism, which would result in hepatic inflammation;
  - raised fibrin may indicate microthrombi in pancreas;
  - hypokalaemia may be caused by fluid losses or nasogastric losses;
  - hypomagnesaemia is also commonly found.
- Abdominal X-ray to identify calcification in the pancreas and perforated viscera.
- Ultrasound to visualize gallstones, dilation of the common bile duct and ascites.
- Chest X-ray to identify bilateral infiltrates indicative of acute respiratory distress syndrome (ARDS).
- Computed tomography (CT) scan to identify pancreatic fluid collections, abscesses and necrosis.

Subsequent management and interventions

- Regular respiratory assessment, including recording of SpO_2 in relation to oxygen administered, is required. ARDS may develop suddenly or over a few days as a result of systemic inflammatory response syndrome (SIRS), and resultant alveolar flooding will cause reduced compliance, dyspnoea and hypoxia. Atelectasis and pneumonia may develop from hypoventilation associated with abdominal pain, ascites and immobility.
- Position the patient to improve ventilation and oxygenation with the patient upright or in a semi-Fowler's position.
- Assess conscious level to monitor for confusion caused by cerebral hypoperfusion or electrolyte abnormalities.
- Intravenous crystalloid and colloids are required to replace volume losses. The rate of administration should be adjusted in response to improvements in peripheral warmth, capillary refill, urine output, tachycardia and blood pressure.
- Potassium and calcium replacement may be required.

- Analgesia is essential. Opiates are normally given by patient-controlled analgesia (PCA), if the patient is able to use it effectively, but may cause pancreatic duct spasm, impeding ductal flow. Fentanyl may be less likely to cause spasm and an epidural may be more effective. Pain causes splinting and abdominal distention causes diaphragmatic elevation leading to atelectasis.
- Treat nausea and vomiting with antiemetics.
- Suppression of pancreatic secretions is achieved by ensuring the patient remains NBM and reduces physical activity, the nasogastric tube is aspirated 4-hourly and remains on free drainage, and histamine H_2 receptor antagonists are administered. Octreotide may also be useful in reducing pancreatic secretions and may inhibit cytokine release.
- Assess blood sugar levels frequently to identify transient hyperglycaemia.
- Oral and enteral feeding is contraindicated during the acute phase, as it increases secretion of pancreatic enzymes and inflammation. Total parenteral nutrition is normally instituted early to improve tissue healing and meet tissue demand for nutrients during the period of critical illness.
- Broad-spectrum antibiotics are recommended (Golub et al 1998).

Discussion

Mrs W's condition improved on the ward after a few hours. Her SpO_2 improved to 96% with the administration of 60% humidified O_2 and her respiratory rate reduced to 20/minute. A central venous cannula was inserted, i.v. fluids were administered at 250 ml/hour and total parenteral nutrition was commenced. A total of 1000 ml Gelofusine was required over the first 3 hours to improve circulating volume and urine output. After 5 days, her pain had settled, she no longer required the PCA, was no longer requiring O_2, her vital signs were stable, her urine output was over 60 ml/hour, nasojejunal feeding was commenced and she was able to tolerate oral fluids. A week later she was discharged from hospital.

PULMONARY EMBOLISM

Case example 9.3 The patient with a pulmonary embolism

Mrs T is a 50-year-old woman who is admitted with a history of a sudden onset of shortness of breath associated with pleuritic chest pain.
The initial impression on seeing Mrs T is that:

- she is breathless, tachypnoeic and looks cyanosed;
- she is restless and looks anxious, with diaphoresis.
  Clinical assessment reveals:
- she has a respiratory rate of 28/minute;
- she has an SpO_2 of 90% on air;
- her heart rate is 118/minute;
- her blood pressure is 90/60 mmHg;
- she has engorged neck veins;

Case example continues

- arterial blood gas analysis reveals pH 7.5, PCO_2 3.2, PO_2 7.5, HCO_3 26, O_2 saturation 79%, BE +3.

  What are your immediate priorities of care?

Interpretation of data and recognition of clinical emergency

This lady is in respiratory distress. Her ABG shows hypoxia and mild hypocapnia secondary to increased minute ventilation. She requires immediate oxygen therapy and medical review.

A pulmonary embolism is an occlusion of the pulmonary artery by a thrombus, fat globule, air bubble or foreign body. Most pulmonary emboli originate in the legs or pelvis, where stagnancy of blood, vessel injury or hypercoagulability promote thrombus formation.

Occlusion of a pulmonary artery branch causes an increase in pulmonary vascular resistance, increased pulmonary arterial pressure and right ventricular workload. In severe cases, pulmonary hypertension and right ventricular failure occur. Impaired gas exchange results in pulmonary ischaemia, infarction and death. The incidence of pulmonary embolism is 60–70 per 100 000. Half of these patients develop venous thromboembolism whilst in hospital or in long term care, and the rest are equally divided between idiopathic cases and those with recognized risk factors. The widespread use of prophylaxis in orthopaedic and general surgery has substantially reduced the incidence of post-operative venous thromboembolism. In-hospital mortality rates range from 6% to 15%. The care and management outlined follows the British Thoracic Society (2003b) guidelines for management of suspected acute pulmonary embolism.

Common symptoms of pulmonary embolism (PE) in decreasing order of frequency are: dyspnoea, tachypnoea, pleuritic pain, apprehension, tachycardia, cough, haemoptysis, leg pain and clinical deep vein thrombosis.

Major risk factors for venous thromboembolism

- Surgery within the previous 12 weeks.
- Immobilization (complete bedrest) of 3 days or more in the previous 4 weeks.
- Previous deep vein thrombosis (DVT) or PE.
- Lower limb fracture requiring immobilization within the previous 12 weeks.
- A strong family history of DVT or PE.
- Cancer treatment within the previous 6 months or palliative care.
- Post-partum.
- Lower extremity paralysis.
- Recent long-distance travel.

Immediate treatment

- High-flow oxygen with a reservoir bag.
- Sit the patient up. If hypoxia is severe, consider turning the patient on to his or her side to find the side associated with best SpO_2. This will

improve the ventilation–perfusion ratio, when the affected lung is uppermost, commonly termed positioning 'good lung down'.
- Ensure a bag-valve face mask is available in case of respiratory collapse and apnoea. Intubation may be required if the patient cannot maintain adequate oxygenation
- Use an early-warning scoring system to alert critical care outreach or ICU assistance.
- Gain i.v. access.
- If shock is present without left ventricular failure, give fluid bolus to increase right ventricular filling pressure, which will improve right heart stroke volume. If there is no response, consider inotropes and ICU.

Investigations

- Blood for urea and electrolytes (U&Es), full blood count (FBC) and clotting.
- Arterial blood gas (typically shows hypoxia and mild hypercapnia secondary to increased minute ventilation).
- Chest X-ray (often normal, excludes other causes). If PE is present, the chest film may show increased heart size, local areas of underperfused lung and an increased density of the main pulmonary artery, although these changes are not easily seen on a portable film.
- ECG (shows tall, peaked, P waves, ST segment changes, T-wave inversion in leads V1–4 and R-axis deviation).

None of the above investigations will unequivocally confirm a diagnosis of PE, but may suggest an alternative diagnosis or assess severity of PE. Further investigations required are the following.

Clinical probability assessment

- Are other diagnoses likely? (If yes, score 1)
- Is a major risk factor present? (If yes, score1)

Clinical probability score explained: 0 = low, 1 = intermediate, 2 = high probability. Patients with a low-probability score should have their plasma D-dimer measured. Patients with intermediate- or high-probability score should not have a D-dimer test, as the result will not affect further management; investigation with CT pulmonary angiography (CTPA) is necessary.

D-dimer test

Venous thromboembolism leads to activation of fibrin degradation, one of the breakdown products of fibrinolysis being plasma D-dimer. Its values are rarely within the normal range in patients with active thromboembolism but are commonly raised in other hospitalized patients, including patients with the following conditions/status: over 70, pregnancy, severe trauma, cancer, sepsis, critically ill, ischaemic heart disease, inflammatory bowel disease and haematological disorders. Normal levels exclude venous thromboembolism.

Isotope lung scanning

This may be carried out if available on site, but PE can only be diagnosed or excluded reliably in a minority of patients.

Computed tomography pulmonary angiography

This is the recommended initial lung imaging for the investigation of PE.

Subsequent management and interventions

- Anticoagulation should be commenced as soon as possible. Thrombolysis with alteplase, unlike streptokinase, does not worsen hypotension.
- Heparin infusion commencing 3 hours after thrombolysis. Heparin should be given to patients with intermediate or high clinical probability prior to imaging.
- Aim for a target international normalized ratio (INR) of 2.0–3.0.
- Monitor and report bleeding from the gums, nose, urinary tract, invasive line sites, surgical wounds or bruising. Observe for joint pain and swelling.
- Brush teeth using a soft toothbrush only, taking care not to cause bleeding.
- Minimize invasive procedures, such as endotracheal suction, manipulation of invasive lines or urinary catheter.
- Encourage patients to shave with a safety razor or electric razor to prevent skin nicks.
- Measure and fit knee-high or thigh-high antiembolism stockings when leg swelling (if present) has decreased. Elevate legs if patient is sitting out in a chair.

Probable massive pulmonary embolism

Massive PE is likely if the patient presents with collapse, is hypotensive, has unexplained hypoxia and has engorged neck veins.

A summary of treatment according to the patient's condition is given in Table 9.3. Thrombolysis is followed 3 hours later by an i.v. heparin infusion.

Table 9.3 Treatment priorities for massive pulmonary embolism according to patient condition

Patient's condition	Treatment
Stable	80 units/kg heparin i.v.
	Urgent echocardiogram or CTPA
	If PE confirmed, give 100 mg alteplase i.v.
	over 90 minutes
Deteriorating	Contact consultant
	50 mg alteplase i.v.
	Urgent echocardiogram or CTPA
Cardiac arrest	Cardiopulmonary resuscitation
	50 mg alteplase i.v.
	Reassess at 30 minutes

PNEUMOTHORAX

Case example 9.4 The patient with a pneumothorax

Mrs S, a 66-year-old woman, is admitted to the ward from the A&E department with a 2-day history of diarrhoea and vomiting. She has a previous medical history of COPD and uses salbutamol and atrovent nebulizers at home.

Since admission, her urine output has been less than 30 ml/hour and she has become hypotensive over the last hour. She has had a right internal jugular vein central line inserted in the A&E department, and has been admitted to the ward for observation and rehydration with i.v. fluids. She is due to have a chest X-ray performed. As you sit her up, she tells you that she is having difficulty breathing and begins to panic.

The initial impression on looking at Mrs S is that:

* she is pale and anxious;
* she is dyspnoeic and tachypnoeic;
* chest movement on inspiration is unequal, with no movement on the right side.

Clinical assessment reveals:

* she has a respiratory rate of 28/minute;
* she has an SpO$_2$ of 88% on air;
* her heart rate is 120/minute.

Can you interpret the above data and identify priorities of care?

Interpretation of data and recognition of clinical emergency
This lady is in respiratory distress, is hypoxic, tachypnoeic, with no chest movement on one side. She requires immediate oxygen therapy and medical review. It is likely that the pleura has been punctured by a needle during the procedure to insert the central venous line. ABG analysis shows: pH 7.2, $PaCO_2$ 7.8 kPa, PaO_2 7.5 kPa, HCO$_3$ 27, BE −3. There is evidence of a primary respiratory acidosis, hypoxaemia and no metabolic compensation. She required oxygen therapy and insertion of a chest drain, and subsequently recovered.

Pneumothorax is defined as air in the pleural space that is between the visceral and parietal pleural membranes. There are four main types of pneumothorax: spontaneous, traumatic, tension and iatrogenic.

Spontaneous Spontaneous pneumothorax is common in two groups of patients: healthy adults who can tolerate a large leak, and older patients with emphysema, in whom a small leak may cause severe respiratory failure.

Traumatic A pneumothorax can occur following blunt chest trauma or a penetrating injury, such as a stab wound. If a fractured rib or other sharp instrument penetrates the parietal and visceral pleura and punctures the lung, a pneumothorax occurs.

Tension Tension pneumothorax occurs when the intrapleural pressure exceeds the atmospheric pressure throughout inspiration as well as expiration. Air is drawn into the pleural space during inspiration through a one-way 'valve' and is not permitted to pass out during expiration. The patient may become rapidly distressed with rapid laboured respiration, cyanosis and diaphoresis. The size of the pneumothorax increases with each breath and causes the affected lung to collapse, causing increased intrathoracic pressure, compression on the myocardium, impaired venous return, reduced cardiac output and compensatory tachycardia. High flow O_2 should be administered and a cannula should be introduced into the pleural space, usually in the second anterior intercostal space mid-clavicular line, followed by an intercostal chest drain when the patient is more stable. Pulseless electrical activity (PEA) cardiac arrest will follow.

Iatrogenic

The incidence of iatrogenic pneumothorax is high and outnumbers spontaneous pneumothoraces (Despars et al 1994). Transthoracic needle aspiration (24%), subclavian vessel puncture (22%), thoracentesis (22%), pleural biopsy (8%) and mechanical ventilation (7%) are the five leading causes (British Thoracic Society 2003c).

Immediate priorities of care

- Move the patient to a bed where she can be closely observed and which has a wall oxygen supply.
- Administer high-flow oxygen to achieve an $SpO_2 > 90\%$.
- Continuously monitor the respiratory rate, SpO_2 in relation to FiO_2, chest movement and respiratory pattern.
- Prepare the patient for intercostal tube drainage by explaining what is happening. Very anxious patients may require a small dose of midazolam to facilitate chest drain insertion.
- Administer analgesia to promote comfort.
- Stay with the patient during insertion of the intercostal drain.
- Following insertion of the drain, observe and record the following.
  - Bubbling in the chest drain bottle (indicating loss of air with each breath and continued presence of pneumothorax) and swinging of fluid in the drainage tubing (indicating correct placement of tube, which is subject to pressure changes during inspiration-expiration) and report any cessation of bubbling and/or swinging.
  - Respiratory rate and pattern to enable early detection of recurring pneumothorax owing to tube displacement.
  - Chest movement, reporting any cessation of chest movement on the affected side, which could indicate a recurrence of the pneumothorax.
  - Chest auscultation to reveal quiet or absent breath sounds on the affected side if the pneumothorax recurs.
- Ensure chest drain tubing is secured to the patient with an appropriate dressing and tape to reduce tension and prevent dislodgement of the drain,
- Perform a chest X-ray to check tube placement.

Signs and symptoms of pneumothorax

The first sign is usually rapid-onset shortness of breath, the severity of which relates to the size of the pneumothorax. This is associated with pleuritic pain, which is also sudden in onset and usually occurs in the lateral chest, radiating to the neck, shoulder or epigastrium. The patient may develop a dry cough, which exacerbates the pain, and may also develop a tachycardia, particularly with large pneumothoraces.

The treatment of iatrogenic pneumothorax tends to be simple, as there is little risk of recurrence and the majority will resolve with observation alone. If required, treatment should be by simple aspiration and repeat aspiration may be appropriate in some cases. However, patients with COPD who develop an iatrogenic pneumothorax are more likely to require intercostal tube drainage, as are mechanically ventilated patients unless immediate weaning is possible.

ACUTE GASTROINTESTINAL BLEED

Case example 9.5 The patient with an acute gastrointestinal bleed

Mrs B is an 81-year-old lady who was admitted 1 week ago following a fall at home. She sustained a fractured neck of her left femur and underwent a total hip replacement under general anaesthetic the day after admission.

Her past medical history includes congestive cardiac failure, atrial fibrillation, hypothyroidism and osteoarthritis. She has a 3-year history of intermittent epigastric pain, was diagnosed with oesophagitis on OGD 2 years ago and takes digoxin, aspirin, sotalol and enalapril tablets. She gave up smoking 20 years ago and drinks occasionally.

She has been recovering on the ward well and is now increasing her mobility with the physiotherapist.

Today you find her in bed whilst doing the drug round. She is drowsy and pale. Further clinical assessment reveals:

* her Glagow Coma Scale (GCS) is 12/15;
* she is pale and diaphoretic;
* her respiratory rate is 30/minute;
* she is peripherally cool;
* her capillary refill is > 3 seconds;
* her pulse is irregular with a rate of 58/minute;
* her blood pressure is 80/60 mmHg;
* she has a distended abdomen;
* she has not passed urine today;

Suddenly, she has a large haematemesis and becomes very frightened.

Can you interpret the above data and identify priorities of care?

Interpretation of data and recognition of clinical emergency

This patient has the clinical signs of shock. She is normally hypertensive and her blood pressure is dangerously low. Note the absence of a tachycardia as part of the compensatory response to shock, which is due to her taking beta-blocker medication.

Patients with upper gastrointestinal (GI) bleeding usually present with haematemesis but this obvious manifestation may not be present. With hypertension and beta-blockade common in the elderly, recognition of shock is more subtle, as these patients have the normal compensatory response of tachycardia blocked and a heart rate within normal range of 60–90 may be observed, even with considerable blood loss.

Acute GI bleeding is a life-threatening emergency resulting from mucosal ulceration, and is usually characterized by haematemesis or melaena. The incidence of acute upper GI haemorrhage in the UK is 103 per 100 000 adults per year with incidence in men double that in women except in the elderly. Overall mortality is 14% (11% in emergency admissions and 33% in-patients), with the elderly and those with severe co-morbidities less likely to survive (Rockall et al 1995). Contributing factors are various, including the existence of cardiac or renal disease, history of alcohol abuse or hepatitis, chronic pain conditions, such as arthritis treated with non-steroidal anti-inflammatory drugs (NSAIDs). Patients with NSAID-related acute GI bleeding often have high compliance with their medication and may ignore warning signs, such as epigastric pain (Wynne & Long 1996), indicating the need for patient education.

Common causes of upper GI bleeding

The most common causes of upper GI bleeding are as follows.

Peptic ulcer disease

Helicobacter is a treatable cause of peptic ulcer disease. Other causes are the use of aspirin and NSAIDs, smoking and alcohol abuse.

Stress ulcers in critically ill patients

Hypotension or sepsis can precipitate ischaemia of the GI tract epithelial calls leading to mucosal barrier breakdown, ulceration and risk of bleeding. The use of vasopressors in the acutely ill, which cause a reduction in blood supply to the GI tract, increases the risk further. For this reason, any patient who has been discharged from ICU to the ward may develop signs of GI bleeding and should be regarded as high risk.

Oesophagitis and gastritis

Oesophagitis can result from gastric reflux into the oesophagus, which causes inflammation and bleeding. Gastritis can develop in patients who regularly take aspirin or NSAIDs. Other risk factors are smoking, excessive stress and use of corticosteroids.

Oesophageal varices

Oesophageal varices result from increased pressure, owing to portal hypertension, typically presenting in patients with end-stage liver disease or cirrhosis.

Signs and symptoms of an upper GI bleed depend on the severity of blood loss. Patients may not complain of any pain, but may feel tired, listless and weak if they are coping with a low haemoglobin for a period of time. Melaena may be reported by the patient; it may be dark red or brown, depending on how long it has spent moving through the GI tract. If the GI bleed is acute with a large blood loss, the melaena may become bright red.

In the presence of blood loss of as much as 30% of the circulating volume (1500 ml), a patient may sustain a normal blood pressure but with compensatory mechanisms activated (i.e. sympathetic stimulation causing peripheral vasoconstriction and tachycardia). Hypotension is a late sign and should be considered an emergency requiring immediate action.

Immediate treatment

The main goals of treatment are to improve organ oxygen delivery: firstly, by maximizing blood oxygenation and, secondly, by increasing oxygen delivery at organ level by volume replacement to restore blood pressure. Identification and management of the cause of the bleeding is then the priority once cardiovascular stability has been achieved.

- Psychological support for the patient, who is extremely frightened after vomiting a large amount of blood.
- Give high-flow oxygen to maximize the oxygen-carrying capacity of the remaining red blood cells.
- Insert two wide-bore (e.g. 14G) peripheral intravenous cannulae.
- Take blood for FBC, cross-match, U&Es, LFTs and amylase.
- Start fluid resuscitation with normal saline 0.9% or colloid, monitoring response by frequent assessment of heart rate, pulse volume and regularity, peripheral warmth, capillary refill and urine output. Urinary catheter placement is essential to observe hourly urine volumes.
- Cross-match 6 units of blood and transfuse to a haemoglobin (Hb) of 10 g/dl. Consider platelets, if below 100, and fresh-frozen plasma, if prothrombin > 20.
- An ECG should be performed to ascertain cardiac rhythm. Her pulse is irregular, indicating a dysrrythmia, which may be reversible with volume replacement and/or correction of electrolyte disturbance, particularly hypokalaemia.
- Arrange for chest and abdominal X-rays.
- Call surgical team to review and contact critical care outreach for support and advice. They may refer to the ICU team if circulatory collapse is imminent and there is no swift response to i.v. fluid.
- Insert a central venous line to enable monitoring of the trend of central venous pressure. Peripheral fluid resuscitation should already be established and the administration of i.v. fluid should not be delayed whilst awaiting insertion of a central line.
- If there are still signs of hypovolaemia after 2 litres of i.v. fluid/colloid have been given, then warmed blood should be administered. Cross-matching of blood takes about 1 hour, so O-negative or type-specific blood (the patient's blood group but not cross-matched) may be given before this, which takes 10 minutes.
- Endoscopy should be performed as soon as possible to find the cause of the bleeding.
- Manage according to severity score as follows.
  - *Trivial bleed* (pulse < 90/minute, no postural blood pressure fall, no melaena, Hb > 10 g/dl): allow oral fluids, observe and record vital signs 4 hourly, group and save. OGD should be performed on the next available list.
  - *Significant bleed* (pulse > 100/minute or postural blood pressure fall, or melaena or Hb < 10 g/dl): observe and record vital signs hourly,

use early-warning scoring criteria to alert critical care outreach team for support, cross-match 4 units of blood and transfuse to Hb 10 g/dl to reduce tachycardia, check Hb after 12 hours, give oral pantoprazole 40 mg and refer to surgical registrar. If stable, allow oral fluids; an OGD should be performed on the next list.

- *Severe bleed* (history of collapse or shock; systolic blood pressure < 100 mmHg): fluid resuscitate and keep NBM, observe and record vital signs half-hourly, insert a urinary catheter and observe urine volumes hourly, give oral/i.v. pantoprazole 40 mg o.d., make an urgent referral to the surgical registrar and critical care outreach team. If unstable, an urgent surgical and ICU review and an urgent OGD in theatre, with the possibility of proceeding to laparotomy, are required. All patients over the age of 70 and/or with significant co-morbidity are usually treated as a 'severe bleed'. All suspected variceal bleeds should be treated as 'severe'.

Subsequent management and interventions

After initial fluid resuscitation with 1 litre of 0.9% normal saline and 1 litre of gelofusine, Mrs B's blood pressure rose to 105/80 mmHg, she warmed peripherally slightly and her urine output was 10 ml/hour.

Her haemoglobin was found to be 4.0g/l. Following transfusion with 5 units blood and 2 units of FFP, she underwent an OGD, where she was found to have a gastric ulcer, which was injected with adrenaline. Her Hb subsequently rose to 8 g/l.

On a past outpatient visit, this lady's blood pressure was recorded as 160/95 mmHg. A calculated mean arterial pressure would be around 117 mmHg, the normal pressure perfusing the renal arterial bed. Unsurprisingly, a blood pressure of 105/80 mmHg (calculated mean arterial pressure = 88 mmHg) was insufficient to produce an adequate urine output, an indicator of organ perfusion.

ANAPHYLAXIS

Case example 9.6 The patient who develops anaphylactic shock

Mr C is a 67-year-old man who is undergoing fluorescein angiography within the ophthalmology outpatients department to investigate deterioration in his sight. He is normally fit and well, and takes no regular medications. Thirty seconds following the administration of the intravenous injection of fluorescein, he tells you with a hoarse voice that he feels warm and dizzy, and his chest feels tight.

What do you suspect and what are your priorities of care?

This man has the signs of clinical anaphylaxis, and requires prompt recognition and emergency treatment of laryngeal oedema, bronchospasm and hypotension.

Anaphylactic shock results from a hypersensitivity reaction, and requires prompt recognition and emergency treatment of life-threatening laryngeal oedema, bronchospasm and hypotension that may result. Most immediate reactions will resolve with administration of adrenaline with or without antihistamines, corticosteroids and fluids.

Clinical anaphylaxis is an acute reaction to a foreign substance. The causes fall into two categories:

1. reaction to a substance to which a patient has been previously sensitised (type I sensitivity);
2. reaction of non-immunological origin or, in some cases, where the agent is unknown. This is termed an anaphylactoid reaction, which is clinically indiscernible from anaphylaxis.

Causes of clinical anaphylaxis include:

- injection of drugs;
- blood products;
- plasma substitutes;
- contrast media;
- ingestion of food or food additives;
- insect stings;
- unknown cause.

Type I sensitivity

The pathophysiology of anaphylaxis is a staged event. Sensitization occurs following exposure to an allergic substance and stimulates the synthesis of immnoglobulin E (IgE), which binds to mast cells and basophils. On re-exposure, the antigen combines with IgE and activates basophils, mast cells and eosinophils. These cells are responsible for releasing histamine, leukotrienes, prostaglandins and platelet-activating factor, which cause bronchoconstriction, increased capillary permeability and vasodilation.

Anaphylactoid reaction

The clinical signs are identical to anaphylaxis but the mechanism is uncertain. Typical causes are intravenous hypnotics and contrast media. It is thought that symptoms are caused by activation of complement C3, an inflammatory mediator that triggers a chain reaction of further mediator release. The latent period between exposure and symptoms is variable but symptoms usually occur within 30 minutes.

Features of clinical anaphylaxis are:

- smooth muscle constriction causing bronchoconstriction;
- vasodilatation resulting in a greatly increased intravascular space with resultant hypotension;
- increased capillary permeability leading to loss of fluid from the circulation causing relative hypovolaemia.

The clinical presentation of anaphylaxis varies but, generally, the earlier the symptoms appear following exposure to the trigger substance, the more severe the reaction. Signs include those shown in Table 9.4.

Immediate treatment

The emergency treatment outlined is according to the Resuscitation Council (UK) (2000) guidance. The aim is to provide oxygenation and restore blood pressure.

Table 9.4 Signs of anaphylaxis

Organ	Clinical signs	What the patient may tell you
Respiratory	Dyspnoea	Feeling of tightness in chest
	Bronchospasm	Inability to speak
	Stridor	
Skin	Pallor	Itching
	Cyanosis	
	Erythematous blush	
	Pruritus	
	Urticaria	
	Soft tissue swelling	
Cardiovascular	Tachycardia	Palpitations
	Hypotension	Chest pain
Central nervous system	Agitation	Dizziness
	Anxiety	A sense of impending doom
Gastrointestinal	Nausea	Abdominal cramps
	Vomiting	
	Diarrhoea	

- Stop the drug or infusion.
- Call for help.
- Maintain i.v. access.
- Give 100% oxygen via a face mask.
- Give i.m. adrenaline 500 µg (0.5 ml of adrenaline 1:1000) and repeat at 5-minute intervals to maintain systolic blood pressure above 80 mmHg; or i.v. adrenaline 100 µg/minute (5 ml of dilute adrenaline 1:10 000 at rate of 1 ml/minute). (NB Patients on non-selective beta-blockers may not respond to adrenaline. In such cases, give i.v. salbutamol (250 µg or 4 µg/kg by slow i.v. injection), and repeat if necessary.)
- Give chlorpheniramine 10–20 mg i.v. over 1 minute after the adrenaline (usually in protracted cases only).
- Give 1 litre of fluid i.v. every 20–30 minutes if shock has not responded to adrenaline.
- Closely monitor and record vital signs (airway, breathing, circulation, urine output).

Further management and nursing interventions

- Monitor continuously.
- If stridor or wheeze develops, call an anaesthetist and give:
  - i.v. aminophylline 250–500 mg (5 mg/kg) over 20 minutes, then 500 µg/hour, if bronchospasm is unresponsive to adrenaline alone; or
  - nebulized salbtamol 2.5–5 mg or terbutaline 5–10 mg.
- Consider steroids for refractory bronchospasm, although there is no benefit in the acute phase (hydrocortisone 100–300 mg i.v.).
- Document the patient's response.

STATUS EPILEPTICUS

Case example 9.7 The patient in status epilepticus

David is 28-years-old and has been a known epileptic since the age of 17. He recently returned from a holiday abroad and presents in the A&E department with frequent fits over the weekend. He was unaccompanied in the A&E department and the police are trying to contact his girlfriend. He takes phenytoin 200 mg/day as anticonvulsant medication.

He develops a tonic–clonic seizure, which lasts 8 minutes. When the seizure ends:

- he remains unresponsive to verbal command and begins convulsing again;
- he is centrally and peripherally cyanosed;
- it is difficult to ascertain whether he is breathing;
- he is bleeding from his mouth.

Following treatment for status epilepticus, he stopped convulsing and was subsequently found to have a subtherapeutic blood phenytoin level. With treatment, his seizures stabilized and he returned home.

Status epilepticus is defined as seizures continuing for over 10 minutes or recurrent seizures that do not allow the patient to regain consciousness between episodes. It is considered a medical emergency because, during continued seizures, the lack of oxygen and glucose to meet the metabolic requirements of the brain may lead to irreversible cerebral damage. Impaired respiration leads to hypoxia, acidosis, cardiac arrythmias, hyperthermia and death. About 10% of all epileptics develop this condition (Borchert & Labar 1993), with a mortality of around 30% (Cascino 1996).

The majority of cases of status epilepticus are patients with known epilepsy on withdrawal or who are non-compliant with anticonvulsant medication. Other causes include electrolyte disturbances, hypoglycaemia, sepsis, renal failure, head trauma, hypoxia and alcohol withdrawal.

Immediate priorities of care

- Check that the airway is clear. Inserting an oropharyngeal airway whilst the patient is fitting may result in damage to the patient's teeth and is usually difficult to perform safely. An airway and oropharyngeal suction may be required when the patient has stopped convulsing.
- Give high-flow oxygen through a face mask. If not breathing, ventilate with a bag-valve-mask.
- Maintain patient safety, supporting the patient with pillows placed to prevent injury during the clonic phase of the seizure.
- Remain with the patient at all times.
- Record the pattern of seizures.
- Maintain i.v. access, ensuring the line is well secured to prevent dislodgement.
- Give diazepam 10 mg or midazolam 5 mg intravenously, which may be repeated.
- If fitting continues, give phenytoin 18 mg/kg over 20 minutes. Side effects are hypotension and cardiac arrythmias (particularly at an infusion rate > 50 mg/minute), so cardiac monitoring is required.
- Call for expert help. Intravenous clonazepam or a diazepam or thiopentone infusion may be considered. These drugs cause severe respiratory

depression and should normally only be administered within ICU or, outside ICU, under the direct supervision of an anaesthetist.

- Conduct a full neurological assessment when the patient has stopped convulsing.
- Carry out capillary glucose testing post-seizure.

Investigation of the cause of the episode of status epilepticus will be dependent on whether the patient is a known epileptic. Known epileptics are likely to require a full blood screen, calcium, anticonvulsant levels, arterial blood gas, chest X-ray and swabs/cultures for microbiology. Previously healthy patients may require a more detailed investigation, including a CT scan, to identify an intracerebral cause.

Patient education regarding seizure management, anticonvulsant therapy as well as referral to a specialist epilepsy nurse, where available, is essential before hospital discharge.

DIABETIC KETOACIDOSIS AND HYPERGLYCAEMIC HYPEROSMOLAR NON-KETOTIC SYNDROME

Case example 9.8 The patient with diabetic ketoacidosis

Miss T, a 28-year-old, is brought to the A&E department with a 2-day history of flu-like symptoms, productive cough and vomiting. She is an insulin-dependent diabetic but has not taken any insulin for the past 24 hours, as she has not been able to eat. Clinical assessment reveals:

- her respiratory rate is 32/minute (her respirations are deep and rapid);
- her pulse is 115/minute;
- her blood pressure is 100/60 mmHg;
- she has a pyrexia of 38.0°C;
- she is lethargic;
- she has a very dry mouth and cracked tongue;
- her breath smells 'fruity';
- she has a capillary blood glucose level of 32 mmol/l;
- urinalysis shows glycosuris and ketonuria.

Rapid infusion of 0.9% sodium chloride is commenced, blood is taken for a full blood count and electrolytes, and a chest X-ray and ECG are performed.

Diabetic ketoacidosis (DKA) is a life-threatening complication of diabetes mellitus owing to a relative or absolute insulin deficiency; it is, therefore, confined to people with type 1 diabetes, namely insulin-dependent or juvenile-onset diabetes. It results in severe alterations in the metabolism of carbohydrates, proteins and lipids, coupled with elevation of stress hormones. It is most commonly associated with underlying infection, disruption of insulin treatment and new-onset diabetes, and is characterized by hyperglycaemia, acidosis and ketosis. DKA is confirmed by a blood glucose > 12 mmol/l, the presence of ketonuria and blood pH < 7.35 (Singh et al 1997).

The pathogenesis of DKA

In the absence of insulin, cells are impermeable to glucose and hyperglycaemia develops. As extracellular glucose rises, water moves by osmosis from the intracellular to the extracellular compartment, depleting intracellular water. As the renal threshold for reabsorption of glucose is exceeded, glucosuria develops, with high levels of glucose in the renal tubules exerting an osmotic effect leading to polyuria. This leads to total body dehydration. Potassium follows the fluid shifts from the intracellular space, causing an initial hyperkalaemia in early DKA. In established DKA, however, potassium is lost with water in the polyuric state and severe hypokalaemia results. Sodium is also lost as a result of osmotic diuresis and further losses occur with vomiting, although normal plasma sodium may be seen with dehydration, as it is a measure of concentration.

The body attempts to compensate for lack of intracellular glucose by releasing catecholamines, glucagons, cortisol and growth hormone. Liver glycogen is converted to glucose by glycogenolysis, and glucagon stimulates the formation of glucose from amino acids in the liver by gluconeogenesis. This leads to rising glucose levels, causing blood hyperosmolarity and osmotic diuresis.

An alternative source of energy is muscle protein. This is broken down to amino acids, which are converted in the liver to glucose and fatty acids for oxidation and conversion to ketones (acetoacetic acid, β-hydroxybutyric acid and acetone). Mobilization of fats for energy leads to formation of ketoacids through lipolysis, further increasing ketones. Some ketones are utilized by cells and the remainder accumulate in the blood, with further production in the liver encouraged by the low insulin:glucagon ratio, resulting in ketoacidosis.

Principles of management of DKA

Diabetic ketoacidosis typically develops over 8-72 hours with symptoms of thirst and polyuria, deep sighing Kussmaul respirations, nausea and vomiting, fatigue, and drowsiness or unconsciousness. The most important principles of the management of diabetic ketocidosis are rehydration, correction of hypokalaemia, reduction of hyperglycaemia, and identification and treatment of the precipitating event.

If any of the following poor prognostic features are present, the patient should be admitted to a designated critical care area:

- pH < 7.0;
- oliguria (urine output < 30 ml/hour);
- serum osmolality > 320 (2 × (Na + K) + urea + glucose);
- newly diagnosed diabetic;
- coma (GCS < 14);
- concomitant disease (cardiac or renal).

Priorities of care

1. Rehydration to restore total body water

- Patients with DKA can have fluid deficits of 6–10 litres. Fluid replacement will be related to degree of dehydration as well as cardiac history and age. Intravenous 0.9% sodium chloride 1–2 litres is administered in the first hour followed by 1 litre/hour until fluid deficit is replaced (Charalambos et al 1999). When glucose is < 15 mmol/l, change to 5% dextrose (and continue with dextrose thereafter)
- The patient will require a central venous line to ensure reliable venous access and central venous pressure (CVP) monitoring. Rate of rehy-

dration will be modified according to CVP and clinical assessment of fluid/cardiac status. Target CVP +5–10 cmH$_2$O.

- Insert a urinary catheter and take hourly urine measurements if the patient has not passed urine after the first 4 hours of rehydration or if serum creatinine is raised.

2. **Correction of hypokalaemia**

- Monitor plasma potassium 2 hourly.
- Potassium replacement should be made in all i.v. fluids, according to plasma levels. Insulin administration will shift potassium from the extracellular to the intracellular space as glucose enters cells, resulting in hypokalaemia and life-threatening arrythmias if not corrected.

3. **Reduction of hyperglycaemia**

- Make hourly capillary blood glucose measurements.
- Give initial slow i.v. bolus insulin.
- Adjust continuous i.v. infusion of insulin according to blood glucose levels.
- Test urine for ketones 2 hourly.
- The insulin infusion should not be discontinued until the urine is free of ketones, arterial pH is > 7.3 and bicarbonate > 18, when subcutaneous insulin can be commenced. The half-life of insulin is around 4 hours and, to ensure the smooth transition to subcutaneous insulin, the regimen should be commenced 1–2 hours before discontinuation of the insulin infusion to ensure a relapse of DKA does not occur.

4. **Arterial blood gas**

Arterial blood gas or venous pH and bicarbonate levels should be checked 4 hourly to identify improvements in acid–base balance until there is improvement, or normal pH and bicarbonate levels.

5. **Cardiac monitoring**

Cardiac monitoring is essential to monitor cardiac rhythm and cardiac arrythmias, as hypokalaemia is common.

6. **Continuous observation**

Continuous observation, and hourly recording of respiratory rate, depth of respirations, peripheral warmth, capillary refill, pulse rate, pulse volume, conscious level and urine output should be maintained to monitor the effectiveness of volume replacement, restoration of circulating volume and acid–base status.

7. **Neurological assessment**

This is required to monitor for:

- cerebral thrombosis owing to blood hyperviscosity;
- cerebral oedema, which may occur owing to movement of extracellular water into brain cells. A gradual reduction in plasma glucose and osmolarity can reduce the risk of cerebral oedema, with the use of hypotonic saline an option if improvement in neurological status is not seen.

8. **Identifying and treating the precipitating event**

Infection is the most common precipitator of DKA, especially pneumonia and urinary tract infections. Omission of insulin, myocardial infarction, cerebrovascular accident, GI bleed, trauma, surgery and pancreatitis are amongst other causes. Drugs such as phenytoin, thiazide diuretics, beta-blockers and calcium-channel blockers can also precipitate DKA. Emotional stress is also thought to be a factor, as an underlying cause cannot always be found.

HYPERGLYCAEMIC HYPEROSMOLAR NON-KETOTIC SYNDROME

Hyperglycaemic hyperosmolar non-ketotic syndrome (HONK) is an acute diabetic emergency commoner in type 2 diabetics (those who are non-insulin-dependent or have maturity-onset diabetes). These diabetics usually have sufficient insulin reserves to avoid the extreme metabolic disturbances that contribute to ketoacidosis.

The pathophysiology is similar to DKA, but the hyperglycaemia, hyperosmolarity and dehydration are more severe in HONK. The reason for the lack of ketoacidosis is unclear and patients tend to be less acutely ill initially owing to the absence of its toxic effects. However, presentation is usually late, with a higher associated mortality. Patients with HONK may present with seizures, focal neurological signs and confusion or coma.

SEPSIS

Case example 9.9 The patient with sepsis

Mrs O is a 68-year-old lady who has been admitted to the ward following a laparotomy and bowel resection for a perforated diverticulum. She had been admitted from the A&E department the previous day with a 2-day history of abdominal pain and vomiting. She has a previous medical history of hypertension, and takes atenolol and furosemide tablets at home. She has i.v. fluids running via a peripheral line, a urinary catheter and a nasogastric tube on free drainage.

Overnight her urine output has remained poor, the junior doctor reviewed Mrs O and a fluid challenge of Gelofusine 500 ml was given. Intravenous fluids were increased to 250 ml 0.9% sodium chloride, but her peripheral line insertion site has been leaking and she remains oliguric.

This morning she is very drowsy. Further clinical assessment reveals:

- she is rousable but drowsy;
- her respiratory rate is 30/minute (respirations are deep and laboured);
- she has an SpO_2 of 91% on air;
- her pulse rate is 74/minute, regular and thready in volume;
- her hands and feet are very cold;
- her blood pressure is 100/40 mmHg;
- she has passed only 17 ml of urine over the last 3 hours;
- her abdomen is tender and distended;
- her temperature is 38.6°C;
- her ABG results are pH 7.29, $PaCO_2$ 2.8 kPa, PaO_2 8.9 kPa, HCO_3 12, BE −12.

Interpretation of data and recognition of clinical emergency

The patient is tachypnoeic and hypoxic, drowsy, hypotensive (with systolic and diastolic blood pressure both low), oliguric and pyrexic. Mrs O is extremely unwell and has the clinical signs of shock and organ hypoperfusion. Note that she is normally hypertensive and organ perfusion is severely compromised by a blood pressure of 100/40 mmHg. The ABG shows a severe metabolic acidosis due to lactic acid production through anaerobic cell respiration with respiratory compensation in an attempt to raise arterial pH, lowering $PaCO_2$ to 2.8 kPa. She requires oxygen and fluids urgently.

Case example continues

Case example 9.9 The patient with sepsis—cont'd

It is essential to inform a senior member of the surgical team quickly and contact the critical care outreach team for advice and support.

The incidence of sepsis is rising (Intensive Care National Audit and Research Centre 2001), with many patients developing sepsis whilst on acute general wards. Sepsis is the consequence of an uncontrolled systemic inflammatory response to an infection, which can result in acute organ dysfunction and multiorgan failure. The course of sepsis can develop rapidly, the patient may deteriorate suddenly and mortality is high; therefore, it is essential for nurses to be alerted to the signs of sepsis in order to offer immediate intervention and treatment.

Definitions of sepsis are given in Box 9.2.

Common causative organisms are Gram-negative organisms such as *Escherichia coli*, Gram-positive organisms such as *Staphylococcus aureus* and *Staphylococcus epidirmidis*, and fungi such as *Aspergillus* and *Candida albicans*. Risk factors are twofold, those relating to host defence and also treatment-related factors. Host risk factors include age over 70 years, malnutrition, debilitating cardiac, respiratory or renal disease and immunocompromised states. Treatment-related risk factors include operative procedures, trauma, the use of invasive lines, artificial airways, immunosuppressant drugs and antibiotics.

Any type of cellular damage or infection initiates an acute inflammatory response. The response is an increase in blood flow and increased vascular permeability, which enable immunogenic cells, such as macrophages and white blood cells, to reach the site of inflammation or injury. Chemical mediators are released from immunogenic cells

Box 9.2   Definitions of sepsis (Adapted from Bone et al 1992)

Systemic inflammatory response syndrome (SIRS)	Two or more of the following: • Temperature > 38.0°C or < 36.0°C • Heart rate > 90/minute • Respiratory rate > 20/minute or $PaCO_2$ < 4.3 kPa • WBC > 12 000, *or* < 4000 cells/mm^3 or > 10% immature neutrophils
Sepsis	SIRS with a documented infective organism
Severe sepsis	Sepsis with organ dysfunction or hypotension
Septic shock	Severe sepsis despite fluid resuscitation

and from endothelial cells damaged by endotoxin, injury or hypoxia. These mediators cause vasodilation, increased capillary permeability and myocardial depression. There is an initial hyperdynamic response manifested by:

- increased cardiac output;
- lowered systemic vascular resistance and hypotension;
- tachycardia;
- tachypnoea;
- drowsiness owing to reduced cerebral perfusion;
- oliguria owing to reduced renal perfusion;
- hyperglycaemia owing to increased gluconeogenesis in shock.

Respiratory failure is a common consequence of sepsis as pulmonary oedema develops owing to increased capillary permeability, causing acute respiratory distress syndrome. This requires prompt intervention, as SpO_2 falls despite increasing FiO_2 and the patient is likely to require intubation and mechanical ventilation.

Priorities of care

- Monitor vital signs every 30 minutes:
  - respiratory rate, SpO_2 in relation to FiO_2;
  - pulse rate and volume;
  - blood pressure;
  - peripheral warmth and capillary refill.
- Cardiac monitoring to identify cardiac arrhythmias.
- Give O_2 to maintain $SpO_2 > 95\%$.
- Replace fluid using boluses of 250 ml 0.9% crystalloid and monitor response.
- Measure urine volume hourly.
- Transfer to designated critical care area for respiratory and inotropic support if no improvement seen or if deterioration in SpO_2 or shock progresses.
- Take blood for arterial blood gas analysis, electrolytes, FBC, clotting screen, LFTs.
- Chest X-ray should be performed.
- Take blood cultures, sputum, urine, drainage fluid and invasive line site swabs for microbiology.
- Administer antibiotics.

Patients who develop sepsis on the ward require collaborative management by the multidisciplinary team. Support and advice from the Critical Care team during the initial stage can prevent admission to Intensive Care and should be sought early by ward teams to ensure the patient receives appropriate timely care.

In a survey of all medical admissions to a UK health region, 25% of all admissions were due to respiratory diseases and over half of these were

EXACERBATION OF CHRONIC OBSTRUCTIVE PULMONARY DISEASE (COPD)

Case example 9.10 The patient with acute exacerbation of COPD

Mrs W, 65 years old, has been admitted to the ward from the A&E department with a 2-day history of breathlessness at rest and increased sputum production. She has had COPD for the last 5 years, has suffered progressive disabling breathlessness on minimal exertion over the last 2 years and has had frequent exacerbations requiring hospital admission. She has home nebulizers.

Clinical assessment reveals:

- she is drowsy, but agitated and distressed;
- she is trying to talk but is unable to complete a sentence without taking a breath;
- she has tachypnoea and dypsnoea with a respiratory rate of 44/minute;
- she has central cyanosis;
- she has a flushed appearance with very warm and oedematous peripheries, particularly the feet;
- she is very shaky and has a flapping hand tremor;
- she has tachycardia (128/minute);
- her blood pressure is 190/90 mmHg;
- ABG analysis on 28% O_2 shows pH 7.09, $PaCO_2$ 15.5 kPa, PaO_2 5.9 kPa, HCO_3 33, BE −2.

This lady is clearly in respiratory distress. She is hypoxic, and has signs of hypercarbia: drowsiness, hypertension, flushed appearance and flapping hand tremor. The ABG shows severe respiratory acidosis with hypercarbia (Type II respiratory failure) with hypoxia (Type I respiratory failure).

COPD (Pearson et al 1994). The British Thoracic Society (1997) guidelines on the management of COPD emphasize the importance of correct and early diagnosis using spirometry, give advice on appropriate drug therapy and encourage attempts to stop patients smoking. COPD is a general term that covers many diseases that are now recognized as different aspects of the same problem (e.g. chronic bronchitis, emphysema, chronic obstructive airways disease and some cases of chronic asthma). COPD is largely caused by tobacco smoking and carries significant mortality. It is slowly progressive characterized by airways obstruction (FEV_1 < 80% predicted and FEV_1/FVC ratio < 70%), which gradually worsens. Chronic airflow limitation is largely fixed, but treatment can improve symptoms and airflow limitation. (Forced expiratory volue in one second (FEV) and forced vital capacity (FVC) are measured using a spirometer and have well-defined normal ranges according to age and sex.

Pathology of COPD

Various changes occur in small and large airways. Chronic airflow limitation develops owing to a combination of mechanical obstruction in the small airways and loss of pulmonary elastic recoil owing to emphysema. Redistribution of ventilation away from regions with high airways resistance to regions of lower resistance results in lung units being ventilated well in excess of their perfusion, contributing to hypoxaemia.

In advanced disease, persistent arterial hypoxaemia leads to permanent pulmonary vascular changes with thickening of the medial pulmonary arterial wall, which does not resolve with long-term oxygen therapy. This causes increased resistance, which causes an increased pulmonary artery pressure, resulting in right ventricular hypertrophy or cor pulmonale. Severe COPD is characterized by $FEV_1 < 40\%$ predicted, breathlessness on any exertion/rest, wheeze and cough, lung overinflation, cyanosis, peripheral oedema and polycythaemia.

Acute exacerbations of COPD present as a worsening of the previous stable situation. Significant signs of a deterioration are those of:

- infection, with increased sputum purulence and pyrexia;
- severe airways obstruction, with audible wheeze, tachypnoea and use of accessory muscles;
- fluid retention, with peripheral oedema;
- cyanosis;
- confusion or drowsiness.

Sudden worsening of established COPD is usually caused by infection but other causes need to be excluded, such as pneumonia, pneumothorax, left ventricular failure, pulmonary embolus, lung cancer or upper airway obstruction.

Priorities of care

Oxygen therapy
- Give 24–28% oxygen via a Venturi mask or 2 litres/minute via nasal cannulae.
- ABG should be checked within 60 minutes of starting oxygen and within 60 minutes of a change in inspired oxygen concentration.
- If the PaO_2 is improving and the acidosis is not worsening, increase the inspired oxygen until the PaO_2 is above 7.5 kPa.
- Closely monitor respiratory rate, depth, accessory muscle use, SpO_2 in relation to FiO_2. Respiratory depression owing to loss of hypoxic drive when oxygen is administered, may be evident by a fall in respiratory rate and depth.
- Ensure the patient is nursed on an electric frame bed, for ease of positioning to reduce the work of breathing, with a wall oxygen supply.

Bronchodilatation and mobilization of secretions
- Administer a nebulized β-agonist (salbutamol 2.5–5 mg or terbutaline 5–10 mg) and an anticholinergic (ipratropium bromide 0.25–0.5 mg) driven by compressed air.
- Continue oxygen during nebulizer administration at 2 litres/minute via nasal cannulae in order to prevent hypoxia during nebulizer therapy.
- If the patient is not responding, intravenous aminophylline 0.5 mg/kg per hour should be considered. Theophylline levels should be measured every 24 hours.
- Adequate hydration should be provided. Intravenous fluids may be required if the patient is dehydrated owing to mouth breathing and lack of oral intake.
- Encourage the patient to cough and expectorate. Send sputum for microbiology.

- Antibiotics may be appropriate if there is increased sputum volume or sputum purulence in addition to increased breathlessness.
- Physiotherapy is usually not well tolerated in acute on chronic respiratory failure but may be useful when acidosis improves. It may induce cardiac arrhythmias if the patient becomes hypoxic during treatment.

Corticosteroids
- Prednisolone 30 mg/day orally or i.v.
- Hydrocortisone, if oral route is not possible, continued for 7–14 days.

Anticoagulants
Prophylactic subcutaneous heparin is recommended (British Thoracic Society 1997).

Investigations

- FBC, U&Es;
- chest X-ray;
- ECG;
- initial peak flow recording and start a serial peak flow chart;
- sputum for culture, if purulent;
- blood cultures if pneumonia is suspected.

Subsequent management

If acidosis worsens and the pH falls further, secondary to a rise in $PaCO_2$, consider alternative management. Non-invasive ventilation (NIV) may be considered.

The aim of oxygen therapy is to achieve a PaO_2 of > 6.6 kPa without a fall in pH to below 7.26 as a result of a rise in $PaCO_2$. The British Thoracic Society (1997) recommends that patients with a history of COPD over 50 years of age should not be administered an FiO_2 of > 28% via a Venturi mask or 2 litres/minute via nasal cannulae until the arterial blood gas tensions are known.

If pH is < 7.26 kPa and $PaCO_2$ is rising, ventilatory support should be considered. Intubation and intermittent positive pressure ventilation or NIV are the options, with NIV best indicated when the pH is > 7.25. NIV may not be appropriate in end-stage disease or when several co-morbidities exist, is contraindicated in the presence of confusion, inability to protect the airway, copious secretions or vomiting, pneumonia and haemodynamic instability. NIV should be used in an appropriate clinical area by appropriately trained staff with support and advice readily available from a respiratory specialist team and/or the critical care team. Age and $PaCO_2$ are not reliable indicators of survival, and the decision not to institute ventilatory support should be made by a senior doctor.

Nebulized bronchodilators should be continued for 24–48 hours or until the patient is improving, when changeover to metered dose aerosol or dry powder inhaler can be used.

The most likely organisms in infective exacerbations of COPD are *Haemophilis influenzae, Streptococcus pneumoniae* and *Moraxella catarrhalis*. The choice of antibiotic depends on local policy but oral antibiotics rather than i.v. are usually indicated, as long as the patient is able to take them reliably.

References

Bone R C, Balk RA, Cerra FB et al 1992 Definitions for sepsis and organ failure and guidelines for the use of innovative therapies in sepsis. Chest 101: 1644–1655

Borchert L D, Labar D R 1993 An organised approach to managing status epilepticus. Journal of Critical Illness 8: 965–972

British Thoracic Society 1997 BTS guidelines on the management of chronic obstructive (pulmonary disease. Thorax 52 (Suppl V) 1–28 British Thoracic Society 2003a British guidelines on the management of asthma. Thorax 58(Suppl 1) 1–94

British Thoracic Society 2003b BTS guidelines for the management of suspected pulmonary embolism. Thorax 58: 470–484

British Thoracic Society 2003c BTS guidelines for the management of spontaneous pneumothorax. Thorax 58(Suppl II): 39–52

Cascino G D 1996 Generalised convulsive status epilepticus. Mayo Clinic Proceedings 71(8): 787–792

Charalambos C, Schofield I, Malik R 1999 Acute diabetic emergencies and their management. Care of the Critically ill 15. 4:132–134

Despars J A, Sassoon C S, Light R W 1994 Significance of iatrogenic pneumothoraces. Chest 105: 1147–1150

Fiorianti J, Sullivan T, Lowenfels A B 2003 Rising incidence of hospitalization for acute pancreatitis in New York State from 1991 to 2001. Abstracts submitted to the American Pancreatic Association. Pancreas 27(4): 368–420

Golub R, Siddiqi F, Pohl D 1998 Role of antibiotics in acute pancreatitis: a meta-analysis. Journal of Gastrointestinal Surgery 2(6): 496–503

Intensive Care National Audit and Research Centre (ICNARC) 2001 Case mix programme database. ICNARC, London

McArthur-Rouse F 2001 Critical Care outreach services and early warning scoring systems: a review of the literature. Journal of Advanced Nursing 36(5): 696–704

Norman J, Cook A 2000 Medical emergencies. In: Sheppard M, Wright M (eds) Principles and practice of high dependency nursing. Baillière Tindall, London

Pearson M G, Littler J, Davies P D O 1994 An analysis of medical workload by speciality and diagnosis in Mersey. Journal of the Royal College of Physicians 28: 230–234

Resuscitation Council (UK) 2000 Emergency treatment of severe anaphylactic reactions. British National Formulary no. 40 British Medical Association Royal Pharmaceutical Society, London

Rockall T A, Logan R F, Devlin H B, Northfield T C 1995 Incidence and mortality from acute upper gastrointestinal haemorrhage in the United Kingdom. British Medical Journal 311: 222–226

Singh R, Perros P, Frier BM 1997 Hospital management of ketoacidosis: are guidelines implemented effectively? Diabetic Medicine 14.7: 482–486

Smith G 2000 ALERT: acute life-threatening events recognition and treatment, 1st edn. University of Portsmouth, Portsmouth

Wynne H, Long A 1996 Patient awareness of the adverse effects of non-steroidal anti-inflammatory drugs. British Journal of Clinical Pharmacology 42(2): 253–256

Chapter 10

Fluid and electrolytes

Wayne Large

KEY LEARNING OBJECTIVES

In relation to maintaining fluid and electrolyte balance, this chapter aims to identify:
- The underpinning physiological principles.
- Specific causes of fluid and electrolyte excess and deficit.
- Specific patient assessment data required in fluid and electrolyte excess and deficit.
- Specific nursing interventions required in fluid and electrolyte excess and deficit.

INTRODUCTION

In high dependency care, a patient's fluid and electrolyte status can change rapidly, and the need to be vigilant and alert to these changes is of paramount importance. Methodical collection of patient assessment information is vital for quick and efficient intervention at any stage of patient care. Fluid and electrolyte imbalance can occur insidiously, without obvious presenting problems. To be alert to these requires the use of invasive and non-invasive measurement techniques, acute patient observation skills, interpretation of biochemical indicators and prioritization of patient care needs.

In health, fluids and electrolytes are finely tuned and constantly maintained by various physiological processes. In ill health, there are many sources of fluid and electrolyte loss and gain, which can result in an overall imbalance. It is crucial that the nurse is aware of these sources of loss and gain. Furthermore, the nurse should appreciate the need to accumulate accurate information in order to identify trends and patterns that indicate subtle changes in fluid balance. The aim of this chapter is to provide relevant information and underpinning principles that may inform assessment and intervention in maintaining fluid and electrolyte balance. For the purpose of organization, fluid and electrolytes will be considered separately.

FLUID AND ELECTROLYTE BALANCE

Evidence that a balance is maintained between the intake and output of body fluids in a healthy person is shown by the fact that body weight remains constant from day to day. If this balance is altered, the consequences will depend on the degree of imbalance incurred. A reduction of 5% in body fluids will cause thirst, a reduction of 8% will result in illness and a 10% reduction will result in death.

Sources of fluid intake and loss are shown in Box 10.1.

BODY FLUID COMPARTMENTS

With age, the body increases its fat content and loses a significant amount of muscle mass. Because muscle holds 40% of total body water, the water content of the older person reduces to around 45–50%, mostly owing to the loss of muscle mass. Any stressor or disease will, therefore, more easily lead to dehydration in the older person. An ageing population is likely to make this issue become increasingly important as years go by.

Total body water constitutes approximately 60% of body weight in males and 52% in females, the latter being slightly less owing to the higher fat content. Total body water is less in obesity and in the elderly. These are important factors for consideration when estimating overall fluid balance in individuals. Body fluids are distributed between two compartments: the intracellular fluid (ICF) and extracellular fluid (ECF) compartments.

The *intracellular fluid* is contained within the cells and accounts for two-thirds of total body water (40% body weight). The *extracellular fluid* surrounds the cells and accounts for one-third of total body water (20% total body weight). The ECF is distributed between:

- the interstitial space (i.e. fluid outside the vessels) bathing the cells – this compartment accounts for three-quarters of total ECF volume;
- the plasma compartment, which constitutes 'plasma volume' (i.e. the 'vascular space' – fluid within the vessels). This compartment accounts for one-quarter of total ECF volume. Adult blood volume is approximately 5 litres, 75 ml/kg.

Box 10.1   Sources of fluid intake and fluid loss

Fluid intake	Fluid loss
Fluid intake is derived from three main sources:	Water is lost from the body in three main ways:
• Ingested fluids = 1500 ml/ 24 hours	• Urine output = 1500 ml/ 24 hours
• Water in food = 500 ml/ 24 hours	• Evaporation (via lungs and skin) = 800 ml/24 hours
• Metabolic water resulting from oxidation of food amounts to approximately 400 ml/24 hours	• Alimentary tract = 100 ml/ 24 hours
Total fluid intake = 2400 ml/ 24 hours	Total fluid output = 2400 ml/ 24 hours

Other examples of 'third space' include peritonitis, burns, crush injuries and increased capillary permeability states. The development of a third space can represent a hidden site of circulating volume, causing signs of ECF loss without any obvious external loss.

Expansion or contraction of either of these compartments will result in presenting clinical features detailed in Table 10.7 (see page 297). Any infused intravenous fluids will directly enter the ECF compartment, primarily the vascular space, and will then be distributed into the respective fluid compartments, according to their composition. When considering fluid balance in the highly dependent patient, it is important to be aware of the potential development of a 'third space' that is, movement of fluid into body cavities (e.g. in paralytic ileus fluid pools into the bowel).

The various fluid compartments are separated by semi-permeable membranes; continuous exchange of water and solutes occurs within the body, transported by diffusion and osmosis to maintain constant balance.

Composition of body fluid compartments

The composition of the fluid compartments varies in relation to their respective electrolyte content (Table 10.1). An electrolyte is defined as a substance that develops an electrical charge when dissolved in water; ions are collectively referred to as electrolytes. Electrolytes that develop a positive charge are cations, for example, sodium (Na^+), potassium (K^+) calcium (Ca^+) and magnesium (Mg^{2+}). Electrolytes with a negative charge are anions, for example, chloride (Cl^-) and bicarbonate (HCO_3^-). In all body fluids, anions and cations are always present in equal amounts, as positive and negative charges must be equal – an electromechanical fact (Metheny 2000).

A summary of the major electrolyte functions is given in Table 10.2.

MECHANISMS INVOLVED IN THE REGULATION OF FLUID AND ELECTROLYTE BALANCE

Movement and maintenance of fluid compartments

Movement of water and solutes between fluid compartments is continuous. In health, the actual concentration of solutes and amount of water in each compartment remains relatively unchanged. In order that movement can take place, cell membranes have to be crossed, and these membranes are described as partially permeable or semipermeable. Water and small electrolyte molecules pass easily, larger colloid substances and proteins are held back. Body fluids are maintained at a constant level by several

Table 10.1   The ionic concentration of body fluids in a typical 70 kg man

Solute	Plasma	ECF	ICF
Sodium (mmol/l)	142	145	12
Potassium (mmol/l)	4	4.1	150
Chloride (mmol/l)	103	113	4
Bicarbonate (mmol/l)	25	127	12
Proteins (g/l)	60	0	25
Osmolality (mosmol/kg)	280	280	280

ECF, extracellular fluid; ICF, intracellular fluid.

Table 10.2 Summary of major electrolyte functions (Metheny 2000)

Electrolyte and plasma level	Functions of electrolytes
Sodium (135–145 mmol/l)	Major cation in ECF, maintains osmotic pressure and volume in this compartment Essential for nerve impulses and muscle contractions Influences acid–base balance, chloride and potassium levels
Potassium (3.5–5.0 mmol/l)	Major cation in the ICF compartment, maintains osmotic pressure and volume in this compartment Essential for transmission and conduction of nerve impulses, for the contraction of skeletal, cardiac and smooth muscles Necessary for movement of glucose into cells
Calcium (4.5–5.5 mmol/l)	Promotes normal nerve and muscle activity Increases contraction of the myocardium Maintains normal cellular permeability and promotes blood clotting Necessary for bone development and healing
Chloride (96–106 mmol/l)	A major anion in the ECF; helps maintain ECF osmotic pressure and water balance Influences neutrality between cations and anions Digestion – essential for production of hydrochloric acid
Phosphate (0.8–1.4 mmol/l)	A vital component in the structure of bone tissue and teeth Essential in the metabolism of all cells As a buffer – maintains acid–base balance
Magnesium (1.5–2.5 mmol/l)	A major ICF cation closely related to potassium Vital for ICF enzyme reactions involving ATP Implicated in neural control, neuromuscular transmission and cardiovascular tone

homeostatic mechanisms, namely osmosis, diffusion and active transport. Movement of water is governed by two principal forces as follows.

1. Osmotic pressure: the pressure that must be applied to a solution on one side of a membrane to prevent osmotic flow of water across the membrane from a compartment of pure water (Vander et al 2004); pressure is exerted by electrolytes and blood proteins.
2. Hydrostatic pressure of blood: the pressure exerted by fluid against the wall of its container.

Small molecular solutes diffuse passively through cell membranes either across a selectively permeable membrane or down a concentration gradient within cells. Their continuous random movement results in transfer in both directions; the net movement tends to be to the compartment having the lower solute concentration. The end result of diffusion is the equilibrium of substances on both sides of the membrane (Figure 10.1).

Active transport

Sodium is the most important electrolyte for the maintenance of osmotic pressure and volume in the ECF compartment. Any change in

Figure10.1 Movement of water between body fluid compartments by osmosis in dehydration.

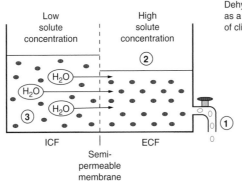

Low solute concentration   **High solute concentration**

Dehydration commonly occurs as a result of a multitude of clinical scenarios (see Box 10.2)

1. Excessive loss of water from ECF compartment
2. Osmotic pressure increases in the ECF compartment
3. Water leaves ICF compartment by osmosis, moving into ECF, thereby maintaining osmolarity and ECF volume (total body fluid volume is reduced)

ICF   ECF

Semi-permeable membrane

sodium concentration will lead to fluid volume changes (water follows sodium). Potassium is the main intracellular cation and maintains the ICF osmotic pressure. Electrolytes do not move between the cell walls and capillaries as easily as water. Na$^+$ and K$^+$ concentrations in ECF and ICF are nearly opposite (Table 10.1). This reflects the activity of the chemical substance known as adenosine triphosphate (ATP) on dependent Na$^+$/K$^+$ pumps. ATP is released from the cell wall, which gives the electrolyte the energy required to pass through semipermeable membranes. The membrane is selectively permeable, so that what is transported in or out of the cell at any time depends on the body's current metabolic condition. Renal mechanisms reinforce this distribution, regulating Na$^+$ excretion. As Na$^+$ is reabsorbed from the filtrate, K$^+$ is secreted. In spite of an enormous variation in dietary intake, K$^+$ levels are kept constant. This is achieved by the renal tubular absorption of potassium and the secretion of variable amounts of potassium. Movement of potassium across cell membranes regulates plasma potassium levels. When potassium is lost from the body (e.g. in urine) potassium moves out of the cells into the ECF to maintain potassium equilibrium between ICF and ECF.

In the ECF compartment, there is exchange of water and electrolytes between the interstitial fluid compartment and the intravascular compartment (Figure 10.2). The principal difference in composition between these compartments (highlighted in Table 10.1) is the presence of proteins in the plasma. Proteins cannot pass the capillary membrane; therefore, they function as osmotically active substances holding fluid in blood vessels. The osmotic pressure exerted by plasma proteins is referred to as oncotic pressure at approximately 20–30 mmHg. With Na$^+$, the plasma proteins control intravascular volume.

Osmolality

Water balance disorders are manifested by alterations in plasma osmolality. Osmolality refers to the number of dissolved particles per kilogram of solvent. Normal plasma osmolality is 280–290 mosmol/kg of water and this provides an environment that is favourable for cellular activity. The major determinant of plasma osmolality is sodium. The

Figure 10.2 Basic principles controlling solute and fluid exchange between compartments.

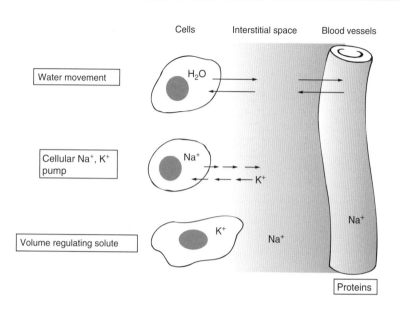

There is a diminution in thirst perception with age so that, even in the face of volume depletion or hyperosmolality, which serve as stimuli for the intake of fluid, these stimuli are less effective.

In the normal ageing individual, the release of ADH appears to be increased in response to a variety of stimuli, which can result in the retention of fluid.

osmolality of the ICF compartment must balance that of the ECF compartment in order to maintain a correct and orderly distribution of fluid between the cell and its environment.

- Osmolality is regulated so precisely that ± 3 mosmol/kg water will activate the body's osmolality-regulating mechanisms.
- Changes in plasma osmolality are detected by osmoreceptors located in the hypothalamus. These receptors regulate the release of antidiuretic hormone (ADH) from the posterior pituitary, as well as having an effect on thirst (Table 10.3).
- The two primary regulators of ADH are osmotic (plasma osmolality) and haemodynamic (blood volume and pressure).
- ADH is removed from the plasma by the liver and kidneys.
- Electrolytes are the major factor in maintaining the osmolality of body fluids, upon which the integrity of the body fluid compartments depends.

Table 10.3   Plasma osmolality and antidiuretic hormone (ADH) response

Plasma osmolality	ADH response	Physiological effect
Normal	Present	Maintenance of normal balance
Lowered – in fluid excess Plasma osmotic pressure reduced	Reduced stimulation of osmoreceptors – inhibited release of ADH	Increased kidney tubule excretion of water, large volumes of dilute urine produced
Increased – in fluid loss/excessive intake of electrolytes Plasma osmotic pressure increased	Stimulation of osmoreceptors – increased release of ADH	Increases kidney tubule reabsorption of water, fluid retained in circulation, small volumes of concentrated urine produced

Antidiuretic hormone, aldosterone and the renin–angiotensin system

Antidiuretic hormone, aldosterone and the renin–angiotensin system play major and interrelated roles in the maintenance of fluid and electrolyte balance (Table 10.4, Figure 10.3).

Acid–base balance

Metabolism results in the production of waste products, necessitating the maintenance of acid–base balance within body fluids. The respiratory system is responsible for this, as are the blood and the kidneys. Blood is normally alkaline at a pH range of 7.38–7.42. This range is essential for the function of processes, such as enzyme function, muscle contraction and blood clotting. The maximum deviation from this range that is compatible with life is 6.8 (extreme acidosis) to 7.8 (extreme alkalosis). The hydrogen ion concentration of blood is measured as pH. These parameters reflect the level of alkalinity or acidity.

Three interrelated and well-integrated mechanisms work within the body to preserve the appropriate pH of blood and maintain acid–base balance: chemical buffer systems in ECF and within cells, removal of carbon dioxide by the lungs and renal regulation of hydrogen ion concentration.

Physiological buffers

A buffer is a substance that accepts hydrogen ions from an acidic solution and donates hydrogen ions to an alkaline solution, thus minimizing a change in pH. In essence, blood buffers (present in all body fluid) provide the means for hydrogen ions to be transported from their site of production to their site of elimination with a minimum alteration of blood pH. These consist chiefly of bicarbonate, phosphate and protein, particularly haemoglobin (Table 10.5).

Table 10.4   Hormones involved in the maintenance of fluid and electrolyte balance

Hormone	Trigger for response	Actions
Aldosterone secreted by the adrenal glands	Stimulated by ↑ K^+ levels and ↓ Na^+ levels Major trigger for release is renin–angiotensin mechanism	Promotes reabsorption of sodium by the distal tubules in the kidney, and from the colon Promotes hydrogen ion secretion, and responds to changes in potassium levels
ADH secreted by the pituitary gland	↓ Plasma osmolality inhibits ADH release ↑ Plasma osmolality stimulates ADH production	Increases kidney tubule excretion of water Increases kidney tubule reabsorption of water
Renin → angiotensin Released by juxtaglomerular cells in kidney nephrons	↓ Blood pressure/circulating volume Change in solute concentration	Vasoconstriction ↑ Peripheral resistance Na^+ and H_2O retention
Parathyroid hormone Produced by parathyroid gland	↓ Calcium levels ↑ Calcium levels	Parathyroid hormone secreted and depressed Maintains level of ionized calcium in plasma

↑, increased; ↓, decreased.

Figure 10.3 Flow diagram outlining the interrelated roles of antidiuretic hormone (ADH), aldosterone and renin–angiotensin. JGA, juxtaglomerular apparatus.

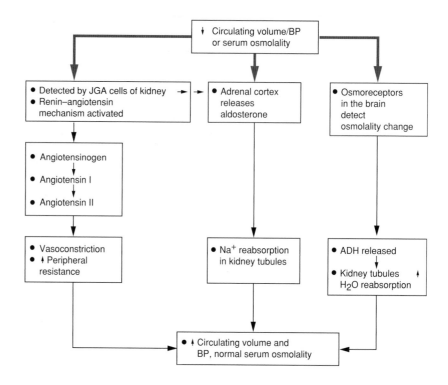

The bicarbonate buffering system is of primary importance and is well described in texts such as Metheny (2000). It precisely regulates the concentration of carbon dioxide by the lungs and the kidneys by the following reaction sequence:

$$CO_2 + H_2O = H_2CO_3 = H^+ + HCO_3^-$$

A change in ECF hydrogen will stimulate peripheral chemoreceptors, resulting in an increased respiratory rate and depth. In the lungs, oxygen will associate with haemoglobin, resulting in the release of hydrogen, which then combines with bicarbonate to form carbonic acid. Carbonic acid dehydrates to form carbonic anhydrase, releasing carbon dioxide, which diffuses out of the erythrocytes and into the alveoli. In this way, carbon dioxide elimination removes hydrogen ions from the blood. A change in hydrogen ion concentration in the blood will also cause the kidneys to excrete acidic or alkaline urine, which helps restore the normal pH balance. Respiratory compensation restores normal pH within minutes, whereas renal restoration is a slow process, which may take hours or days to achieve. The largest source of buffer capacity in

Table 10.5 The main physiological buffers

Buffer	Body compartment		
Bicarbonate	Blood	ICF	ECF
Plasma protein	Blood	ICF	ECF
Haemoglobin	Blood	–	–
Phosphate	Blood	ICF	ECF

the body is found in the tissues and plasma proteins; haemoglobin is of particular importance.

In the vascular compartment, carbon dioxide dissolves in water producing carbonic acid that dissociates to release hydrogen ions, which is buffered by haemoglobin. The amount of bicarbonate produced in this way depends on the partial pressure of carbon dioxide (PCO_2) in the blood. Once the bicarbonate is produced, it leaves the red blood cells by passive diffusion across the cell membrane into the plasma. As bicarbonate is an anion, its movement out of the cell is compensated by the inward movement of chloride. This movement is called the chloride shift. In this way, the buffering capacity of haemoglobin greatly assists in the maintenance of a normal plasma pH. These acid/bases provide a source of one of the most predominant buffers in the ICF – phosphate. Two forms of phosphate are involved:

- NaH_2PO_4, which is a weak acid;
- Na_2HPO_4, which is weakly alkaline.

Buffering occurs when the alkaline phosphate combines with hydrogen to form the acid phosphate. This process takes place in the kidneys and is probably more important during chronic disturbances, such as renal failure. If the mechanisms and buffer systems fail, the resultant changes in blood pH will become life-threatening.

FLUID VOLUME LOSS AND GAIN

Fluid volume loss

Many clinical situations threaten fluid and electrolyte balance. The results of such a loss can be sudden and acute, or gradual. In either case, assessment is the key to effective intervention.

Most clinical situations potentially threaten an individual's fluid and electrolyte balance: water imbalance rarely occurs alone and is usually accompanied by sodium imbalance. Loss of fluid volume may be sudden and acute, requiring immediate resuscitation, or gradual and insidious as a consequence of disease, infirmity or surgical intervention. This can result in fluid loss owing to reduced input, increased output or both. Dehydration (depletion of body water) results from fluid deprivation or loss of water. Individuals who are otherwise healthy may become dehydrated if deprived of water. Clinically significant volume loss results from loss of water, sodium and other electrolytes. Fluid volume loss is usually described in terms of serum sodium concentration: that is, hyperosmolar, isosmolar or hypo-osmolar volume depletion (Box 10.2).

In response to reduced fluid volume, homeostatic mechanisms will attempt to compensate for fluid loss. Antidiuretic hormone will reduce water loss from the body by retaining fluid and consequently reducing urine volume. The kidneys will also attempt to expand volume through activating the renin–angiotensin–aldosterone mechanism, resulting in sodium and water retention.

How fluid volume loss will manifest itself will depend on the severity of loss and how quickly it has occurred. Irrespective of the cause of fluid loss, cardiac output will be impaired because of diminished pre-load. Presenting patient problems will reflect the effects of reduced cardiac

Box 10.2   Fluid loss and possible causes

Type of fluid deficit

Hyperosmolar (due to body water losses)
The ECF compartment is depleted, initially increasing the osmolality (creating an osmotic gradient) – fluid becomes hypertonic. In response, fluid moves out of the ICF compartment into the ECF compartment, thereby maintaining intravascular volume.

Isosmolar (due to loss of fluids and electrolytes)
Water and electrolytes are lost in equal proportions. ECF remains isosmolar, but volume decreases in all fluid compartments, if not replaced.

Hypo-osmolar (solute loss in excess of water excretion)
Reduced serum sodium and osmolality cause the ECF to become hypotonic. This results in an osmotic shift of fluid from the ECF compartment into the ICF compartment.

Possible causes

- Food and water deprivation
- Increased body or environmental temperature
- Diabetes mellitus with hyperglycaemia
- Hyperalimination
- Diuresis in diabetes insipidus
- Loss of body fluids containing salt, e.g. gastrointestinal loss from vomiting, diarrhoea, nasogastric loss
- Haemorrhage, burns, peritonitis
- Excessive use of diuretics, causing solutes to be lost in excess of water, and hypertonic urine
- Gastrointestinal secretion loss

output, disruption of normal cellular metabolism and the resulting activation of homeostatic mechanisms to compensate.

Hypovolaemic shock

When fluid loss is due to a shortage of extracellular fluid (Hudak et al 1998) from any cause, such as bleeding both internally and externally, hypovolaemia develops and causes onset of shock. There are discrete stages of hypovolaemic shock (Table 10.6) as the body tries, at first, to compensate for the loss of circulating blood volume. An untreated loss of significant amounts of blood with ultimately lead to death.

The symptoms of hypovolaemia include:

- a weak ('thready') pulse;
- a marked sinus tachycardia;
- tachypnoea;
- pale-coloured cool skin;
- hypotension;

Table 10.6 The stages of hypovolaemic shock

Stage of shock	Compensatory mechanisms and characteristics
Compensatory stage	Blood pressure triggers ↑ baroreceptor and chemoreceptor reflexes ↑ Ischaemia within the medulla oblongata → sympathetic responses leading to ↑ vasoconstriction and ↑ heart rate ↓ Blood renal blood flow leads to ↑ renin release causing ↑ angiotensin II formation This leads to ↑ vasoconstriction and ↑ aldosterone release ↑ Aldosterone promotes water and salt retention by the kidneys These measures restore blood pressure and blood volume
Progressive stage	Compensatory mechanisms are not adequate to restore blood pressure and blood volume ↓ Blood pressure, ↑ heart rate Cardiac and other tissue deterioration in response to poor blood flow Medical treatment to restore blood flow will rectify this situation
Irreversible stage	Absence of medical treatment leads to irreversible hypovolaemic shock Results in death, regardless of the amount of medical treatment given

↑, increased; ↓, decreased.

- decreased or no urine output;
- anxiety and restlessness.

The treatment of hypovolaemia is to restore an adequate circulating volume as soon as possible. The use of plasma substitutes, such as dextran, Haemaccel and Gelofusine, are suitable to expand blood volume until a blood transfusion is available. However, plasma substitutes should not be used to expand plasma volumes in conditions such as burns or septicaemia. In these cases, albumin solution is recommended (British National Formulary 2002). There is some debate on the use of colloid versus crystalloid solutions. There are claims that the use of colloids is associated with increased mortality. However, Moretti et al (2003) and Bradley (2001) are both in agreement that there is little evidence that any specific fluid therapy is associated with increased mortality. Bunn et al (2004) go on to say that a review of the literature shows no evidence that one colloid is safer than any other.

Fluid volume excess

Excess fluid volume (overhydration) is usually iatrogenic, but may be exacerbated by certain diseases, and in the presence of impaired heart, renal or liver function (Box 10.3).

Oedema is defined as the accumulation of abnormal quantities of fluid in the interstitial tissues. However, the presence of oedema does not always indicate true fluid overload. A loss of albumin from the vascular compartment can cause peripheral oedema, yet the patient may be hypovolaemic (Oh et al 2003).

Box 10.3   Fluid gain and possible causes

Type of fluid excess

Hypertonic
Can result from increased solutes in the ECF compartment, leading to water being drawn out of the cells.

Isotonic
Resulting from increased fluid and electrolyte gains. Expansion of both ICF and ECF compartments occurs.

Hypotonic (water intoxication)
Excess water in the ECF compartment has a dilutional effect, reducing the osmotic gradient (sodium content is normal but excess water is present leading to hyponatraemia). Water moves from the ECF, causing overhydration and swelling of cells.

Possible causes

- Excessive administration of sodium bicarbonate (a greater proportion of sodium and protein) and of glucose (in hyperglycaemia)
- Excessive infusion of isotonic solutions
- Congestive heart failure, acute renal failure, nephrotic syndrome, liver cirrhosis
- Excessive fluid intake, orally or infusion of 5% dextrose
- Renal impairment, retention of irrigation fluid (urological surgery)
- Physiological stress, e.g. as a result of trauma or surgery (ADH production is affected and increases rapidly, overriding normal regulation). This can result in reduced urine output and osmolality, leading to water retention and hyponatraemia

NURSING ASSESSMENT IN FLUID AND ELECTROLYTE BALANCE

Fluid balance may be viewed as a dynamic entity, where assessment and intervention overlap, and where there are no clearly distinguishable boundaries as to where one starts and the other ends. It is the findings of assessment that inform nursing intervention and, therefore, through efficient analysis of assessment findings, interventions can be anticipated and promptly instigated. Identification of sources of fluid and electrolyte loss and gain in the highly dependent patient are imperative for continuous safe and effective monitoring (Box 10.4). Loss or gain of relatively small amounts of fluid and electrolytes can tip a very delicate balance in an unstable patient.

COLLECTION OF ASSESSMENT DATA

Records of fluid intake and output

All fluid losses and gains need to be recorded on a fluid balance chart to provide a comprehensive record of fluid balance over a period of time. The time of day, and the volume and nature and sources of loss and gain need to be clearly identified. It is crucial that the previous status of the patient is taken into account when collecting accurate assessment data.